Preface

The greatest resource that a clinician has is his ability to establish an accurate diagnosis, for it is only upon such a diagnosis that he can formulate effective treatment, prognosis, and disease prevention. In most instances specific diagnoses can be established only by the use of reasoning and logic based on facts rather than beliefs. Careful evaluation of the history and physical examination are essential prerequisites to diagnostic accuracy. Although the information obtained from the history and physical examination may not be sufficiently precise to allow one to make a specific diagnosis, it often allows one to formulate a logical approach to the establishment of a specific diagnosis. The infinite number of diagnostic possibilities can thus be reduced to those few which comprise reasonable diagnostic probabilities. Laboratory, radiographic, and biopsy procedures should be selected on the basis of tentative diagnoses formulated from evaluation of the history and physical examination, with the purpose of confirming or eliminating diagnostic probabilities. Obviously, if the differential diagnoses can be reduced to a relatively small number of probabilities, confirmation by various laboratory tests, radiographic techniques, and biopsy procedures becomes economically feasible.

This book has been prepared for students and practitioners of veterinary medicine who have not specialized in urology, but whose clinical practice requires familiarity with diagnostic and therapeutic techniques which are available for the management of diseases of the urinary system of the dog and cat. The primary objective of the book is to provide information about urinary diseases in a simplified, systematic, and readily accessible outline form. The scope of the book has therefore been limited to a discussion of the clinical findings, diagnosis, treatment, and prognosis of urinary diseases.

Our concept of urology differs from that used in human medicine because we have literally accepted the term in its purest sense, a study of all diseases of the urinary system. In contrast, human urology is a surgically oriented specialty that ignores nonsurgical diseases of the kidney but encompasses diseases of the genital tract. To us, the only things that the genital and urinary systems have in common are embryologic development, a common pathway to the exterior, and an external orifice.

Throughout the book we have tried to emphasize logic and common sense. Where possible, basic principles of physiology and pathology have been correlated with clinical manifestations and treatment of disease in order to emphasize their interrelationships. It is our conviction that adequate patient care is best provided by individuals with a conceptual understanding of the pathophysiology of various disease processes.

The book does not provide an exhaustive review of veterinary urology, and should be supplemented wherever necessary with standard textbooks of anatomy, physiology, pharmacology, pathology, clinical pathology, clinical medicine, and clinical surgery. A list of references has been included at the end of each section for the benefit of those who are interested in obtaining additional information about diseases of the urinary system. If used in conjunction with reference lists included at the end of published works cited herein, one should be able to survey the majority of important contributions to clinical and experimental canine and feline urology.

Many arbitrary restrictions concerning subjects included in the book have been made. In an effort to conserve space and minimize expense, we have attempted to keep repetition to a minimum by including cross references to guide the reader to available information about a particular subject. Excessive detail, theories, and less commonly encountered urinary diseases have been allotted minimal space. For the sake of clarity and teaching, some controversial concepts and disease entities have been oversimplified by generalities. Often one view is advocated, even though existing controversy would allow several. We have endeavored to support facts and concepts which are based on experimental and clinical evidence and on principles of clinical medicine. Because knowledge about various urinary diseases in the dog and cat is in its infancy, many of the generalities that follow may be expected to change or undergo modification in the months and years ahead. If they do not, the outlook for future progress is dismal.

CARL A. OSBORNE
DONALD G. LOW
DELMAR R. FINCO

Canine and Feline Urology

CARL A. OSBORNE, D.V.M., Ph.D.
College of Veterinary Medicine
University of Minnesota
St. Paul, Minnesota

DONALD G. LOW, D.V.M., Ph.D.
College of Veterinary Medicine
Colorado State University
Fort Collins, Colorado

DELMAR R. FINCO, D.V.M., Ph.D.
College of Veterinary Medicine
University of Georgia
Athens, Georgia

W. B. SAUNDERS COMPANY   PHILADELPHIA · LONDON · TORONTO

W. B. Saunders Company: West Washington Square
Philadelphia, Pa. 19105

12 Dyott Street
London, WC1A 1DB

833 Oxford Street
Toronto, Ontario M8Z 5T9, Canada

Canine and Feline Urology   ISBN 0-7216-7019-9

© 1972 by W. B. Saunders Company. Copyright under the International Copyright Union. All rights reserved. This book is protected by copyright. No part of it may be reproduced, stored in a retrieval system, or transmitted in any form or by any means, electronic, mechanical, photocopying, recording, or otherwise, without written permission from the publisher. Made in the United States of America. Press of W. B. Saunders Company. Library of Congress catalog card number 72-80792.

Print No.:   9   8   7   6   5   4

RHEAL (RAY) J. BOUCHARD
Student '76

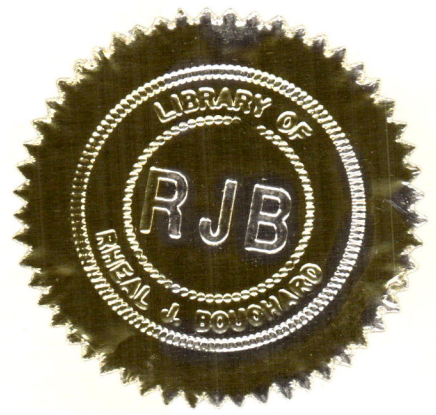

Acknowledgments

The authors express sincere appreciation and thanks to all who have helped to make this book possible. We are especially grateful to the staff and students of the Colleges of Veterinary Medicine at the University of Minnesota, the University of Georgia, and Colorado State University for their assistance in gathering information about diseases of the urinary system of the dog and cat.

Grateful acknowledgment is extended to the Schering Corporation, Bloomfield, New Jersey, for their encouragement and financial support in initiating the preparation of this book.

Special thanks are extended to Mrs. Lynn Osborne and Mrs. Susan Mathews for their help in typing the manuscript.

We acknowledge our indebtedness to Mr. Carroll C. Cann and the staff at W. B. Saunders Company for their efforts, patience, and cooperation in our behalf.

C.A.O.
D.G.L.
D.R.F.

Table of Contents

Part I
DIAGNOSIS OF URINARY DISEASES

Chapter 1 / APPLIED ANATOMY OF THE
URINARY SYSTEM 3

Chapter 2 / APPLIED PHYSIOLOGY OF THE
URINARY SYSTEM 11

Chapter 3 / EVALUATION OF THE CLINICAL HISTORY
IN DISEASES OF URINARY SYSTEM...................... 20

Chapter 4 / PHYSICAL EXAMINATION OF THE
URINARY SYSTEM 23

Chapter 5 / COLLECTION OF URINE 25

Chapter 6 / LABORATORY FINDINGS IN DISEASES OF
THE URINARY SYSTEM 39

    HEMOGRAM 39
    BUN, CREATININE, AND NONPROTEIN NITROGEN 40
    INTERPRETATION OF URINALYSIS 40
    BACTERIAL CULTURE OF URINE 55
    SERUM ELECTROLYTES 56
    BLOOD pH 59
    SERUM AMYLASE 59
    ALKALINE PHOSPHATASE 59
    CHOLESTEROL 59
    SERUM PROTEINS 60

Chapter 7 / TESTS OF RENAL FUNCTION 62

    PERSPECTIVE OF RENAL FUNCTION TESTS 62
        Urine Specific Gravity 63
        Osmolality 64
        Urine Concentration Test 66
        Exogenous Antidiuretic Hormone Concentration Test 68
        Urine Dilution Test 69
        Phenolsulphonphthalein Excretion Test 70
        Blood Urea Nitrogen 73
        Creatinine 76
        Nonprotein Nitrogen 78
        Excretory Urography 79
        Renal Clearance and Glomerular Filtration Rate 79
        Simultaneous Determination of PSP Excretion and
        Endogenous Creatinine Clearance 82

viii   CONTENTS

Chapter 8 / RADIOGRAPHIC EVALUATION OF THE
URINARY SYSTEM 85

    PRE-RADIOGRAPHIC CONSIDERATIONS 85
    RADIOGRAPHIC ESTIMATION OF KIDNEY SIZE OF DOGS 85
    PATIENT PREPARATION 87
    SURVEY RADIOGRAPHY 88
    CONTRAST RADIOGRAPHY OF THE URINARY SYSTEM 91

Chapter 9 / PERCUTANEOUS RENAL BIOPSY 107

Chapter 10 / CYSTOSCOPY 118

Chapter 11 / SUMMARY OF DIAGNOSTIC ASPECTS
OF URINARY DISEASE 121

Part II
DISEASES OF THE UPPER URINARY SYSTEM

Chapter 12 / PATHOPHYSIOLOGY OF RENAL FAILURE 127

Chapter 13 / EXTRARENAL MANIFESTATIONS OF
UREMIA 135

Chapter 14 / CAUSES OF POLYURIA—POLYDIPSIA
COMPLEX 147

Chapter 15 / CONGENITAL AND INHERITED
RENAL DISEASE 153

    Renal Aplasia 153
    Renal Hypoplasia 153
    Polycystic Disease 155
    Renal Cortical Hypoplasia 156
    Horseshoe Kidneys 157
    Primary Renal Glucosuria 158
    Cystinuria 159
    Familial Renal Disease in Norwegian Elkhound Dogs 160
    Familial Renal Disease in Lhasa Apso Dogs 161
    Congenital and Inherited Renal Diseases in
    Dogs and Cats 162

Chapter 16 / ACUTE RENAL DISEASE 165

Chapter 17 / ISCHEMIC AND CHEMICAL NEPHROSIS 169

    RENAL ISCHEMIA VERSUS NEPHROTOXINS 169
    ETIOPATHOGENESIS OF ISCHEMIC NEPHROSIS 170
    ETIOPATHOGENESIS OF NEPHROTOXIC NEPHROSIS 172
    CLINICAL FINDINGS 172
    LABORATORY FINDINGS 174
    RADIOGRAPHIC FINDINGS 174
    RENAL BIOPSY FINDINGS 174
    DIAGNOSIS 175
    TREATMENT 175
    PROGNOSIS 179

Chapter 18 / CHRONIC INTERSTITIAL NEPHRITIS 182

Chapter 19 / PYELONEPHRITIS 184

Chapter 20	/	END—STAGE KIDNEYS	189
Chapter 21	/	RENAL CYSTS	196
Chapter 22	/	HYDRONEPHROSIS	198
Chapter 23	/	DIOCTOPHYMA RENALE	209
Chapter 24	/	MISCELLANEOUS PARASITES OF THE URINARY SYSTEM	213
Chapter 25	/	PRIMARY DISEASES OF GLOMERULI	214

    GLOMERULONEPHRITIS 214
    SCLEROSING GLOMERULAR DISEASE 218
    GLOMERULAR LIPOIDOSIS 219
    INFARCTION 219

Chapter 26	/	RENAL AMYLOIDOSIS	220
Chapter 27	/	NEPHROTIC SYNDROME	228
Chapter 28	/	RENAL DISEASES ASSOCIATED WITH POLYSYSTEMIC DISEASES	232

    BACTERIAL ENDOCARDITIS 232
    DIABETES MELLITUS 234
    INFECTIOUS CANINE HEPATITIS 238
    LEPTOSPIROSIS 238
    MALIGNANT LYMPHOMA 241
    POLYARTERITIS NODOSA 248
    PYOMETRA 249
    SYSTEMIC LUPUS ERYTHEMATOSUS 253
    SYSTEMIC MYCOSES 254

Chapter 29	/	NEOPLASMS OF THE KIDNEY	255
Chapter 30	/	PROGNOSIS OF RENAL FAILURE	261
Chapter 31	/	TREATMENT OF RENAL FAILURE	266
Chapter 32	/	FLUID THERAPY IN RENAL FAILURE	291
Chapter 33	/	DRUG THERAPY IN RENAL FAILURE	310

Part III
DISEASES OF THE UPPER AND LOWER URINARY SYSTEM

Chapter 34	/	UROLITHIASIS	319
Chapter 35	/	DISEASES OF THE URETER	330

    OBSTRUCTIVE URETEROPATHY 331
    TRAUMA 332
    CALCULI 332
    NEOPLASIA 332
    VESICO-URETERAL REFLUX 332
    ECTOPIC URETERS 334

CONTENTS

Chapter 36 / PHYSICAL INJURIES 338

    RENAL TRAUMA 338
    TRAUMATIC RUPTURE OF THE URETER AND
    RENAL PELVIS 342
    TRAUMA TO THE URINARY BLADDER 343

Chapter 37 / OBSTRUCTIVE UROPATHY 350

Part IV
DISEASES OF THE LOWER URINARY SYSTEM

Chapter 38 / BACTERIAL CYSTITIS 355

Chapter 39 / CYSTITIS—URETHRAL OBSTRUCTION
                    COMPLEX IN THE CAT 361

Chapter 40 / CAPILLARIA PLICA 372

Chapter 41 / NEOPLASMS OF THE URINARY BLADDER 374

Chapter 42 / PATENT URACHUS 386

Chapter 43 / ABNORMAL LOCATIONS OF THE
                    URINARY BLADDER 389

Chapter 44 / URINARY INCONTINENCE 394

Chapter 45 / DISEASES OF THE URETHRA 400

    CONGENITAL ANOMALIES 400
    TRAUMA TO THE URETHRA 401
    NEOPLASMS OF THE URETHRA 401

APPENDICES 403

GENERAL REFERENCES 407

INDEX 409

DIAGNOSIS OF URINARY DISEASES

Chapter 1
APPLIED ANATOMY OF THE URINARY SYSTEM

I. **Kidneys**

   A. *Location and gross appearance*
1. The right kidney of the dog is located approximately between the thirteenth thoracic and the second lumbar vertebrae; the left kidney is located about one half kidney length caudal to the right.
2. The kidneys are retroperitoneal. The cranial part of the dorsal surface of each organ is variably covered with peritoneum, but the ventral surface of the organ is consistently covered.
3. The attachment of both kidneys to the body wall is relatively loose. The right kidney of the dog is more firmly attached to the body wall than the left, but the right kidney can be displaced cranially or caudally by other structures. The left kidney is freely movable and is commonly pushed caudally by the distended stomach.
4. Both kidneys lie in an oblique direction and are tilted cranioventrally.
5. The anatomic relationship of the kidneys of the cat to adjacent structures, and to each other, is the same as in the dog. The kidneys of the cat are even more loosely attached to the body wall than are those of the dog.
6. The kidneys of the dog and cat are bean-shaped, but the kidneys of the cat are slightly more spherical. The renal artery enters the kidney at the hilus. The renal vein and ureter leave the kidney at the hilus.
7. The kidneys of both species are enveloped by a fibrous capsule which normally can be easily peeled from the cortical surface.
8. Superficial subcapsular veins are prominent in the cat.
9. Kidney size.
   a. In both species, the right and left kidneys are nearly the same size and weight (Fig. 1–1).
   b. Kidney size in both species is variable, depending not only on variation in body weight, but also on other factors.
   c. Mean values and standard deviations for 27 normal mongrel dogs are:
     (1) Body weight—18.1 ± 7.5 kg.
     (2) Right kidney length—6.5 ± 1.06 cm.
     (3) Right kidney weight—47.4 ± 18.8 Gm.
   d. In adult cats, kidney weight varies from 0.6 to 1.0 per cent of body weight, with large males having slightly heavier kidneys.

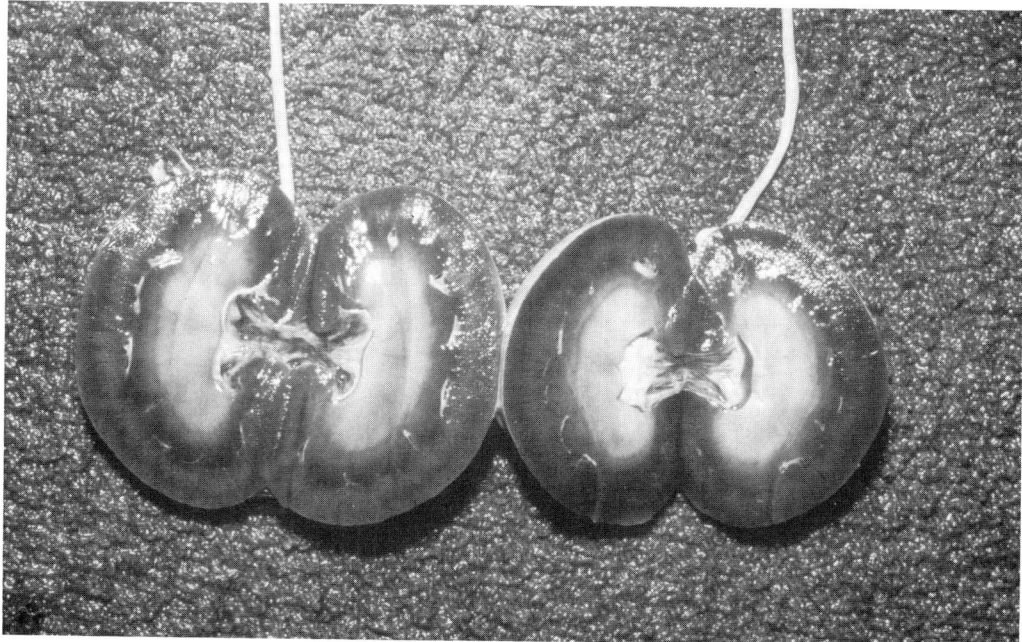

Figure 1–1. The cut surface of normal kidneys obtained from an adult male dog. Both kidneys are of similar size and have a smooth outline and regular contour. The cortex is sharply demarcated from the medulla at the corticomedullary junction.

B. *The nephron and collecting duct system*

All the nephrons are similarly constructed, but vary markedly in overall measurements and proportionalities, depending on their location within the kidney and on the size of the dog or cat.
1. Parts of the nephron.
    a. Bowman's capsule.
    b. Glomerulus.
    c. Proximal tubule.
    d. Loop of Henle.
    e. Distal tubule.
2. Numbers of nephrons.
    a. Glomeruli counts in 27 normal mongrel dogs indicate that there are 415,000 ± 130,000 glomeruli per kidney.
    b. There are approximately 190,000 glomeruli per kidney in the cat.
    c. There appears to be no correlation between glomeruli numbers and body size in the dog.
    d. It is generally assumed that the presence of a glomerulus is an indication of the presence of the remainder of the nephron and thus glomeruli numbers are synonymous with nephron numbers.
3. Collecting duct system.
    a. Each distal tubule empties into a collecting duct.
    b. Several collecting ducts unite to form progressively larger ducts.
    c. Urine is eventually emptied into the renal pelvis through large papillary ducts.
4. Formation of urine.
    a. An ultrafiltrate of blood passes through the glomerular capillaries and proceeds down the lumen of the proximal tubule, the loop of Henle,

the distal tubule, and the collecting duct system to reach the pelvis of the kidney.

C. *Gross organization of the kidney*
 1. Bisection of the kidney along its long axis and through the hilus reveals many of the anatomic features of the kidney of the dog and cat (Fig. 1–1).
 2. The cortex is the red-brown granular peripheral area.
    a. Close visual inspection of the cortex allows visualization of renal corpuscles (glomeruli and Bowman's capsules). Glomeruli are not present in the medulla or within 2 mm. of the capsular margin of the cortex.
    b. The remaining cortical tissue is composed predominantly of proximal and distal tubules. Collecting ducts, blood vessels, and supporting tissues are also present.
    c. Projections of medullary substance (medullary rays) into the cortical area may be observed. Medullary rays are composed of collecting ducts, descending and ascending limbs of loops of Henle, and distal tubules.
 3. The medulla is lighter in color than the cortex and is normally striated in appearance.
    a. It is composed of loops of Henle, collecting ducts, papillary ducts, interstitial tissue and small blood vessels (vasa recta) which originate from juxtamedullary glomeruli.
    b. The long loops of Henle and the vasa recta originate in the juxtamedullary portion of the cortex, descend into the medulla, then loop back to the cortex.
    c. The close proximity of the loop of Henle and the blood vessels is significant in the countercurrent system of urine concentration (see Applied Physiology of the Urinary Tract).
 4. The renal pelvis.
    a. The renal pelvis is a funnel-shaped structure that collects urine from the papillary ducts of the kidney.
    b. The pelvis is entirely intrarenal.
    c. The kidneys of the dog and cat are unipyramidal.
    d. Several (five to six) diverticula extend from the pelvis into the renal parenchyma. The diverticula are formed as a result of pelvic mucosal reflection around large arteries and veins.
    e. The pelvis is lined with transitional cell epithelium.

D. *The renal circulation*
 1. Arterial circulation. The arterial system of the kidneys is composed of end arteries without significant collateral blood supply.
    a. The renal arteries arise from the dorsal aorta. The right renal artery usually arises about 2 cm. cranial to the left, and lies dorsal to the postcava.
    b. The left renal artery is a complete double structure in about 13 per cent of dogs. The right renal artery is rarely multiple in dogs. Multiple renal arteries are rare in cats.
    c. Branching of the renal artery usually occurs 1 cm. outside the hilus. Further subdivisions occur, providing separate vessels called the interlobar arteries. In the dog, three to four interlobar arteries arise from each branch of the renal artery, resulting in a total of six to eight interlobar arteries. These arteries supply the renal cortex in a symmetrical manner.

d. Arcuate arteries branch from the interlobar arteries at the corticomedullary junction and radiate toward the periphery of the cortex.
e. There they divide into interlobular arteries. These arteries give off branches at wide angles on every side, which are termed intralobular arteries.
f. Intralobular arteries give rise to the afferent vessels of the glomeruli (afferent arterioles). Cells of the terminal portion of the afferent arterioles are modified (juxtaglomerular cells) to secrete the enzyme renin.
g. Afferent arterioles give rise to glomerular capillary tufts.
h. Glomerular capillaries drain into efferent arterioles.
   (1) Efferent arterioles from glomeruli in the outer cortex empty their blood into capillary beds (peritubular capillaries) that surround the proximal and distal convoluted tubules in the cortex.
   (2) Efferent glomerular arterioles from deeper in the cortex yield long straight vessels (vasa recta) that parallel the loops of Henle and contribute to the countercurrent mechanism for urine concentration.
i. Most of the blood which supplies the renal tubules via the peritubular capillaries must first pass through glomeruli.
2. Venous circulation.
   a. Single renal veins per kidney occur in 99 per cent of dogs, but multiple right renal veins occur in over 44 per cent of cats.
   b. In the dog, the main renal vein divides into 2 branches which supply halves of the kidney depicted by a longitudinal sectioning through the hilus.
   c. Abundant interconnections occur between arcuate veins.
   d. Both the dog and the cat have rather extensive capsular veins which drain into the renal vein at the hilus.
3. Cortical and medullary circulation.
   a. Special techniques for monitoring intrarenal circulation indicate that blood flow through the cortex is much more voluminous and rapid than through the medulla.
   b. No conclusive evidence exists for shunting of cortical blood to the medulla during such abnormal conditions as shock.

E. *The juxtaglomerular apparatus*
1. The juxtaglomerular apparatus consists of:
   a. Juxtaglomerular cells in the media of afferent arterioles.
   b. The macula densa of the distal convoluted tubules. Cells of the latter are located in the portion of the distal tubule which is adjacent to the afferent arteriole.
2. The juxtaglomerular apparatus is involved with production and release of a proteolytic enzyme called renin.
   a. Renin initiates several reactions which convert a circulating α-globulin to angiotensin.
   b. Angiotensin is a vasoconstrictor, but its most important function is to stimulate the release of aldosterone from the adrenal cortex.

II. Ureters

A. *Location*
1. The ureters are retroperitoneal structures that carry urine from the renal pelvis to the bladder.

2. They run parallel and adjacent to the postcava and dorsal aorta in the cranial part of the abdomen.
3. They enter between the two layers of peritoneum forming the lateral ligament of the bladder and reach the dorsolateral surface of the bladder just caudal to its neck (trigone).

B. *Structure*
1. The diameter of a distended ureter is 0.6 to 0.9 cm. in the dog.
2. Ureter length varies with body size, but is 12 to 16 cm. in a 35 pound dog.
3. The right ureter is longer than the left because of the more cranial position of the right kidney.
4. The ureteral wall is composed of three layers of smooth muscle and is lined with transitional cell epithelium.
5. Anatomical ureterovesical valves are not present; however, the oblique course of the ureters through the bladder wall normally prevents retrograde flow of urine from the bladder.

III. Urinary bladder

A. *Location*
1. The location of the urinary bladder depends upon the degree of distention.
2. When empty, the bladder lies within or just ahead of the bony pelvis.
3. When distended, the bladder assumes a more cranial and more ventral position within the abdominal cavity.
4. Location may be altered by increase in size or change in location of adjacent organs, such as the prostate gland.

B. *Shape*
1. The bladder is normally pear-shaped with a rounded vertex when slightly to moderately distended.
2. It becomes almost spherical when markedly distended.

C. *Structure*
1. Three layers of muscle (detrusor muscle) are present in the bladder wall.
   a. Outer and inner longitudinal layers.
   b. Thick middle circular layer.
   c. The muscle fibers all take on a circular or oblique appearance at the urethra-bladder junction, forming a functional sphincter.
2. The triangular area near the neck of the bladder is called the trigone. The urethral orifice and the two ureteral openings make up the boundaries of this triangular area.
3. Lateral umbilical ligaments connect the lateral surface of the bladder to the lateral pelvic wall.
4. The bladder is lined with transitional cell epithelium.

IV. Urethra

A. *Male*
1. Canine.
   a. For purposes of description, the urethra of the male dog may be divided into 3 parts.
      (1) The prostatic urethra extends from the urinary bladder to the

posterior end of the prostate. It passes through and is completely surrounded by the prostate gland.
- (2) The membranous urethra extends from the posterior aspect of the prostate gland to the urethral bulb of the penis.
- (3) The penile urethra begins at the entrance of the membranous urethra into the penis and extends to the tip of the penis. The urethral groove of the os penis surrounds approximately two thirds of the dorsal circumference of the penile urethra.
 b. Except for a short distance adjacent to the external urethral orifice, the urethra is lined by transitional cell epithelium. A short segment adjacent to the external urethral orifice is lined by stratified squamous epithelium.
 c. The urethral muscle is composed of an inner layer of longitudinal smooth muscle fibers and an outer layer of transverse striated muscle fibers.
 d. The length and diameter of the urethra are variable. Only that portion of the penile urethra which passes through the urethral groove of the os penis is limited in expansion by extrinsic structures.
2. Feline.
 a. The urethra of the male cat may also be divided into 3 parts.
  (1) The preprostatic urethra extends from the urinary bladder to the prostate gland. Proportionately, this segment of the urethra is longer in the cat than in the dog.
  (2) The pelvic or membranous urethra extends from the prostate gland to the bulbourethral glands which are located at the caudal aspect of the bony pelvis. This portion of the urethra is surrounded by a thick layer of striated muscle.
  (3) The penile urethra extends from the bulbourethral glands to the tip of the penis. The os penis, when present, is not grooved to accommodate the penile urethra. The diameter of the penile urethra is smaller than that of the pelvic urethra.

B. *Female*
1. The urethra of the female dog and cat is much shorter than the urethra in the male of either species and has a larger diameter.
2. The urethra originates at the urinary bladder and enters the ventral floor of the vagina.
 a. In the dog, the urethra opens on a tubercle which is located cranial to the clitoris, approximately 4 to 5 cm. from the ventral commissure of the vulva. A voluntary muscle (external sphincter) is present at the junction of the urethra with the vagina.
 b. The dorsal aspect of the urethra lies in close proximity to the ventral wall of the vagina.
3. The urethra is lined by transitional cell epithelium.
4. The urethral muscle in the dog is composed of inner and outer longitudinal layers and a middle transverse layer of smooth muscle.

REFERENCES

Anderson, A. C.: Renal system. *In* The Beagle as an Experimental Dog. Edited by A. C. Anderson and L. S. Good. Ames, Iowa, Iowa State University Press, 1970.

Anderson, A. C., and Goldman, M.: Growth and development. *In* The Beagle as an Experimental Dog. Edited by A. C. Anderson and L. S. Good. Ames, Iowa, Iowa State University Press, 1970.

Arnautovic, I.: Distribution of the renal artery in the kidney of the dog. Brit. Vet. J., *115*:446–448, 1959.
Barger, A. C., and Herd, J. A.: The renal circulation. New Eng. J. Med., *284*:482–490, 1971.
Bell, R. D., Keyl, M. J., Shrader, F. R., Jones, E. W., and Henry, L. P.: Renal lymphatics: The internal distribution. Nephron, 5:454–463, 1968.
Bharadwaj, M. B., and Calhoun, M. L.: Histology of the urethral epithelium of domestic animals. Amer. J. Vet. Res., *20*:841–851, 1959.
Bradley, W. E., and Fletcher, T. F.: Innervation of the mammalian bladder. J. Urol., *101*:846–853, 1969.
Calhoun, M. L.: Comparative histology of the ureters of domestic animals. Anat. Rec., *133*:365–366, 1959.
Cass, A. S., and Hinman, F.: Constant urethral flow in female dog. I. Normal vesical and urethral pressures and effect of muscle relaxant. J. Urol., *99*:442–446, 1968.
Chein, K. C. H., and Bradley, J. E.: The relationship between proximal and distal convoluted tubules in the dog. Fed. Proc., *27*:742, 1968.
Christensen, G. C.: The urogenital system and mammary glands. In Anatomy of the Dog. Edited by Miller, M. E., Christensen, G. C., and Evans, H. E., Philadelphia, Pa., W. B. Saunders Co., 1964.
Christensen, G. C.: Circulation of blood through the canine kidney. Amer. J. Vet. Res., *13*:236–245, 1952.
Christie, B. A.: The ureterovesical junction in dogs. Invest. Urol., *9*:10–16, 1971.
Cowgill, G. R., and Drabkin, D. L.: Determination of a Formula for the Surface Area of the Dog Together with a Consideration of Formulae Available for Other Species. Amer. J. Physiol., *81*:36–61, 1927.
Ferber, R., Evans, H., and Amador, E.: The renal veins of the dog. J. Urol., *95*:318–322, 1966.
Fletcher, T. F., and Bradley, W. F.: Comparative morphologic features of urinary bladder innervation. Amer. J. Vet. Res., *30*:1655–1662, 1969.
Foote, J. J., and Graffdin, A. L.: Quantitative measurements of the fat-laden and fat-free segments of the proximal tubule in the nephron of the cat and dog. Anat. Rec., *72*:169, 1938.
Gairns, F. W., and Morrison, S. D.: Lipid in the nephron of the cat. J. Physiol., *110*:17P–18P, 1949.
Gerard, P.: Comparative histology of the vertebrate nephron. J. Anat., *70*:354–379, 1936.
Gordon, N.: Surgical anatomy of the bladder, prostate gland and urethra in the male dog. J.A.V.M.A., *136*:215–221, 1960.
Grahame, T.: The pelvis and calyces of the kidneys of some mammals. Brit. Vet. J., *109*:51–55, 1953.
Gramiak, R., and Ross, P.: Determination of transported ureteric volume in dogs by cineroentgenologic analysis. Am. J. Roentgen., *104*:366–371, 1968.
Helmholz, H. F.: Presence of tubular epithelium within the glomerular capsule in mammals. Proc. Staff Meet. Mayo Clin., *10*:110–212, 1935.
Helmy, F., and Longley, J. B.: Chromatographic analysis of lipid in kidney of the cat and dog. Anat. Rec., *151*:360, 1965.
Hodson, N.: On the intrinsic blood supply to the prostate and pelvic urethra in the dog. Res. Vet. Sci., *9*:274–280, 1968.
Hoorens, J., Thoonen, J., and Cloet, G.: Intranuclear crystals in liver and kidney cells of dogs. Vlaams Diergeneesk Tijdschr., *34*:265–270, 1965.
Horster, M., Kemler, B. J., and Valtin, H.: Intracortical distribution of number and volume of glomeruli during postnatal maturation in the dog. J. Clin. Invest., *50*:796–800, 1971.
Hull, V. E., and MacGregor, W. W.: Relation of kidney weight to body weight in the cat. Anat. Rec., *69*:319–331, 1937.
Jackson, B., and Capiello, V. P.: Ranges of normal organ weights of dogs. Toxicol. Appl. Pharm., 6:664–668, 1964.
Klapproth, H. J.: Distribution of renal arterial circulation in the dog. J. Urol., *82*:417–423, 1959.
Kunkel, P. A.: The number and size of the glomeruli of several mammals. Bull. Johns Hopkins Hosp., *47*:285–291, 1930.
Latimer, H. B.: The prenatal growth of the cat. VIII. The weights of the kidneys, bladder, gonads and uterus with weights of the adult organs. Growth, *3*:89–108, 1939.
Latimer, H. B.: The growth of the kidneys and bladder in the fetal dog. Anat. Rec., *109*:1–12, 1951.
Latimer, H. B.: Changes in relative organ weights in the fetal dog. Anat. Rec., *153*:421–428, 1965.
Lobban, M. C.: Some observations on the intracellular lipid in the kidney of the cat. J. Anat., *89*:92–99, 1955.
MacNider, W. deB.: The occurrence of stainable lipoid material in the renal epithelium of animals falling in different age segments. Proc. Soc. Expt. Biol. Med., *58*:326–328, 1945.
Mattenheimer, H., Pollak, V. E., and DeBruin, H.: Quantitative histochemistry of the nephron. IX. Distribution and activity of various enzymes in the kidneys of the dog. Enzymol. Biol. Clin., *4*:107–126, 1964.
Mayer, E., and Ottolenghi, J. H.: Protrusion of tubular epithelium into the space of Bowman's capsule in dogs and cats. Anat. Rec., *99*:477–510, 1947.
Modell, W.: Observations on the lipoids in the renal tubule of the cat. Anat. Rec., *57*:13–28, 1933.
Moore, R. D., and Calhoun, M. L.: Comparative histology of the bladder and proximal urethra of domestic animals. Anat. Rec., *127*:338, 1957.
Movat, H. Z., and Steiner, J. W.: Studies of nephrotoxic nephritis. I. The study of the fine structure of the glomerulus of the dog. Amer. J. Clin. Path., *36*:289–305, 1961.
Mullink, J. W. M. A., and Feron, V. J.: Intraglomerular epithelial reflux as a post mortem phenomenon in the kidneys of the dog and rat. Path. Vet. *4*:366–377, 1967.

Oliver, J.: Nephrons and Kidneys. A quantitative study of developmental and evolutionary mammalian renal architectonics. New York, N. Y., Harper and Row, 1968.

Pfeiffer, W. E.: Comparative anatomical observations of mammalian renal pelvis and medulla. J. Anat., *102*:321–331, 1968.

Pierce, E. C.: Renal lymphatics. Anat. Rec., *90*:315, 1944.

Ratzlaff, M. H.: Lymphatics. *In* The Beagle as an Experimental Dog. Edited by A. C. Anderson and L. S. Good, Ames, Iowa, Iowa State University Press, 1970.

Reis, R. H., and Tepe, P.: Variations in patterns of renal vessels and their relation to the type of posterior vena cava in the dog (Cania familiaris). Amer. J. Anat., *99*:1–16, 1956.

Rytand, D. A.: The number and size of mammalian glomeruli as related to kidney and to body weight with methods for their enumeration and measurement. Amer. J. Anat., *62*:507–520, 1938.

Sellwood, R. V., and Verney, E. B.: Enumeration of glomeruli in the kidney of the dog. J. Anat., *89*:63–68, 1955.

Smith, C., and Freeman, B. L.: Distribution of lipids, lipase and alkaline phosphatase in renal tubule of the cat. Proc. Soc. Exptl. Biol. Med., *86*:775–778, 1954.

Stewart, G. N.: Possible relations of the weight of the lungs and other organs to body weight and surface area in dogs. Amer. J. Physiol., *58*:45–52, 1922.

Swann, H. G., and Railey, M. J.: Weights of right and left kidneys in dogs. Texas Rep. Biol. Med., *17*:256–258, 1959.

Thompson, S. W., Cook, J. E., and Hoey, H.: Histochemical studies of acidophilic, crystalline intranuclear inclusions in the liver and kidney of dogs. Amer. J. Path., *35*:607–623, 1959.

Thompson, S. W., Weigand, R. G., Thomassen, R. W., Harrison, M., and Turbyfill, C. L.: The protein nature of acidophilic crystalline intranuclear inclusions in the liver and kidney of dogs. Amer. J. Path., *35*:1105–1115, 1959.

Vaughan, J. A., and Adams, T.: Surface area of the cat. J. Appl. Physiol, *22*:956–958, 1967.

Vimtrup, B.: On the Number, Shape, Structure and Surface Area of the Glomeruli in the Kidneys of Man and Mammals. Amer. J. Anat., *41*:123–151, 1928.

Yadava, R. P., and Calhoun, M. L.: Comparative histology of the kidney of domestic animals. Amer. J. Vet. R., *19*:958–968, 1958.

Chapter 2
APPLIED PHYSIOLOGY OF THE URINARY SYSTEM

I. **Functions of the kidney**

   A. *Conservation of water and electrolytes in order to maintain a constant extracellular environment.*

   B. *Excretion of waste products of metabolism, and water and electrolytes in instances of excessive ingestion or production.*

   C. *Elaboration of hormones involved in the regulation of hematopoiesis, blood pressure, and sodium reabsorption.*
      1. Erythropoietin.
      2. Renin.

   D. *Metabolism of vitamin D to its active form (1,25 dihydroxycholecalciferol).*

II. **Requirements for normal kidney function**

   A. *Adequate perfusion with blood*
      Inadequate renal perfusion may cause prerenal uremia initially, and primary ischemic renal failure if prolonged.
      1. Normally the kidneys of the dog receive about 10 to 20 per cent of the cardiac output.
      2. Blood pressure provides the force necessary for glomerular filtration.
      3. When the canine kidney is perfused at pressures between 90 and 220 mm. Hg, renal vascular resistance varies with pressure so that renal blood flow is relatively constant (autoregulation). Changes in renal vascular resistance associated with autoregulation tend to stabilize filtration pressure. When mean systemic arterial blood pressure falls below 90 mm. Hg, however, a marked decrease in glomerular filtration rate occurs. Perfusion of the kidneys with blood at a pressure sufficient to perform filtration requires:
         a. An adequate blood volume.
         b. Cardiac function capable of maintaining blood pressure above the minimum pressure necessary for filtration.
      4. Inadequate renal perfusion with blood may lead to prerenal uremia. Some causes of prerenal uremia are:

12 DIAGNOSIS OF URINARY DISEASES

      a. Heart disease (valvular insufficiency, valvular stenosis, myocardial disease, congenital defects, dirofilariasis, cardiac tamponade).
      b. Shock due to any cause.
      c. Severe dehydration due to any cause.
      d. Hypoadrenalcorticism.
   5. Clinical signs and the results of tests of renal function are similar in prerenal uremia, primary renal uremia, and postrenal uremia.
      a. BUN and creatinine concentrations are elevated due to decreased glomerular filtration rate.
      b. Phenolsulfonphthalein (PSP) dye excretion may be decreased due to lack of perfusion of tubules with blood containing PSP.
      c. Unlike primary renal uremia, the kidneys retain their capacity to concentrate urine in prerenal uremia.

B. *Normal renal function also requires a sufficient quantity of functional renal tissue. Sufficient loss of functional renal tissue causes primary renal uremia.*
   1. The kidney has considerable functional reserve, and death may not occur even after destruction of three fourths or more of the functional renal parenchyma of both kidneys (see Chapter 12, Pathophysiology of Renal Failure).
   2. A decrease in the quantity of functional renal tissue below this level is associated with primary renal failure and uremia. If the loss of functional tissue is gradual, however, compensatory change often permits survival with much less than one fourth of the total functional renal tissue (see Chapter 12, Pathophysiology of Renal Failure).

C. *Adequate expulsion of urine from the urinary tract*
   A defect in passage of urine may cause postrenal uremia. Primary renal lesions (hydronephrosis) may develop if obstruction to urine outflow exists for a sufficient period of time.
   1. Impairment of urine flow from the kidneys by obstruction in the lower urinary tract results in:
      a. An initial increase in pressure in the renal pelves and duct system due to continued production of urine.
      b. Development of "back pressure" which counters the force of blood pressure responsible for glomerular filtration.
      c. Diminished renal function and oliguria or anuria.
      d. Development of postrenal uremia.
   2. Postrenal uremia can be caused by obstructive uropathy whenever both kidneys are affected by the site(s) of obstruction.
   3. Tests of renal function (PSP, BUN, creatinine) alone do not distinguish between prerenal, renal, and postrenal causes of uremia.
   4. Some causes of postrenal uremia are:
      a. Urethral obstruction due to calculi or debris.
      b. Neoplasms of the urinary bladder, urethra, or adjacent structures which obstruct urine outflow.
      c. Rupture of both ureters, the bladder, or the proximal urethra.

III. Mechanisms of kidney function

Several mechanisms characterize the overall function of the kidney. An ultrafiltrate of blood (glomerular filtrate) passes through the glomeruli and into the tubules. As the filtrate traverses the renal tubules, its volume is reduced and its composition is modified by tubular reabsorption and tubular secretion.

A. *Glomerular filtration*
   1. Glomerular filtration is a passive process for the kidneys since energy is transmitted to the kidneys in the form of blood pressure.
   2. The volume of glomerular filtrate in the dog is normally about 4 ml. per minute per kg. of body weight or 80 ml. per minute per square meter of body surface area. In the cat, glomerular filtration rate is reported to be about the same.
   3. Glomerular filtrate is an ultrafiltrate of blood and contains all components of the blood except significant quantities of cells and protein.
   4. Factors impairing glomerular filtration include:
      a. Inadequate perfusion of the kidney with blood (see IIA, renal physiology).
      b. Altered permeability of glomerular membranes due to generalized glomerular disease.
      c. Factors which increase resistance to the flow of glomerular filtrate through the tubule, including:
         (1) Intrarenal edema.
         (2) Inflammation of renal interstitial tissue.
         (3) Obstruction.
            (a) Intrarenal (casts or debris in the tubules and collecting ducts).
            (b) Ureteral obstruction.
            (c) Urethral obstruction.

B. *Tubular reabsorption*
   1. Tubular reabsorption of many substances (sodium, potassium, phosphate, glucose, amino acids, and others) is an active process that requires energy. Other substances (water, chloride) are reabsorbed by passive diffusion along osmotic, concentration, or electrical gradients.
   2. The quantities of substances that are reabsorbed from glomerular filtrate are dependent upon several factors, including:
      a. The physiologic capacity of normal tubules.
      b. The needs of the body for the substance in question.
      c. Functional alterations which occur as a result of renal diseases.
   3. Other organs produce hormones that influence tubular reabsorption of specific substances.
      a. Antidiuretic hormone (ADH) from the posterior pituitary gland promotes reabsorption of water from the distal tubules and collecting ducts.
      b. Aldosterone from the adrenal glands stimulates sodium reabsorption by the renal tubules.
   4. Many substances (e.g., glucose, amino acids, water soluble vitamins) are "threshold substances" that are almost completely reabsorbed until a certain concentration in the blood and glomerular filtrate is exceeded. The maximal rate at which an active transport system can transport a particular solute is called its transport maximum (Tm). The amount of a particular solute reabsorbed (transported) by the tubules is proportional to the quantity of the solute present in tubular filtrate, up to the Tm for the solute. At higher tubular concentrations, the tubular transport mechanism is saturated and there is no significant increase in the quantity of the solute transported. Then overflow into urine occurs. Glucose is used as an example.

a. If the plasma concentration of glucose is 100 mg. per 100 ml. and GFR = 4.0 ml. per minute per kg., then about 4 mg. of glucose per minute per kg. of body weight is delivered to the tubules. Essentially all of the glucose is reabsorbed; none can be detected in the urine.
b. When the blood glucose concentration is high (about 180 mg. per 100 ml. or greater) the reabsorptive capacity of the renal tubules is exceeded and overflow of glucose in urine occurs. The glucose carries an increased volume of water with it because of its osmotic effect.
c. Administration of the plant glycoside phlorhizin specifically inhibits the enzyme system responsible for reabsorption of glucose. As a result of tubular impairment, glucosuria occurs at normal blood glucose concentrations.
d. Primary renal glucosuria is a defect in the mechanism of glucose reabsorption. Overflow of glucose into the urine occurs at normal blood glucose concentrations (see Chapter 15, Congenital and Inherited Renal Diseases).
e. Significant glucosuria rarely occurs as the result of naturally occurring renal disease. When detected, usually only small amounts of glucose are present.
f. Renal tubular transport of glucose is unaffected by insulin.
5. Many substances are reabsorbed in relation to the body's needs. Sodium, potassium, and bicarbonate are examples. In the case of sodium:
a. Most is reabsorbed in the proximal tubules without regard for body needs.
b. Absorption in the distal tubules is dependent upon body requirements and is influenced by aldosterone.
c. Normally, sodium is regulated by balancing the amount of sodium excreted with the amount ingested.
d. In instances of generalized chronic nephritis in the dog, sodium reabsorption is altered and a negative body balance of sodium eventually occurs.
6. Bicarbonate reabsorption.
a. In the dog, the normal blood concentration of bicarbonate is 25 to 28 mEq/L..
b. If the blood concentration of bicarbonate falls below this amount, an increased amount of bicarbonate is reabsorbed by the renal tubules.
c. If the blood concentration exceeds the normal range, bicarbonate is excreted by the kidney.
d. Bicarbonate plays an important role in acid-base balance, since it acts as a buffer which can minimize blood pH changes due to alterations in hydrogen ion production or retention.
e. In uremia, impaired excretion of hydrogen ions occurs, and bicarbonate utilization exceeds renal bicarbonate conservation. Therapy with alkalinizing agents such as sodium bicarbonate or sodium citrate orally, or sodium bicarbonate, sodium lactate, or sodium acetate parenterally, helps alleviate the acidosis (see Chapter 31, Treatment of Renal Failure).
7. Potassium reabsorption and excretion.
a. A large quantity of filtered potassium is removed from tubular fluid by active reabsorption in the proximal tubules.
b. Potassium is also excreted into tubular fluid by distal tubular cells.

c. In the healthy adult dog and cat, the quantity of potassium excreted is approximately equal to the quantity of potassium ingested, and potassium balance is maintained.
d. Since the kidneys provide the major route of excretion of potassium, the concentration of potassium in the body may become abnormally elevated in the presence of oliguria or anuria.
e. In instances of total body potassium deficit caused by inadequate intake or excessive excretion, the kidneys are unable to conserve all of the potassium filtered. Hypokalemia may be associated with hyposthenuria.

8. Water reabsorption.
   a. Obligatory water reabsorption occurs in the proximal convoluted tubules regardless of the body's actual need for water. Reabsorption is passive as it accompanies active reabsorption of glucose, sodium and other solutes. About 80 per cent of the water is absorbed from the tubules by obligatory reabsorption.
   b. Facultative reabsorption of water:
      (1) Occurs in the distal tubules and collecting ducts and is regulated according to the needs of the body.
      (2) Is regulated by antidiuretic hormone of the hypothalamoneurohypophyseal system. Antidiuretic hormone is synthesized in the hypothalamic nuclei and is transported by axoplasmic flow to the neurohypophysis. There it is stored in specialized cells called pituicytes. Antidiuretic hormone release occurs predominantly in response to increased plasma osmolality. Decreased extracellular fluid volume and pain may also cause its release. Antidiuretic hormone increases the permeability of the distal tubules and collecting ducts to water and thus enhances water reabsorption. In the absence of antidiuretic hormone, the distal convoluted tubules and collecting ducts become relatively impermeable to water, and water diuresis results (see Diabetes insipidus, in Chapter 14).
      (3) In renal diabetes insipidus, the distal tubules and collecting ducts do not respond to antidiuretic hormone even though it is present.
      (4) In the presence of generalized renal disease, the ability of the tubules to dilute or concentrate glomerular filtrate is often impaired. Eventually the specific gravity becomes fixed at that of glomerular filtrate (1.008 to 1.012) (see Chapter 12, Pathophysiology of Renal Failure).
   c. The countercurrent system
      (1) A countercurrent system is a system in which inflow runs parallel to, in close proximity to, and opposite to outflow.
      (2) The ability of the kidneys to concentrate urine is dependent upon a gradient of increasing osmolality from the renal cortex to the tip of the renal papilla.
      (3) This osmotic gradient is established and maintained by active transport mechanisms in the loops of Henle (countercurrent multipliers), and passive diffusion in the vasa recta (countercurrent exchangers). Reduced volume and rate of blood flow in the renal medulla, as compared to the renal cortex, contributes to maintenance of hyperosmolality in the medulla.
      (4) Before the concept of a countercurrent mechanism in the kidney was established, the formation of concentrated urine was explained by theories which were physiologically improbable.

(a) One explanation was the active transport of water across renal tubules. The latter was a poor hypothesis since in all other biological systems, water transport is known to be passive.

(b) An alternative explanation was the presence of an unusually large osmotic gradient between the tubular lumen and interstitial tissue.

(5) Although there is a large osmotic gradient in the kidneys, the countercurrent system distributes this gradient along the entire length of the renal tubules, rather than across a single layer of tubular cells a few micromillimeters thick.

C. *Tubular secretion*

1. Tubular secretion is very important in regulation of acid-base balance.
    a. An exchange mechanism in the distal tubules is concerned with secretion of hydrogen ions. Secreted hydrogen ions may be bound by phosphate and excreted.
    b. The formation and secretion of ammonia (NH_3) facilitates excretion of hydrogen ions. Ammonia readily diffuses from cells into the tubular lumen where it combines with hydrogen ions to form ammonium ions (NH_4^+). Ammonium ions are incapable of being reabsorbed by tubular cells and thus are excreted in the urine.
2. Tubular secretion is of minor importance in the elimination of metabolic waste products.

D. *Elaboration of hormones*

1. Erythropoietin.
    a. Erythropoietin is a circulating glycoprotein which acts on bone marrow stem cells at several stages of maturation to stimulate erythrocyte production.
    b. Current evidence indicates that erythropoietin is formed by the action of a substance secreted by the kidneys, renal erythropoietic factor (REF), on a globulin in plasma.
        (1) The production of REF is increased by renal hypoxia and androgens.
        (2) In dogs, REF production is confined to the kidneys.
        (3) In man, rats, and rabbits, a significant quantity of erythropoietin can be produced following removal of the kidneys. It is thought that extrarenal sites of REF production exist in these species.
    c. In chronic generalized renal disease, a progressive nonregenerative anemia develops. This anemia is thought to be related to, at least in part, lack of a sufficient quantity of erythropoietin.
    d. In man, neoplasms of the kidneys are sometimes associated with polycythemia. The polycythemia is thought to occur as a result of excessive quantities of erythropoietin in the body. Polycythemia associated with a renal carcinoma has been observed in 2 dogs* (see Chapter 29, Neoplasms of the Kidney).
2. Renin.
    a. Renin is produced by cells of the juxtaglomerular apparatus. The primary stimulus for its release is renal ischemia.

---

*Personal communication, Dr. Richard C. Scott and Dr. Richard Greene, 1971. The Animal Medical Center, 510 East 62nd Street, New York, New York 10021.

b. Renin is a proteolytic enzyme that reacts with a plasma globulin. Eventually an octapeptide, angiotensin II, is produced.
c. Angiotensin II stimulates aldosterone secretion by the adrenal cortex.
d. The renin-aldosterone system plays a significant role in the regulation of extracellular sodium content and blood volume.
e. Experimental production of renal ischemia in the dog will cause renin release; hypertension is a consequence of the procedure (so-called Goldblatt kidneys).
f. The prevalence of spontaneous disease in the dog due to abnormalities in the renin-aldosterone system has not been adequately examined.

E. *Renal function is also modified by hormones of nonrenal origin*
1. Antidiuretic hormone (see III, B, 8).
2. Aldosterone (see III, B, 3).
3. Urinary excretion of calcium and phosphorus are regulated by parathormone and thyrocalcitonin.
4. Somatotrophic (growth) hormone, thyroid hormone and androgens stimulate renal hypertrophy.

IV. Physiology of micturition

A. *Normal micturition requirements*
1. Anatomically normal ureters, bladder and urethra.
2. Physiologically normal smooth and skeletal muscle of the urinary tract.
3. Physiologically normal neural reflexes between:
   a. The bladder and spinal cord.
   b. The spinal cord and brain.

B. *Muscles involved in micturition*
1. The external sphincter of the urethra is skeletal muscle.
2. The detrusor muscle of the bladder, trigone, and proximal urethra is smooth muscle.

C. *Nerves involved in micturition*
1. Motor nerve fibers to the bladder and urethral sphincter are located in the pudendal, pelvic, and hypogastric nerves.
   a. The pudendal nerve innervates the external sphincter (somatic fibers).
   b. The pelvic nerve carries motor fibers via the parasympathetic system to the bladder wall. These fibers originate in the sacral portion of the spinal cord.
   c. The hypogastric nerve carries sympathetic fibers to the bladder wall. These fibers originate in the lumbar portion of the spinal cord.
2. Sensory fibers also pass from the bladder and sphincters to higher centers in pudendal, pelvic, and hypogastric nerves. Fibers synapse in the lumbosacral spinal cord, and pass from there to the brain.

D. *Mechanism of micturition*
1. Filling of the urinary bladder is accommodated by relaxation of detrusor muscle of the bladder.
   a. A certain amount of filling occurs without a significant increase in intravesical pressure. This occurs because of accommodation by muscle

fibers and central inhibition of parasympathetic fibers which stimulate contraction of the bladder.

   b. At a critical level of volume there is a sudden increase in pressure in the bladder lumen.

2. The increase in intravesical pressure stimulates the release of impulses which travel to the brain, where they are integrated to provide coordination of the contractile system.
3. Efferent impulses which travel via the parasympathetic system (pelvic nerve) stimulate contraction of the detrusor muscle.
4. Simultaneous relaxation of the external sphincter is mediated by impulses which travel via the pudendal nerve.
5. Complete evacuation of the bladder requires maintenance of detrusor contraction and sphincter relaxation.

   a. Receptors in the bladder wall continue to send impulses to higher centers in order to maintain contraction.

   b. Receptors in the wall or mucosa of the urethra, stimulated by the flow of urine, maintain impulses causing persistent relaxation of the sphincters and contraction of the bladder.

E. *Cystometry*

1. The relationship between intravesical pressure and intravesical volume can be studied by cystometry.
2. Following removal of residual urine from the bladder lumen, recordings of pressure are made as the bladder is filled with appropriate quantities of fluid or air.
3. Graphs depicting the relationship of intravesical pressure to intravesical volume are called cystometrograms.
4. Cystometrograms are frequently used in humans with bladder disease as an aid to diagnosis and treatment.

REFERENCES

Alexander, R. S.: Mechanical properties of the urinary bladder (cat). Amer. J. Physiol., *220*:1413–1421, May, 1971.

Bell, R. D.: Experimental study of sites of lymph formation in the canine kidney. Invest. Urol., *8*:356–362, Nov., 1970.

Bennett, C. M., Clapp, J. R., and Berliner, R. W.: Micropuncture study of the proximal and distal tubule in the dog. Amer. J. Physiol., *213*:327–333, 1959.

Blumentals, A. S.: Acid-base balance. Arch. Int. Med., *116*:647–742, 1965.

Bradley, S. E., Laragh, J. H., Wheeler, H. O., MacDowell, M., and Oliver, J.: Correlation of structure and function in the handling of glucose by nephrons of the canine kidney. J. Clin. Invest., *40*:1113–1131, 1961.

Bradley, W., Clarren, S., Shapiro, R., and Wolfson, J.: Air cystometry. J. Urol., *100*:451–455, 1968.

Busuthl, R. W.: The cytological localization of erythropoietin in the human kidney using the fluorescent antibody technique. Proc. Soc. Exp. Biol. Med., *137*:327–330, 1971.

Chinard, F. P., Taylor, W. R., Nolan, M. F., and Enns, T.: Renal handling of glucose in dogs. Amer. J. Physiol., *196*:535–544, 1959.

Clapp, J. R., and Robinson, R. R.: Osmolality of distal tubular fluid in the dog. J. Clin. Invest., *45*:1847–1853, 1966.

Dicker, S. E.: Mechanisms of Urine Concentration and Dilution in Mammals. London, Edward Arnold, 1970.

Dirks, J. H., Clapp, J. R., and Berliner, R. W.: The protein concentration in the proximal tubule of the dog. J. Clin. Invest., *43*:916–921, 1964.

Eggleton, M. G., and Shuster, S.: Glucose and phosphate excretion in the cat. J. Physiol., *124*:613–622, 1954.

Ganong, W. F.: Review of Medical Physiology. 5th edition, Los Altos, California, Lange Medical Publications, 1971.

Gans, J. H.: The kidneys. *In* Duke's Physiology of Domestic Animals. 8th ed. Edited by Melvin J. Swenson. Ithaca, N.Y., Cornell University Press, 1970.

Goldstein, M. H.: Urea reabsorption in the nephron of man and dog. Mount Sinai J. Med., N.Y., *37*:396–403, July–Aug., 1970.

Gottschalk, C. W.: Osmotic concentration and dilution of the urine. Amer. J. Med., *36*:670–685, 1964.

Hook, J. B.: Development of Canine Renal Function Related to Drug Excretion in Puppies. 20th Gaines Veterinary Symposium Proc. Gaines Dog Research Center, White Plains, N.Y., 1970.

Horster, M., and Valtin, H.: Postnatal development of renal function. Micropuncture and clearance studies in the dog. J. Clin. Invest., *50*:779–795, 1971.

Keyes, J. L., and Swanson, R. E.: Dependence of glucose Tm on GFR and tubular volume in dog kidney. Amer. J. Physiol., *221*:1–7, 1971.

Kleiman, L. I., and Lubbe, R.: Factors affecting GFR and RBF in newborn puppies. J. Pediatrics, *76*:961, June, 1970.

Lathem, W., and Davis, B. B.: Renal tubular reabsorption of protein. Demonstration and localization of egg albumin and B-lactoglobulin reabsorption in the dog. Amer. J. Physiol., *199*:644–648, 1960.

Lemieux, G., Warren, Y., and Gervais, M.: Characteristics of potassium conservation of the dog kidney. Amer. J. Physiol., *206*:743–749, 1964.

MacConnachie, H. F.: An old fashioned approach to acid-base balance. Amer. J. Med., *49*:504–518, 1970.

Millerschoen, N. R.: Homeostatic control of plasma osmolality in the dog and the effect of ethanol. Amer. J. Physiol., *217*:431–437, 1969.

Mitchell, A. R.: Protons, pH, and survival. J.A.V.M.A., *157*:1540–1548, 1970.

Murphy, G. P., Mirand, E. A., Takita, H., Schoonees, R., and Groenewald, J. H.: The effects of hypoxia and ischemia on erythropoietin and renin release in dogs. Invest. Urol., *8*:521–525, 1971.

Navar, L. G.: Minimal preglomerular resistance and calculation of normal glomerular pressure. Amer. J. Physiol., *219*:1658–1664, 1970.

Orloff, J., Wagner, H. N., and Davidson, D. G.: The effect of variations in solute excretion and vasopressin dosage on the excretion of water in the dog. J. Clin. Invest., *37*:458–464, 1958.

Park, R., and Rabinowitz, L.: Effect of reduced glomerular filtration rate on the fractional excretion of urea in the dog. Proc. Soc. Exp. Biol. Med., *132*:27–29, 1969.

Pitts, R. F.: Physiology of the Kidney and Body Fluids. 2nd edition. Chicago, Ill., Year Book Medical Publishers, Inc., 1968.

Santos-Martinez, J., and Selkurt, E. E.: Renal lymph and its relationship to the countercurrent multiplier system of the kidney. Amer. J. Physiol., *216*:1548–1555, 1969.

Smith, H. W.: Principles of Renal Physiology. 3rd edition. New York, Oxford University Press, 1957.

Symposium on antidiuretic hormone. Amer. J. Med., *42*:651–827, 1967.

Webber, W. A., and Campbell, J. L.: Effect of amino acids on renal glucose reabsorption in the dog. Canad. J. Physiol. Pharmacol., *43*:915–923, 1965.

Chapter 3
EVALUATION OF THE CLINICAL HISTORY IN DISEASES OF THE URINARY SYSTEM

I. **Introduction**

    The history should be taken by a veterinarian responsible for establishing the diagnosis, for it is he who must evaluate the owner's remarks and place them in proper perspective. Misconceptions due to ignorance on the part of the owner may be misleading if accepted, and the latter is most likely to occur when someone other than a veterinarian obtains the history. Incomplete or erroneous histories are often responsible for erroneous diagnostic conclusions. The veterinarian must determine the difference between observations made by the owner and interpretations which the owner may place on those observations. The owner's observations may be accurate, but his interpretations may be erroneous. Lay personnel and owners tend to pay insufficient attention to some aspects of the problem, and exaggerate the importance of other aspects. This history may suggest a definitive diagnosis, as, for example, when the owner observes passage of calculi during micturition. More often, the history suggests certain diagnostic possibilities which must be confirmed by physical examination, laboratory data, radiography, or other diagnostic techniques.

II. **Questions related to water consumption**

    The history related to water consumption is especially important because, as a generality, polyuria and compensatory polydipsia are the first clinical manifestations of chronic progressive renal diseases. The following are examples of questions which should be routinely asked about patients with possible renal disease.

    A. *Does your pet drink more or less water than formerly?*
        1. An answer of no is not pursued further. Depending on the circumstances, however, such an answer does not eliminate the possibility of significant changes in water consumption.
        2. An answer indicating that the patient drinks more water than usual may be related to many possible causes, including:
            a. All generalized chronic renal diseases.
            b. The polyuric phase of acute generalized nephrosis.

EVALUATION OF THE CLINICAL HISTORY IN DISEASES OF THE URINARY SYSTEM

     c. Vomition.
     d. Diarrhea.
     e. Pyometra.
     f. Hyperadrenocorticism.
     g. Diabetes mellitus.
     h. Diabetes insipidus.
     i. Renal diabetes insipidus.
     j. Administration of certain drugs including:
        (1) Diuretics.
        (2) Glucocorticoids.
        (3) Sodium chloride.
     k. Psychogenic polydipsia.
     l. High environmental temperature.
     m. Heavy exercise.
     n. Some diseases of the liver.
     o. Others.

  B. *Further questioning may help to confirm or eliminate non-urinary causes of polydipsia without the necessity of laboratory data.*

III. Questions related to urine output

  A. *Does your pet micturate more than usual?*
    1. If micturition has not increased, but the patient has polydipsia, obviously there must be a greater than normal loss of water through another system such as the respiratory system or gastrointestinal system. If not, the owner may be mistaken about the quantity of water consumed by his pet.
    2. If the volume of urine excreted is increased, the diseases mentioned in association with polydipsia must be considered.

  B. *Can your pet go through the night without micturating?*

  Some owners are more impressed by nocturia than by polyuria. If nocturia exists, causes of polyuria and polydipsia must be considered. It is important to define accurately the period of time during which the pet is deprived of the opportunity to micturate. Depending on the circumstances, this period may be as short as a few hours or as long as 12 to 14 hours.

IV. Questions related to frequency of micturition

  A. *Does your pet void a greater volume of urine, or are frequent attempts made to micturate?*
    1. When polyuria is present, large amounts of urine are passed often. Many of the diseases previously mentioned in association with polydipsia should then be considered as diagnostic possibilities.
    2. If the patient makes frequent attempts to micturate, but the quantity of urine passed is small, the problem is likely to be related to a disease process causing irritation of the bladder or urethra.

  B. *Does your pet have a normal stream of urine during micturition?*

  A "no" answer implies partial occlusion of the urethra, which may be caused by a variety of diseases, the most common of which are urethral calculi and stricture of the urethra (see Chapter 45, Diseases of the Urethra).

C. *Does your pet strain during micturition?*

Straining associated with micturition occurs as the result of diseases which cause irritation to the bladder or urethra.

V. Questions related to the gross appearance of urine

A. *Do you observe the act of micturition by your pet? If so, how frequently?*

If the answer is no, the veterinarian cannot learn much about the appearance of the urine from the owner.

B. *Is any blood passed in the urine?*

A negative answer does not eliminate the possibility of hematuria since owners often do not closely observe micturition by their pets. Positive information, however, is of great value.

C. *When, during the process of micturition, is blood observed?*
   1. Blood originating from the uterus or vagina in the female, or from the prostate gland or urethra in the male, may be the source of hemorrhage flushed through the passageway by urine. Blood originating from these areas is often passed at the onset of micturition, or independent of micturition.
   2. Clinical experience has revealed that gross hematuria is more likely to be associated with diseases of the bladder than with diseases of the kidney.
   3. Blood associated with diseases of the bladder is commonly passed during the end of micturition. The specific gravity of red cells often exceeds the specific gravity of urine, thereby favoring precipitation of red cells in dependent portions of the bladder when the patient is inactive. Active patients with gross hematuria usually pass urine which contains blood throughout the entire period of micturition.

Chapter 4
PHYSICAL EXAMINATION OF THE URINARY SYSTEM

I. **Physical examination of the urinary system is limited to inspection and palpation.**

   A. *Kidneys*

   Both kidneys are usually palpable in cats. In dogs, the left kidney is often palpable, but the right kidney can rarely be palpated, even in the presence of disease (see Chapter 1, Applied Anatomy of the Urinary System for a review of the size and position of the kidneys).
   1. Technique of kidney palpation.
      a. Placing the patient in different positions is helpful in locating the kidneys. The following positions are recommended:
         (1) Standing.
         (2) Lateral recumbency (right and left).
         (3) Dorsal recumbency.
      b. Tranquilization, sedation, or anesthesia may be indicated to facilitate palpation of the kidneys of uncooperative patients.
   2. When either or both of the kidneys can be palpated, one should attempt to determine:
      a. Size.
      b. Consistency.
      c. Smoothness of surface.
      d. Shape.
      e. Presence or absence of pain.
         (1) The presence of pain in renal disease has been grossly exaggerated by some authors. Most diseases of the kidneys do not result in increased sensitivity to pain by the kidneys. In addition, pain in the area usually occupied by the kidneys can be caused by nonrenal disorders (e.g., intervertebral disc disease).
         (2) Pain associated with renal disease only occurs when there is swelling of the renal parenchyma and resultant stretching of the renal capsule.
         (3) If pain is present in the area of the kidneys, more reliable methods of detecting renal disease should be employed.

   B. *Ureters*

   Normal ureters cannot be evaluated by physical examination in the dog and cat. With rare exceptions, the same is true for abnormal ureters.

C. *Urinary Bladder*
   1. The bladder can be palpated in most dogs and cats. The position and size vary with the degree of distention. The bladder moves cranially and ventrally into the abdomen when distended with urine and contracts to near the pubis when empty.
   2. One should be able to determine by abdominal palpation:
      a. The position of the bladder.
      b. The consistency of the bladder.
      c. The degree of bladder distention.
      d. The thickness of the bladder wall.
      e. Spasms of the bladder musculature.
      f. Presence or absence of cystic calculi.
      g. Abnormal masses in or adjacent to the bladder.
D. *Urethra*
   1. The urethra cannot be evaluated by physical examination in female dogs or cats.
      a. The external urethral orifice may be inspected with the aid of a vaginal endoscope.
      b. The urethral lumen of medium- and large-sized dogs may be examined with a cystourethroscope (see Chapter 10, Cystoscopy).
   2. Physical examination of the urethra in male cats is usually limited to inspection of the distal portion of the penile urethra.
   3. The urethra of male dogs can be examined by inspection and palpation.
      a. The external urethral orifice may be inspected by exteriorizing the penis from the prepuce.
      b. The perineal portion of the urethra may be palpated just beneath the skin.
      c. The pelvic urethra may be examined by digital palpation through the wall of the rectum.

REFERENCES

Bovee, K. C.: Physical examination of the urinary system. Vet. Clin. No. Amer., *1*:119–128, 1971.
Low, D. G.: General examination of dogs. Vet. Clin. No. Amer., *1*:3–14, 1971.
Osborne, C. A.: Diagnostic accuracy—the veterinarian's most important resource. J. Amer. Anim. Hosp. Assoc., *4*:159–164, 1968.
Osborne, C. A.: Urologic logic—Diagnosis of renal disease. J.A.V.M.A., *157*:1656–1666, 1970.

Chapter 5
COLLECTION OF URINE

I. Regardless of technique employed, all manipulations associated with urine collection must be gentle in order to prevent trauma to the urethra or urinary bladder.

II. Urine may be removed from the bladder by one of four methods.

    A. *Collection during spontaneous micturition.*

    B. *Manual compression of the urinary bladder.*

    C. *Catheterization.*

    D. *Cystocentesis.*

III. **Collection of samples during spontaneous micturition**

    A. *When possible, the first part of the urine stream of noncatheterized urine samples should not be used for urinalysis or bacterial culture because it may contain debris, bacteria, or exudate flushed from the urethra or genital tract.*

    B. *A collection device which holds a container can easily be made from aluminum splint rod.* Construction of the device so that it has a long handle will facilitate collection of the urine sample from the patient.*

    C. *This technique is not associated with any risk of complications to the patient (i.e., bacterial infection, trauma to the urinary system).*

IV. **Manual compression of the urinary bladder**

    A. *Compression of the urinary bladder by application of digital pressure through the abdominal wall may be used to collect urine samples from dogs and cats.*

    B. *The first portion of noncatheterized urine samples should not be used for urinalysis or bacterial culture since it may be contaminated with debris, bacteria, or exudate flushed from the urethra or genital tract.*

    C. *The success of this technique is dependent on the quantity of urine in the bladder. As a generality the technique will not be successful unless the bladder contains at least 10 ml. of urine.*

    D. *Success in obtaining urine by this method is usually greater in female than male dogs because of the greater ease in overcoming urethral resistance in females.*

    E. *Technique*

        1. Outline the urinary bladder by abdominal palpation.
        2. The patient may be in a standing or recumbent position.

---
*Haver Lockhart Labs., Shawnee, Kansas 66201.

DIAGNOSIS OF URINARY DISEASES

3. Exert moderate digital pressure over as large an area of the bladder as possible with the fingers and thumb of one hand, or with the fingers of both hands.
    a. Steady continuous pressure should be applied rather than forceful intermittent squeezing motions.
    b. Sustain the digital pressure until the urethral sphincters relax and urine is expelled from the body. It may be necessary to apply pressure for several minutes before urethral sphincter resistance is overcome.
    c. Avoid vigorous palpation as it may traumatize the bladder and induce hematuria.
    d. If the bladder is overdistended with urine, extreme caution must be be used to avoid rupture of the bladder.

F. *Complications*
 1. This technique is not associated with a significant risk of bacterial infection.
 2. If poor technique is used, trauma or rupture of the bladder may occur.

V. Catheterization

A. *Indications*

Catheterization of the urinary bladder may be performed for one or more of several reasons.
 1. Diagnostic catheterization may be indicated to:
    a. Collect bladder urine for urinalysis or bacterial culture.
    b. Collect accurately timed volumes of urine for renal function studies.
    c. Instill contrast media prior to contrast radiography.
    d. Evaluate the urethral lumen for the presence of calculi, space-occupying lesions, or strictures.
 2. Therapeutic catheterization may be indicated to:
    a. Relieve obstruction to urine outflow.
    b. Instill medications into the urinary bladder. The value of this mode of therapy is questionable.
    c. Facilitate surgical repair of the urethra or surrounding structures.

B. *Size, composition, and type of urinary catheters*
 1. Size.
    a. The scale of measurement commonly used for calibrating diameter is the French scale (abbreviated as F.). Each French unit is equal to one third mm. For example, a 9F. catheter has an external diameter of 3 mm.
    b. Catheters are available in a variety of diameters and lengths.
 2. Composition.
    a. Urinary catheters are fabricated from a variety of materials including rubber, plastic, metal, and woven silk.
    b. Catheters impregnated with radiopaque material are of value when used in conjunction with radiographic evaluation of the urinary system.
 3. Types.
    a. Catheters.
       (1) Depending on their size and shape, urinary catheters may be classified as urethral or ureteral catheters.
       (2) The openings in the distal end of catheters are called "eyes." Most catheters have two eyes.
       (3) Canine urinary catheters.

(a) Flexible catheters* similar in diameter and length to human ureteral catheters may be used to catheterize male or female dogs. Flexible human ureteral catheters** may also be used to catheterize dogs.

(b) Rigid metal catheters designed for use in female dogs are also available. Because of their rigid structure, the use of these catheters is frequently associated with urethral and vesical trauma.

(4) Feline urinary catheters.

(a) Disposable tom cat catheters (3½ to 5F.) can be obtained from commercial manufacturers.***

(b) Infant feeding tubes† and other types of synthetic tubing†† may be used to catheterize cats.

(c) Straight lacrimal cannulas are often used to catheterize the distal urethra of tom cats. These instruments must be used with caution in order to prevent trauma to the urethra.

(d) The use of rigid metal tom cat catheters is not recommended since they often cause trauma to the urethral and bladder mucosa.

(5) Catheters with inflatable balloons are called Foley catheters.

(a) By inflating the balloon following insertion of the catheter into the bladder, the catheter is fixed in position.

(b) These catheters are designed to be used as indwelling catheters.

b. Filiforms and followers.

(1) Filiforms and followers are instruments commonly used in human medicine to locate and dilate urethral strictures.

(2) Filiforms are solid structures made of pliable woven silk or plastic material. They have a variety of different types of tips (i.e., coudé and corkscrew).

(3) Followers are made of woven silk or metal. They may be solid or hollow. Hollow followers permit catheterization.

c. Sounds.

(1) Sounds are special instruments made of metal that may be used instead of catheters to explore the urethra for stenoses and in the treatment of urethral strictures.

(2) Sounds are available in a wide variety of designs for use in man.

d. Consult human textbooks of urology for specific details about filiforms, followers, and sounds. Many of these instruments may be of benefit in dogs.

C. *Care of urinary catheters*

1. Only catheters which are in excellent condition should be used.

a. Catheters weakened by damage to their walls may break apart while in the patient.

b. The wall of flexible catheters usually weakens first in the area of the "eye."

---

*Disposable rubber catheters for small animals. Brunswick Labs., Inc., St. Louis, Mo. Disposable polypropylene catheters for small animals, Haver Lockhart Labs., Shawnee, Kansas 66201.
**American Cystoscope Makers, Inc., Pelham Manor, N.Y. 10803.
***Tom cat catheter, Sherwood Medical Industries Inc., St. Louis, Mo. 63103.
†Brunswick sterile disposable feeding tube and urethral catheter, Brunswick Labs., Inc., St. Louis, Mo.
††Intramedic polyethylene tubing, PE60 to 90, Clay Adams Inc., New York, N.Y.

28 DIAGNOSIS OF URINARY DISEASES

  c. Catheters that have a rough external surface may traumatize the mucosa of the urethra or bladder.
 2. Catheters should be individually packaged prior to use. Use of packaging material that is transparent allows visualization of the catheter.
 3. Sterilization.
  a. Nonsterile catheters should never be used because:
   (1) They may cause infection of the urinary system.
   (2) They may contaminate urine that is to be used for bacterial culture.
  b. Catheters must be thoroughly cleaned prior to sterilization.
  c. Catheters may be sterilized with steam under pressure (autoclaving), chemical sterilizing solutions, or ethylene oxide gas.
   (1) Repeated autoclaving of nonmetal catheters significantly reduces their longevity.
   (2) Ethylene oxide sterilization is the procedure of choice.
   (3) Chemical sterilizing solutions containing quaternary ammonia compounds may be used, but are less effective than sterilization with steam under pressure or ethylene oxide gas.
  d. Disposable catheters which are prepackaged in sterilized wrappers may be obtained from commercial manufacturers.

D. *Technique of catheterization in all species*
 1. Regardless of the specific procedure employed, meticulously aseptic and gentle atraumatic technique should be used.
 2. Conscious patients should be restrained by an assistant in order to minimize contamination of the catheter as well as trauma to the urethra.
 3. Use the smallest diameter catheter which will permit the objective of catheterization.
 4. If a stylet is used in the catheter, it should be lubricated before it is inserted into the lumen of the catheter. If it is not lubricated, difficulty may be encountered in removing the stylet after the catheter has been placed in the patient.
 5. Regardless of species or sex, the approximate distance from the external urethral orifice to the neck of the bladder should be determined and mentally transposed to the catheter. This step will minimize the likelihood of traumatizing the bladder wall due to insertion of an excessive length of catheter, and will prevent the catheter from reentering the urethra from the bladder (see catheterization of the male dog in this chapter).
 6. The distal end of the catheter should be lubricated with a liberal quantity of sterilized aqueous lubricant. Proper lubrication of the catheter will minimize discomfort to the patient and catheter-induced trauma to the urethra.
 7. Although usually unnecessary, local anesthesia of the urethra may be induced with a topical anesthetic such as lidocaine hydrochloride.*
 8. Maintain asepsis during insertion of the catheter into the bladder.
  a. Cleanse periurethral skin with soap and water.
  b. Do not contaminate the catheter by allowing it to contact hair or skin of patient or clinician.
  c. The catheter may be manipulated:
   (1) Through the packaging material in which it is contained.
   (2) With the aid of sterilized surgical gloves.
   (3) With the aid of sterilized forceps.

---
*Anestacon, Conal Pharmaceuticals Inc., Chicago, Ill. 60640.

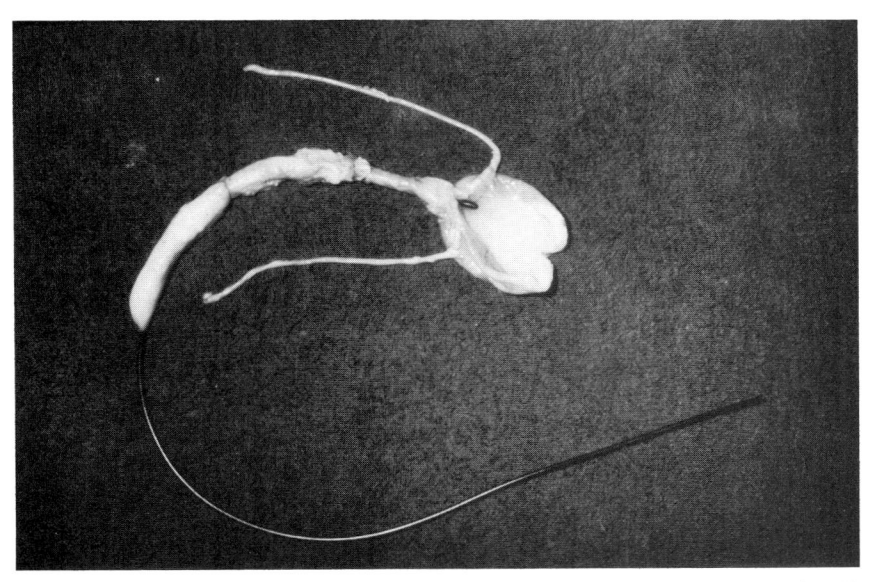

Figure 5–1. Photograph of the urethra and urinary bladder obtained from a male dog illustrating correct placement of a catheter in the urethra and bladder.

9. Never force the catheter through the urethra! If difficulty is encountered in inserting the catheter into the bladder, withdraw the catheter for a short distance and insert it again with a rotating motion. If this does not permit catheterization, a smaller diameter catheter should be used.
10. The tip of the catheter should be positioned so that it is located just beyond the junction of the neck of the bladder with the urethra (Fig. 5–1).
    a. Verification of this position may be accomplished by injection of a known quantity of air through the catheter. Inability to remove all of the air indicates improper positioning of the catheter.
    b. Proper positioning of catheters facilitates removal of all of the urine from the bladder.
11. Urine may be aspirated from the bladder with the aid of a syringe and two-way valve. Aspiration must be gentle in order to prevent trauma to the bladder mucosa as a result of sucking it into the eye of the catheter.
12. The first few milliliters of urine obtained via the catheter should not be used for urinalysis or bacterial culture since it may be contaminated with debris, bacteria, or exudate from the urethra or genital tract.
13. Catheters that are to remain in the bladder for some time but that are not designed to permit self-retention may be sutured to the skin. Suture material should be anchored to a piece of adhesive tape which has been placed around the catheter.

E. *Potential complications associated with catheterization in all species*
   1. Analysis of catheterized urine samples frequently reveals the presence of microscopic hematuria. Although the hematuria is usually self-limiting, it may interfere with interpretation of the results of urinalysis.
   2. Because of the risk of inducing infection of the bladder as a result of catheterization indiscriminate use of this technique is condemned. This generality must be kept in perspective, however. When necessary for

diagnostic or therapeutic purposes, catheterization of the urinary bladder should be performed without hesitation.
- a. Potential sources of bacterial infection of the bladder associated with single catheterization include:
  - (1) Inadequate preparation of the periurethral skin.
  - (2) Use of a nonsterile or contaminated catheter.
  - (3) Catheter-induced trauma to the urethral or vesical mucosa.
- b. The risk of bacterial infection caused by single catheterization is dependent on the integrity of the urinary bladder.
  - (1) Normal urinary bladders are inherently resistant to infection because of the mechanical washout action of frequent and complete voiding of urine, and because of intrinsic antibacterial defense mechanisms of the urethral and bladder mucosa.
  - (2) Provided proper technique is utilized, the risk of bacterial infection following catheterization of a normal urinary bladder is low.
  - (3) Catheterization of urinary bladders with pre-existing abnormalities is more likely to be complicated by bacterial infection.
- c. Repeated catheterization or indwelling catheterization should be avoided when possible since the risk of bacterial infection associated with these procedures is enhanced.

3. Procedures which may be used to reduce the incidence of infection following catheterization include:
   - a. Strict adherence to principles of asepsis.
   - b. Administration of oral or parenteral antibiotics. As a generality, the risk of infection associated with single catheterization of a patient with a normal bladder is too low to warrant routine prophylactic antibacterial therapy.
   - c. Catheters impregnated with antibacterial agents have been designed for use in man.
   - d. Irrigation of the bladder with antibacterial solutions such as neomycin or Furacin.
     - (1) Although commonly used, this technique is of unproven and doubtful value.
     - (2) Irrigation of human bladders with antibacterial solutions has provided only a transient antibacterial effect.
     - (3) Only solutions known to be sterile should be used.
     - (4) The volume of solution instilled into the bladder should be sufficient to allow contact with all portions of the bladder mucosa.

F. *Catheterization of the male dog*
  1. See discussion of technique of catheterization of all species.
  2. The length and diameter of the catheter selected will vary with the size of the patient.
     - a. Catheter diameters ranging from 4 to 10 F. are selected in most instances.
     - b. The length of the canine urethra varies from approximately 10 to 35 cm., and is approximately 25 cm. in an adult weighing 25 lbs.
     - c. Difficulty in passing the catheter through the urethral lumen may be encountered at the level of the os penis and at the site where the urethra curves around the ischial arch.
  3. The external urethral orifice should be exposed by reflecting the prepuce away from the penis.

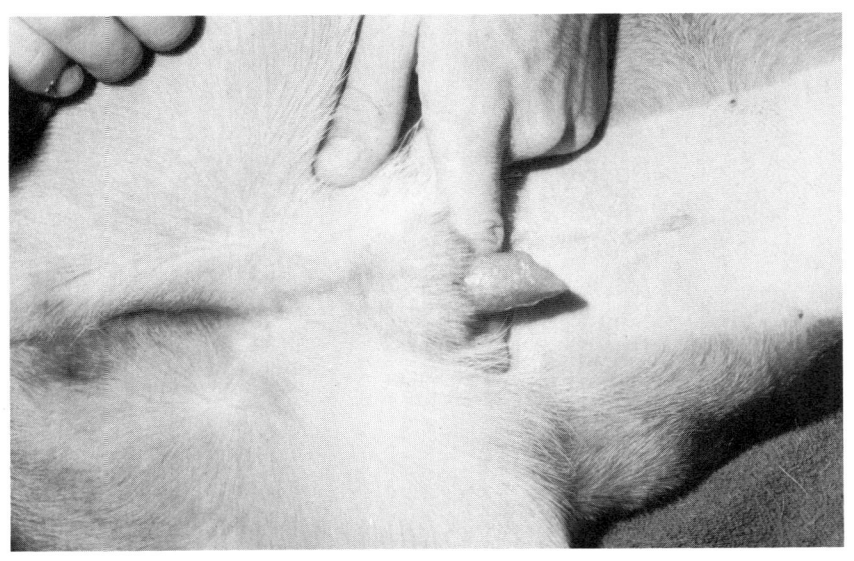

Figure 5–2. Photograph of a male dog illustrating exposure of the penis by digital pressure applied to the portion of the prepuce immediately adjacent to the ventral abdominal wall.

    a. This may be easily accomplished by placing the thumb or index finger just cranial to the prepuce and against the ventral abdominal wall. Digital pressure in a caudal direction will consistently expose the penis (Fig. 5-2).
    b. It is helpful to place the dog in lateral recumbency and to flex his back rather than to have his back and extremities extended.
    c. Once exposed, the tip of the penis and the external urethral orifice should be thoroughly cleansed with soap and water.
    d. Once reflected, the prepuce must not be allowed to contact the catheter as it is being advanced through the urethral lumen.
4. Care must be used not to insert an excessive length of the catheter because it may follow the curvature of the bladder wall, double back on itself, and reenter the urethral lumen (Fig. 5-3). As the catheter is withdrawn, the loop of the catheter becomes progressively smaller until a point is reached where the wall of the catheter bends. The catheter often bends at the eye since it is the weakest point of the catheter wall. As the bent catheter is withdrawn, it usually lodges at the caudal end of the os penis. If a catheter does become lodged in the wall of the urethra as a result of bending on itself, the following procedures, listed in order of priority, should be considered.
    a. Advance the catheter back into the bladder lumen with the objective of releasing the tight bend in the catheter wall.
    b. Apply a liberal quantity of sterilized lubricant to the outside wall of the catheter, and inject a dilute solution (2 parts lubricant to 1 part water) of sterilized lubricant into the catheter lumen. Apply gentle, steady pressure to the catheter with the objective of dilating the urethral lumen ventral to the os penis. Do not apply pressure of such force as to tear the urethral mucosa.

32   DIAGNOSIS OF URINARY DISEASES

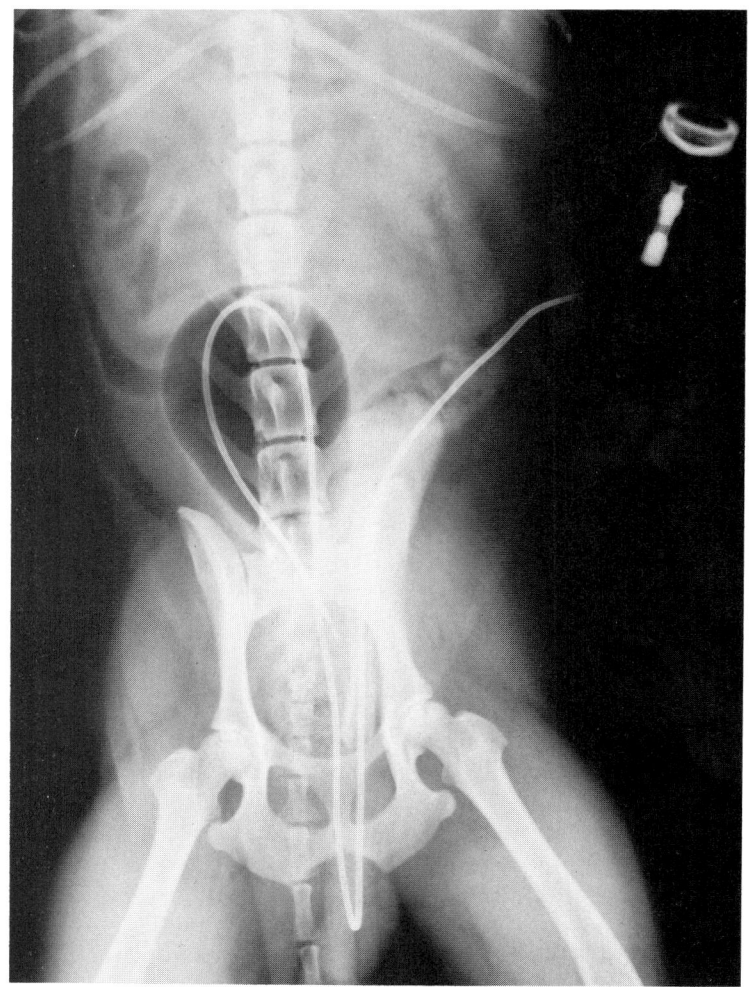

Figure 5–3. Overinsertion of a flexible catheter into the urinary bladder of a 9-year-old male mixed breed dog. The tip of the catheter has reentered the urethra.

    c. Inject a liberal quantity of dilute sterilized aqueous lubricant through and around the catheter. An assistant should then occlude the lumen of the pelvic urethra by applying digital pressure against the ischium through the ventral wall of the rectum. Next a teat cannula, with attached syringe loaded with sterilized saline, should be placed in the penile urethra via the external urethral orifice. The external urethral orifice should be compressed around the teat cannula and catheter by digital pressure. As a result of these maneuvers, a portion of the urethra from the external urethral orifice to the bony pelvis becomes a closed system. Saline should then be injected into the urethra until a definite rebound is perceived through the syringe plunger. This rebound should be associated with a palpable increase in the diameter of the pelvic urethra. At this point, another assistant should grasp the catheter and attempt to remove it with gentle but steady pressure. If

COLLECTION OF URINE 33

the portion of the urethral lumen ventral to the os penis dilates sufficiently, the catheter may be removed from the patient.
d. Inject aqueous organic iodinated material* into and around the catheter with the objective of visualizing the exact nature of the problem via contrast radiography. Anesthetize the patient and repeat step b or c. Stretching the urethral lumen with the catheter will induce a lesser degree of injury than a urethrotomy.
e. If all of the above steps are unsuccessful, the catheter must be removed by urethrotomy.
5. If the length of the catheter is similar to that of the urethra, only a catheter with a flared end should be used. If the end is not flared, the catheter may migrate into the urethra and be inaccessible for withdrawal from the patient.

G. *Catheterization of the female dog*
1. See discussion of technique of catheterization of all species.
2. Cleansing of the external genitalia and vagina.
  a. The vulva and perivulvar skin should be cleansed with soap and water.
  b. Vaginal debris should be rinsed to the outside with sterilized saline prior to catheterization.

---

*Hypaque-50, Winthrop Labs., New York, N.Y.

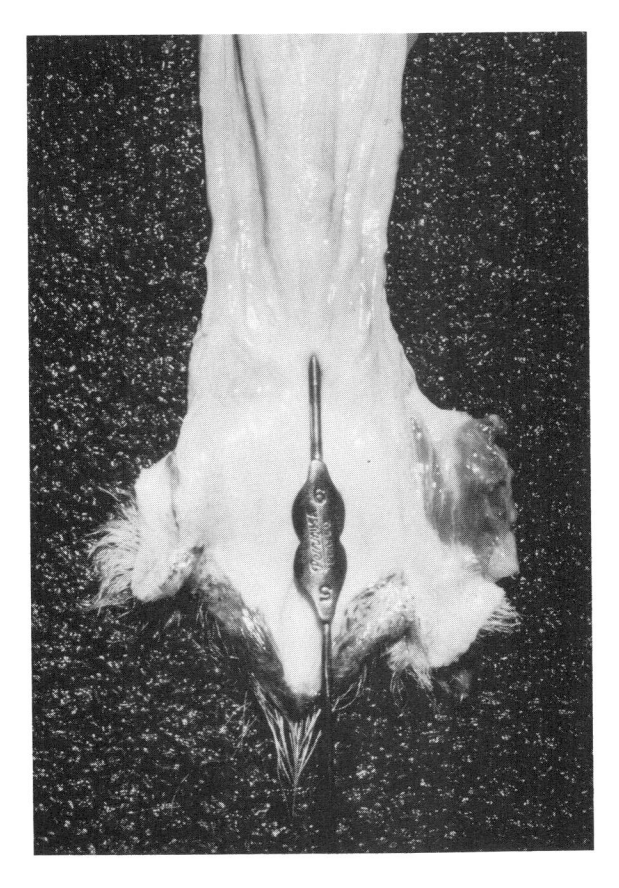

Figure 5–4. Photograph of a normal canine vagina illustrating the position of the external urethral orifice on the ventral floor of the vagina. A metal probe has been inserted into the urethra via the external urethral orifice.

34   DIAGNOSIS OF URINARY DISEASES

   3. The external urethral orifice is located on a tubercle in the ventral wall of the vagina.
      a. The external urethral orifice is approximately 3 to 5 cm. cranial to the ventral commissure of the vulva (Fig. 5–4).
      b. The clitoral fossa lies just caudal to the external urethral orifice. Catheters to be placed in the urethra must be passed dorsal to this structure.
   4. Flexible catheters similar to those recommended for male dogs may be used. Use of rigid metal catheters often results in trauma to the mucosa of the vagina, urethra, and bladder.
   5. Catheterization using endoscopes.
      a. A variety of endoscopes may be used in the vagina to visualize the external urethral orifice, including:
         (1) Human nasal specula.
         (2) Brincker-Hoff's human rectal speculum (small size).
         (3) Homemade specula fashioned from disposable syringe cases (Fig. 5–5).
         (4) Otoscopic cones.
      b. For patients too small to permit visualization of the external urethral orifice with an endoscope, a Foley catheter (8 to 14 F.) with inflatable balloon may be used.
         (1) Insert the Foley catheter into the vagina as far as possible and inflate the balloon.
         (2) Insert a small Killian nasal speculum into the vagina and open the blades.
         (3) Gently pull the Foley catheter outward.
         (4) The urethral orifice can be visualized as a small opening in the ventral floor of the vagina.
         (5) Insertion of the urethral catheter will usually not be hindered by the Foley balloon. If it is, however, the balloon should be deflated.

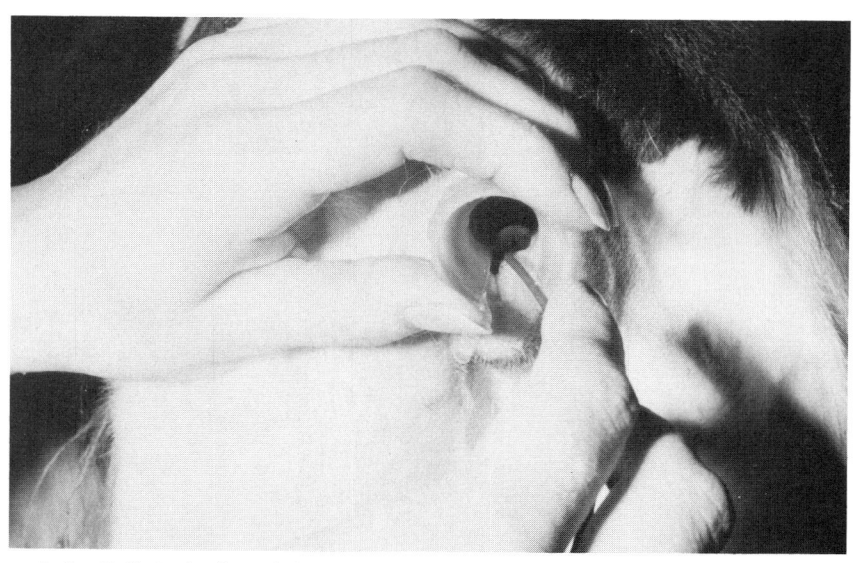

Figure 5–5. Catheterization of the urethra of a female dog with the aid of an endoscope made from a disposable plastic syringe container. The endoscope was made by removing a rectangular section from the side of the syringe container.

c. All techniques requiring direct visualization of the vagina are dependent on a good light source.
6. Female dogs large enough to permit digital palpation of the vagina may be catheterized without the use of endoscopes. Direct visualization of the urethra is unnecessary.
    a. The dog should be in the standing position as this facilitates anatomical orientation.
    b. Using sterilized gloves, a finger should be lubricated and inserted into the vagina.
    c. A sterilized flexible catheter should be inserted into the vagina and guided to the external urethral orifice with the finger.
    d. Entry of the catheter into the urethra is indicated when the tip of the catheter disappears into the ventral floor of the vagina.
    e. The most common error of individuals inexperienced in this technique is to insert the tip of the catheter too far into the vagina.
7. "Blind" catheterization.
    a. This technique is not recommended if other techniques are feasible.
    b. This technique may be useful in catheterization of patients in which visualization of the external urethral orifice is not feasible because:
        (1) The patient is uncooperative.
        (2) The vulvar orifice is too small.
    c. Because the position of the portion of the catheter inside the patient cannot be visualized, this procedure must be performed with caution in order to avoid trauma to the genital tract.
    d. Technique.
        (1) With the patient in the standing position, the lips of the vulva should be parted.
        (2) A sterilized, lubricated catheter should be inserted into the vagina and passed over the clitoral fossa.
        (3) With the long axis of the catheter directed in a cranioventral position with respect to the long axis of the vagina, the catheter should be cautiously directed along the ventral floor of the vagina.
        (4) The tip of the catheter must be kept on the ventral midline of the vaginal floor.
        (5) Detection of increased resistance to insertion of the catheter indicates that it has bypassed the external urethral orifice and encountered the cervix. In the latter instance:
            (a) The catheter should be withdrawn to the vulva and the procedure repeated.
            (b) The procedure may be abandoned.
        (6) If the urinary bladder contains sufficient urine, successful catheterization will be indicated by the passage of urine through the catheter.

H. *Catheterization of the male cat*
1. See discussion of technique of catheterization of all species.
2. Depending on the disposition of the patient, sedation or anesthesia may be required.
3. Catheters which are 3.5 to 5 F. in diameter are satisfactory for use in the majority of cats (see V.B.3., types of catheters, in this chapter).
    a. Catheters made from synthetic tubing should be prepared by cutting

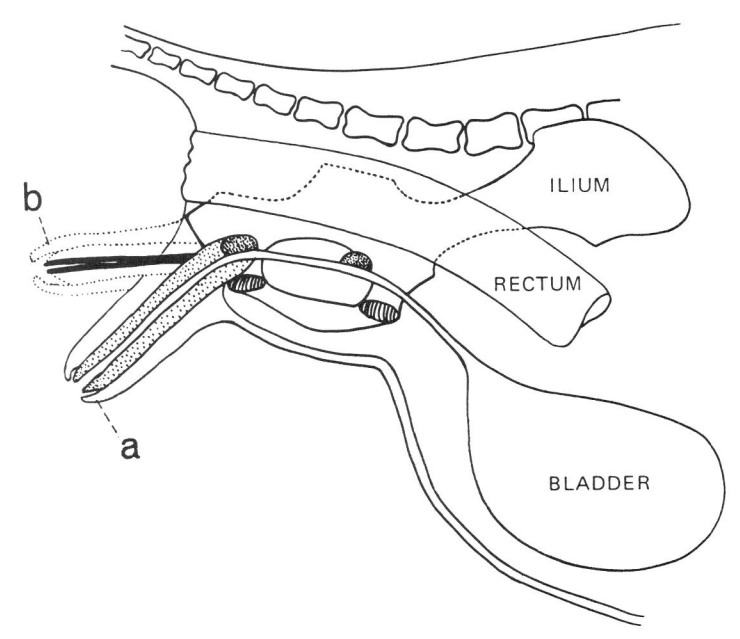

Figure 5–6. Normal position of the feline penis (a), and the position for catheterization (b). (Archibald, J., Sumner-Smith, G., and Dingwall, J.: Surgical management of urethral obstruction in male cats. Modern Veterinary Practice, 52:55–61, 1971.)

one end at a 45° angle and flaring the other end with the heat from a burning match. If this modification is not made, the catheter may migrate into the urethra.
   b. Rigid metal catheters should be avoided if possible as they often traumatize the urethra and vesical mucosa.
4. Extend the penis from the preputial sheath by pulling it in a caudal direction. Then displace the extended penis in a dorsal direction with the objective of getting the long axis of the urethra approximately parallel with the vertebral column. This maneuver will reduce the natural curvature of the caudal portion of the urethra and will facilitate atraumatic catheterization (Fig. 5–6).
5. Wash the distal end of the penis and urethral orifice with soap and water.
6. Gently insert the catheter into the bladder. Variable degrees of resistance may be encountered in normal cats because a large portion of the urethra is surrounded by voluntary skeletal muscle.

I. *Catheterization of the female cat*
   1. See catheterization of the female dog and discussion of technique of catheterization of all species.
   2. Flexible catheters similar to those recommended for male cats should be used.
   3. Depending on the disposition of the patient, sedation or anesthesia may be required.

VI. Cystocentesis

A. *Cystocentesis may be performed for diagnostic or therapeutic objectives*
   1. Diagnostic cystocentesis may be indicated to obtain urine samples for bacterial culture.

2. Therapeutic cystocentesis may be indicated to provide temporary decompression of the excretory pathway of the urinary system in instances of urethral obstruction to urine outflow.

B. *Equipment*
1. Twenty-one to 24 gauge needles which are 1½ to 2 inches in length.
2. Syringe (6 to 35 ml.).
3. Two-way or three-way valves.

C. *Technique*
1. Cystocentesis should not be performed unless the bladder contains a sufficient volume of urine to permit needle puncture without significant risk of damage to the bladder or adjacent structures.
2. The abdominal skin penetrated by the needle should be aseptically prepared each time cystocentesis is performed. The portion of the bladder wall through which the needle is inserted is not critical, although the ventral midline provides the least risk of damage to vessels.
3. Following immobilization of the bladder by abdominal palpation, the hypodermic needle with attached syringe should be inserted through the abdominal wall into the bladder lumen.
    a. If possible, the needle should be placed a few centimeters cranial to the neck of the bladder in order to facilitate removal of as much urine as possible. If the needle is placed in the vertex, it may not remain in the bladder lumen as the bladder decreases in size.
    b. By directing the needle through the wall of the bladder at an acute angle, small openings in the bladder wall may be occluded by the elasticity of the vesical musculature, and the interlacing arrangement of individual muscle contracts.
4. Urine should be removed by gentle suction with the syringe. The bladder should be emptied as completely as is consistent with atraumatic technique in order to minimize leakage of residual urine into the peritoneal cavity.
5. Digital pressure should not be applied to the bladder for several hours following cystocentesis.
6. Use of prophylactic antibacterial therapy following cystocentesis must be determined on the basis of clinical judgment.

REFERENCES

Buchanan, J. W.: Kinked catheters in pneumocystography. J. Amer. Vet. Rad. Soc., *8*:31–35, 1966.
Cohen, S. N., and Kass, E. H.: A simple method for quantitative urine culture. New Eng. J. Med., *277*: 176–180, 1967.
Froe, D. L., and Williams, B. J.: An evaluation of anti-microbial sensitivity testing. Mod. Vet. Pract., *52*: 45–49, 1971.
Gregory, J. G., Wein, A. J., Sansone, T. C., and Murphy, J. J.: Bladder resistance to infection. J. Urol., *105*:220–222, 1971.
Hinman, F., and Belzer, F. D.: Urinary tract infection and renal homotransplantation. I. Effect of antibacterial irrigations on defenses of defunctionalized bladder. J. Urol., *101*:477–481, 1969.
Hogle, R. M.: Antibacterial-agent sensitivity of bacteria isolated from dogs and cats. J.A.V.M.A., *156*: 761–764, 1970.
Kalinske, R. W., Yelderman, J. J., Weaver, R. G., and Hoeprich, P. D.: Cold sterilization of ureteral catheters with ethylene oxide gas. J. Urol., *96*:31–35, 1966.
Masih, B. K., Drouin, G., and Hinman, F.: Voiding and intrinsic defenses of the lower urinary tract of the female dog. I. Effects of episiotomy, colostomy, dilatation, and urinary diversion. J. Urol., *104*:130–136, 1970.

Moore, E. S.: Catheterization of the urinary bladder in young female animals. Biol. Neonate, *16*:256–259, 1970.
Moyad, R. H., and Persky, L.: Vesical irrigation and urosepsis. Invest. Urol., *6*:21–25, July, 1968.
Riggins, A. P.: Ethylene oxide as a sterilizing agent. Comments and cautions. J. Amer. Animal Hosp. Assoc., *7*:202–205, 1971.
Singleton, W. B.: Catheterization of the bitch. Vet. Rec., *71*:106, 1959.
Thompson, I. M., and Baker, J. J.: The histological effects of dilation and internal urethrotomy on the canine urethra. J. Urol., *103*:168–173, 1970.

Chapter 6
LABORATORY FINDINGS IN DISEASES OF THE URINARY SYSTEM

I. **Hemogram**

   A. *Erythrocyte numbers (RBC per cmm.) Packed cell volume (PCV) and Hemoglobin (Hb.)*

   1. A progressive normocytic, normochromic, nonregenerative anemia is a common finding in patients with chronic generalized progressive irreversible renal disease. Because the kidneys are the primary source of erythrocyte stimulating factor in dogs, generalized destruction of the renal parenchyma is commonly associated with bone marrow hypoplasia and nonregenerative anemia. The nonregenerative anemia associated with uremia may also be related to decreased red blood cell (RBC) survival time.
   2. PCV, Hb, and RBC numbers are increased above the actual level in clinically dehydrated patients. If the patient is anemic and dehydrated, the PCV, Hb, and total number of RBC may appear to be within normal limits. In order to avoid erroneous interpretation of such findings, the results of the hemogram should always be evaluated in association with the results of a physical examination. Evaluation of the serum concentration of total protein may also aid in evaluating the state of the patient's hydration (see Chapter 32, Fluid Therapy in Renal Failure).
   3. Uncommonly, a nonregenerative anemia associated with severe and prolonged infection of the urinary system may develop (anemia of infection). The cause of nonregenerative anemias associated with prolonged infection has not been established.
   4. If a primary disease of the urinary system is associated with a significant loss of blood, a regenerative anemia may be observed, provided a sufficient quantity of erythropoietin is produced.

   B. *White blood cell count (WBC per cmm.)*

   1. As a generality, primary inflammatory diseases of the urinary system in the dog and cat are not associated with marked alterations in WBC. Because the total amount of tissue involved is small when compared to the body as a whole, there is usually not a great stimulus for the bone marrow to produce a large quantity of leucocytes. Pyonephrosis, generalized

pyelonephritis, and large abscesses involving one or both kidneys are examples of primary renal diseases which often are associated with immature neutrophilia.
2. Polysystemic diseases, such as bacterial endocarditis, pyometra, and leptospirosis, which involve the urinary system in addition to other body systems and tissues, are often associated with leucocytosis (see Chapter 28, Renal Diseases Associated with Polysystemic Diseases).
3. Chronic generalized renal diseases are commonly associated with mature neutrophilia (approximately 20,000 to 30,000$^+$ WBC per cmm.) and lymphopenia. This response is related to the increased output of adrenocortical hormones in response to stress.

II. BUN, creatinine, and nonprotein nitrogen (see Chapter 7, Tests of Renal Function)

III. Interpretation of urinalysis

A. Collecting the urine specimen
1. Use a clean container. Use of a transparent container made of glass or plastic will facilitate observation of macroscopic abnormalities.
2. Collect early morning samples from house-trained pets because they are most likely to contain constituents of diagnostic significance.
3. Avoid the first part of the urine stream of noncatheterized samples because it may contain debris and exudate flushed from the urethra or the genital tract.

B. Timing of the analysis
1. A fresh sample is preferred.
   a. Contamination with urea-splitting bacteria may alter the results if urine is allowed to stand several hours at room temperature.
      (1) Urea is split to ammonia which alkalinizes urine.
      (2) Formed elements dissolve as urine becomes more alkaline.
2. Urine preserved by refrigeration is satisfactory for examination for several hours (a lower temperature will slightly increase specific gravity).
3. A preservative may be used when immediate analysis or refrigeration is impossible.
   a. Toluene. Toluene acts primarily as an antimicrobial preservative.
      (1) Add a sufficient quantity to just cover the surface of the urine.
      (2) The portion to be examined should be pipetted from beneath the surface film of toluene.
      (3) This technique of preservation does not interfere with chemical determination of protein or sugar, and allows preservation of 24 hour urine specimens obtained with the aid of a metabolism cage.
      (4) Toluene has some protective action against the loss of acetone, but the amount used must be limited since acetone is half as soluble in toluene as in water.
   b. Thymol. Thymol acts primarily as an antibacterial preservative.
      (1) Dissolve 100 gm. of thymol in 500 ml. of isopropyl alcohol.
      (2) Add a few ml. to the urine sample.
      (3) Thymol will give false-positive reactions for albumin.

c. Formalin. One drop of 40 per cent formalin per 30 ml. of urine may be used to preserve casts or cellular elements. The use of nonspecific tests for glucose on formalin-preserved urine will result in false-positive reactions.

C. *Quantitative vs. qualitative analysis*
1. Random samples of urine are only suitable for qualitative examination because the concentration of any solute will vary with the quantity of water being excreted at that time.
2. Twenty-four hour specimens are satisfactory for quantitative analysis.

D. *Urine volume*
1. The volume of urine formed per day by normal dogs is dependent on the following variables:
   a. Diet.
   b. Fluid intake.
   c. Environmental temperature and humidity.
   d. Activity.
   e. Size and weight.
2. Normal values for urine volume.
   a. The range of normal values is variable.
   b. A normal dog in a controlled environment will produce approximately 12 to 20 ml. of urine per pound of body weight per 24 hours.
   c. When determining 24 hour urine volumes, collect several 24 hour specimens and use the average value.
3. In health, urine volume is usually inversely related to specific gravity.
   a. A high volume is usually associated with a low specific gravity.
   b. A low volume is usually associated with a high specific gravity.
4. In the presence of generalized renal disease, patients usually have a low urine specific gravity, regardless of urine volume. Exceptions include:
   a. Uncomplicated diabetes mellitus may be associated with a large urine volume of high specific gravity due to glucosuria.
   b. Diseases of the kidney characterized by glomerular damage, but which have not yet caused significant tubular damage, theoretically could be associated with a small urine volume of high specific gravity.
5. Increased urine volume (polyuria).
   a. Non-pathologic causes of increased urine volume which are usually transient in duration include:
      (1) Increased water consumption.
      (2) Diuretic therapy.
      (3) Parenteral fluid administration.
      (4) Corticosteroid or ACTH administration.
   b. Pathological causes of increased urine volume which may be of permanent duration include:
      (1) Diabetes mellitus.
      (2) Primary renal glucosuria.
      (3) Diabetes insipidus.
      (4) Renal diabetes insipidus.
      (5) Nephrotoxic nephrosis, diuretic phase.
      (6) Polyuric phase of generalized acute nephritis.
      (7) Generalized chronic nephritis.

(8) Renal cortical hypoplasia and other inherited generalized progressive renal diseases.
(9) Severe renal amyloidosis.
(10) Generalized pyelonephritis.
(11) Pyometra.
(12) Hyperadrenalcorticism.
(13) Some diseases of the liver.
(14) Compulsive (psychogenic) polydipsia.
(15) Others.
6. Decreased urine volume (oliguria).
 a. Physiological causes of decreased urine volume which are usually transient in duration include:
  (1) Decreased water intake.
  (2) High environmental temperature.
  (3) Hyperventilation (excessive panting).
 b. Pathological causes of decreased urine volume include:
  (1) Dehydration due to impaired intake or excessive loss of water (vomiting, diarrhea, etc.).
  (2) Fever due to any cause.
  (3) Oliguric phase of acute generalized nephritis.
  (4) Edema secondary to circulatory dysfunction.
  (5) Markedly reduced blood pressure.
  (6) Terminal renal disease due to any cause.

E. *Color*
 1. Always consider color in association with specific gravity and urine volume.
 2. Normal urine color is pale yellow to light amber.
  a. Urine color is dependent primarily on the concentration of urochromes, the output of which is relatively constant.
  b. Intensity of urine color varies inversely with urine volume.
   (1) High urine volume is associated with a decreased urochrome concentration per unit volume, which results in a pale yellow to clear color and low specific gravity.
   (2) Low urine volume is associated with an increased urochrome concentration per unit volume which results in a dark yellow color and high specific gravity.
 3. Abnormal urine color.
  a. A yellow-brown or yellow-green urine color is associated with bilirubinuria. Yellow foam forms and persists when urine containing bilirubin is shaken.
  b. Red or red-brown urine color.
   (1) Hematuria causes a cloudy (smoky) urine that becomes clearer after centrifugation. Considerable variation in color occurs depending on the quantity of blood present, the length of time it has been in urine, and the character of the urine.
   (2) Hemoglobinuria causes a transparent, wine red urine color that is unaffected by centrifugation.
   (3) Phenolsulfonphthalein dye or bromsulphalein dye in alkaline urine causes a transparent pink to red urine color.
   (4) Neoprontosil causes a transparent red urine color.

c. Blue-green urine color may be caused by:
   (1) Methylene blue.
   (2) Dizan.*

F. *Transparency*
  1. Normal fresh urine may have a clear transparency.
  2. Cloudy.
     a. Normal urine may have a cloudy transparency. Crystals precipitate in urine allowed to stand and cool to room temperature, especially if the sample is concentrated.
     b. Abnormal urine.
        (1) The presence of large quantities of WBC, RBC, epithelial cells, mucus, or bacteria from the urinary tract may cause cloudiness.
        (2) Contamination of urine with exudate from the genital tract may cause cloudiness of noncatheterized urine samples.
     c. The cause of urine turbidity is best determined by microscopic examination of the sediment.

G. *Specific gravity (S.G.)*
  1. Specific gravity may range from approximately 1.001 to 1.060 in the normal dog and from 1.001 to 1.080 in the normal cat.
     a. Randomly obtained urine samples obtained from normal dogs and cats usually have a specific gravity which encompasses a narrower range (1.015 to 1.045), but an individual urine sample with a specific gravity outside these limits is not reliable evidence of renal disease.
     b. Factors causing variation of S.G. in normal dogs and cats include:
        (1) Diet.
        (2) Fluid intake.
        (3) Climate.
        (4) Activity.
     c. Variation of S.G. in a normal healthy dog or cat consuming a constant diet usually reflects variation in water consumption.
  2. In health, specific gravity is usually inversely related to volume of urine output per day.
  3. In the presence of generalized renal disease, patients usually have a low urine specific gravity, regardless of urine volume. Exceptions include:
     a. Uncomplicated diabetes mellitus is often associated with a large urine volume or high specific gravity due to glucosuria.
     b. Diseases of the kidney characterized by glomerular damage, but which have not yet caused significant tubular damage, theoretically could be associated with a small urine volume of high specific gravity.
  4. Addition of considerable quantities of any type of solid will increase the specific gravity.
     a. Each 0.4 Gm. of protein per 100 ml. of urine increases the specific gravity by approximately 0.001.
     b. Each 0.27 Gm. of glucose per 100 ml. of urine increases the specific gravity by approximately 0.001.
  5. Intepretation of all other components of the routine urinalysis should be considered in association with the specific gravity of the specimen if conclusions are to be meaningful.

---
*3,3' diethylthiadicarbocyanine iodide, Corvel, Inc., Omaha, Nebraska.

a. Most tests are performed on a fixed volume of urine without regard to specific gravity (and thus rate of formation and urine volume) of the specimen.
   (1) Example: 2+ proteinuria in the presence of a low specific gravity implies a heavier loss of protein than 2+ proteinuria in a more concentrated (higher S.G.) sample.
   (2) The same is also true for formed elements of sediment, glucose, bilirubin, etc.
6. The specific gravity reflects the concentrating or diluting ability of the kidney, and metabolic work is required to dilute as well as to concentrate urine.
   a. Glomerular filtrate enters the proximal convoluted tubule at a S.G. of 1.010 ± 0.002.
      (1) A specific gravity above 1.012, in the absence of protein and glucose, indicates that the kidney altered the filtrate and was capable of metabolic work.
      (2) A specific gravity below 1.008 indicates that the kidney altered the filtrate and was capable of metabolic work.
7. Specific gravity of a random urine sample.
   a. Specific gravity varies with water consumption.
      (1) A S.G. in the fixed range (1.008 to 1.012) may be seen in a random urine sample from a normal patient since the ability of the normal kidney to change specific gravity overlaps this fixed range.
      (2) The presence of S.G. of 1.008 to 1.012 in a random urine sample is justification for further evaluation of the functional competence of the kidneys. *It is not pathognomonic of any types of renal disease.* When detected, one should proceed as follows:
         (a) The presence of the following in association with a fixed S.G. indicates that the patient cannot conserve needed body water.
            [1] Clinical signs of dehydration, and/or abnormal elevations in packed cell volume and plasma protein concentration indicating the presence of dehydration. In this circumstance, the stimulus for release of antidiuretic hormone exists and the inability of the patient to concentrate urine indicates:
               [a] Lack of release of antidiuretic hormone (diabetes insipidus).
               [b] Inability of the kidney to respond to antidiuretic hormone (generalized renal disease or renal diabetes insipidus).
            [2] The presence of elevated blood urea nitrogen or creatinine concentration in association with a fixed S.G. indicates the probability of generalized renal disease. In the latter instance, the inability to concentrate or dilute urine is related, at least in part, to obligatory osmotic diuresis.
            [3] When these circumstances exist, a water deprivation test is contraindicated.
         (b) Perform a water concentration or Pitressin test (see Chapter 7, Tests of Renal Function).
8. The ability of the kidneys to regulate S.G. depends upon their functional

competence at the time the urine is formed, and therefore cannot be used as the only means of prognosis.
  a. A S.G. of 1.010 can occur in:
    (1) Normal animals.
    (2) Patients with acute or chronic renal disease.
    (3) Patients with reversible or irreversible renal disease.
9. Causes of increased specific gravity include:
  a. Physiological causes which are usually of transient duration, such as:
    (1) Decreased water intake.
    (2) High environmental temperature.
    (3) Hyperventilation (excessive panting).
  b. Pathological (duration variable) causes such as:
    (1) Dehydration due to any cause (vomiting, diarrhea, etc.).
    (2) Fever due to any cause.
    (3) Edema due to circulatory dysfunction.
    (4) Loss of extracellular fluid and serum associated with burns (rare in dogs and cats).
    (5) The initial stage of acute nephritis due to any cause. Generalized acute nephritis is associated with low urine S.G.
    (6) Diabetes mellitus. A high S.G. is not a constant finding in this disease because the S.G. of the urine is affected by the presence or absence of concomitant renal disease in addition to the degree of glucosuria.
    (7) Primary renal glucosuria.
    (8) Shock, if generalized organic renal disease is not present.
    (9) Any disease state in which abnormally large quantities of particles are added to urine.
      (a) Protein.
      (b) Glucose.
      (c) Inflammatory exudate (minor effect).
10. Causes of decreased specific gravity include:
  a. Non-pathologic (usually of transient duration) causes such as:
    (1) Excessive water consumption (most common cause).
    (2) Diuretics.
    (3) Parenteral fluids.
    (4) Corticosteroids or ACTH.
  b. Pathological causes such as:
    (1) Chronic generalized nephritis (S.G. becomes fixed if severe).
    (2) Acute generalized nephritis (S.G. becomes fixed if severe).
    (3) Nephrotoxic nephrosis, diuretic phase.
    (4) Severe renal amyloidosis.
    (5) Renal cortical hypoplasia and other inherited generalized progressive renal diseases.
    (6) Chronic generalized pyelonephritis.
    (7) Diabetes insipidus.
    (8) Renal diabetes insipidus.
    (9) Pyometra.
    (10) Hyperadrenalcorticism.
    (11) Rapid mobilization and excretion of edema fluid.
    (12) Some generalized diseases of the liver.

46 DIAGNOSIS OF URINARY DISEASES

(13) Psychogenic polydipsia.
(14) Others.

H. *Urine pH*
1. Normal (5.5 to 7.5).
   a. In the normal animal, urine pH varies with the following:
      (1) Diet.
         (a) Metabolism of foods of animal origin, the usual diet of dogs and cats, are associated with acid urine.
         (b) Metabolism of foods of vegetable origin are associated with alkaline urine.
         (c) Urine tends to become less acid after meals as a result of the "alkaline tide" which is associated with gastric secretion of HCl.
      (2) Urine tends to become more alkaline when kept at room temperature because of ammonia formation which occurs as a result of decomposition of urea.
2. Causes of an alkaline urine pH include:
   a. Delay in examination of the specimen and subsequent ammonia formation.
   b. Cystitis associated with urea-splitting organisms.
   c. Administration of alkalinizing drugs such as:
      (1) Sodium bicarbonate.
      (2) Sodium lactate.
      (3) Sodium citrate.
   d. Retention of urine in the bladder and subsequent decomposition of urea to ammonia.
   e. Metabolic or respiratory alkalosis.
3. Causes of an acid urine pH include:
   a. High protein diets.
   b. Administration of acidifying drugs such as:
      (1) Ammonium chloride.
      (2) Calcium chloride given orally.
      (3) Sodium acid phosphate.
      (4) D, L-methionine.
   c. Catabolism of body proteins due to:
      (1) Fever.
      (2) Starvation.
      (3) Diabetes mellitus.
   d. Metabolic or respiratory acidosis due to any cause including:
      (1) Diabetes mellitus.
      (2) Uremia—any cause.

I. *Proteinuria*
1. Always interpret proteinuria in association with specific gravity.
2. Because of significant discrepancies between various laboratory tests for proteinuria (Albustix, Hema-Combistix, Labstix, sulphosalicylic acid test, Heller's nitric acid test), the clinical significance of proteinuria should be interpreted in association with other clinical and laboratory findings. As a generality, reagent-strip tests tend to give false-positive readings at low concentrations of urine protein. If reagent-strip tests are used as screening

LABORATORY FINDINGS IN DISEASES OF THE URINARY SYSTEM

tests, positive findings should be confirmed with more reliable tests such as the sulphosalicylic acid test.

3. Physiologic proteinuria is usually of transient duration.
    a. A small quantity of protein normally passes through the glomerular capillaries, but most is reabsorbed by the proximal tubules.
    b. The small amount of protein which escapes into the urine is composed of globulins and albumin, but it is of insufficient quantity to give a positive reaction with conventional laboratory tests.
    c. A persistent proteinuria of sufficient quantity to allow detection by usual clinical laboratory tests should always be investigated.
    d. Causes of physiologic proteinuria include:
        (1) Strenuous exercise.
        (2) Altered renal function during the first few days of life.
        (3) The following are associated with proteinuria in man and may occur in the dog:
            (a) Immersion in cold water.
            (b) Emotional stress.
4. Pathologic proteinuria.
    a. Care must be used in interpretation of proteinuria since proteinuria may be of renal or nonrenal origin. Detection of proteinuria does not necessarily indicate the presence of renal disease.
        (1) Many diseases of the genito-urinary system may result in proteinuria, and its significance should be considered in association with the history, physical examination, pertinent laboratory data, and other findings in the urinalysis.
        (2) Qualitative tests currently available for detection of proteinuria do not provide information of sufficient specificity to allow one to make a definitive diagnosis of a specific renal disease.
    b. The quantity of proteinuria is not necessarily commensurate with the severity of the causative disease. Terminal stages of many renal diseases (e.g., amyloidosis) may be associated with decreased proteinuria, while earlier stages may have been associated with heavy proteinuria (see Chapter 26, Renal Amyloidosis).
    c. It is difficult to determine the cause of proteinuria on the basis of the amount of protein in the urine. A heavy proteinuria in the absence of hematuria or pyuria usually originates from the kidneys, especially the glomeruli.
    d. Renal proteinuria.
        (1) Renal proteinuria may occur as a result of:
            (a) Leakage of protein through glomeruli at an increased rate.
            (b) Tubular disease with resultant decrease or lack of tubular reabsorption of protein.
            (c) Both of the above.
            (d) Inflammatory exudate in the kidneys.
        (2) Protein losing renal diseases are usually associated with urinary excretion of an increased quantity of albumin, and to a lesser extent, globulins.
        (3) Specific causes of renal proteinuria include:
            (a) Renal amyloidosis (mild to very severe proteinuria).
            (b) Acute nephritis due to any cause (moderate to heavy protein-

uria often associated with casts, RBC, and WBC in the urine sediment).
- (c) Chronic generalized nephritis (absent to mild proteinuria).
- (d) Renal cortical hypoplasia and other inherited generalized diseases of the kidney (absent to mild proteinuria).
- (e) Pyelonephritis (mild to moderate proteinuria, often with RBC, WBC, casts, and bacteria).
- (f) Renal neoplasms (variable degree of proteinuria associated with RBC, WBC, and occasionally neoplastic cells).
- (g) Polycystic kidneys (absent to moderate proteinuria).
- (h) Glomerulonephritis (mild to heavy proteinuria).
- (i) *Dioctophyma renale* (variable degrees of proteinuria associated with RBC, WBC, and eggs).
- e. Postrenal urinary proteinuria.
  - (1) Any marked hematuria, regardless of cause, will be associated with moderate to severe proteinuria.
  - (2) Slight to large amounts of protein may appear in urine as a result of the presence of inflammatory exudate from any location in the urinary tract.
- f. Polysystemic or extraurinary causes of proteinuria include:
  - (1) Chronic passive congestion of the kidneys caused by:
    - (a) Cardiac insufficiency.
    - (b) Increase in intra-abdominal pressure (i.e., ascites, neoplasms).
  - (2) Contamination of urine with inflammatory exudate from the genital tract.
  - (3) Renal infarction.
  - (4) Metastatic neoplasia of the kidneys.
  - (5) Microfilaria of *Dirofilaria immitis.*
- g. Bence Jones proteinuria.
  - (1) Bence Jones proteins are pathognomonic of multiple myeloma.
  - (2) They may be detected by heating urine. Bence Jones proteins may precipitate at 50 to 60° C., although the latter is not a consistent finding.
  - (3) Detection by urine electrophoresis is more reliable.

J. Glucosuria
1. Normal urine contains no detectable glucose because glucose filtered through glomeruli is reabsorbed by the proximal tubules.
2. Glucosuria occurs in dogs when venous blood levels of glucose exceed about 180 mg. per 100 ml.
3. Causes of glucosuria include diseases:
   a. Associated with hyperglycemia:
      (1) Diabetes mellitus is usually associated with heavy glucosuria, and is often accompanied by ketonuria.
      (2) Hyperadrenalcorticism (not a frequent finding).
      (3) Severe acute pancreatic necrosis causing hypoinsulinism.
      (4) Parenteral treatment with dextrose or fructose solutions.
      (5) Ingestion of excessive quantities of sugar or carbohydrate.
      (6) Parenteral administration of epinephrine.
   b. Not associated with hyperglycemia:
      (1) Primary renal glucosuria (not associated with acetonuria. See Chapter 15, Congenital and Inherited Renal Diseases).

(2) Renal disease may be associated with a small quantity of urine glucose, although the latter is relatively uncommon.
(3) Drugs such as phlorhizin or morphine.

K. *Ketonuria (acetonuria)*
  1. Ketonuria occurs as the result of increased blood concentrations of acetoacetic acid, beta-hydroxybutyric acid, and acetone, with subsequent excretion of these compounds in the urine.
  2. Causes of ketonuria include:
    a. Diabetes mellitus.
      (1) Diabetes mellitus is the most common cause of ketonuria in the dog.
      (2) Diabetic ketonuria is associated with altered lipid catabolism, and is related to defective carbohydrate metabolism.
    b. Starvation.
      (1) Adult dogs seldom develop ketonuria, but occasionally it is associated with prolonged inanition.
      (2) Infrequently ketonuria is encountered in young malnourished puppies.
      (3) Lipid is utilized as an energy source because carbohydrate stores are depleted.

L. *Bilirubinuria*
  1. Always interpret bilirubinuria in association with the specific gravity.
  2. The renal threshold for bilirubin in the normal dog is low. Urine obtained from normal dogs often contains some bilirubin, especially when the specimen has a high specific gravity. Tests for bilirubinuria are frequently positive in the absence of detectable liver disease.
  3. Pathologic bilirubinuria.
    a. Bilirubin must be conjugated by the liver to pass through normal glomeruli.
    b. Conjugated bilirubin may spill into urine following excessive accumulation in blood.
    c. Causes of pathologic bilirubinuria include:
      (1) Hepatocellular disease:
        (a) Infectious canine hepatitis.
        (b) Leptospirosis.
        (c) Cirrhosis.
        (d) Neoplasia.
        (e) Toxicities.
        (f) Others.
      (2) Obstruction of bile ducts due to any cause.

M. *Occult blood*
  1. Routine laboratory tests do not distinguish between hematuria, hemoglobinuria, and myoglobinuria.
    a. The use of tablets to detect occult blood will give positive results:
      (1) Whenever intact RBC are present in numbers greater than 10 per high power field.
      (2) Whenever free hemoglobin or myoglobin is present.
    b. The use of sticks to detect occult blood will give positive results when-

ever free hemoglobin or myoglobin is present. The results will be negative (or less positive) when only intact RBC are present.
   2. Interpretation (see hematuria and hemoglobinuria in this chapter).
N. *Urine sediment*
   1. Noncatheterized urine samples may be contaminated with debris or exudate from the genital tract. The latter is less likely to occur with samples obtained by catheterization.
   2. Always examine a fresh or preserved urine sample. Cellular elements and casts may be destroyed in urine allowed to stand at room temperature.
      a. Sediment for microscopic examination should be obtained by centrifugation of 10 to 15 ml. of urine in a conical-tip centrifuge tube. The sample should be centrifuged at a low rate of speed (1000 rpm) for approximately five minutes in order to prevent fragmentation of organized components of the sediment.
      b. The use of special stains such as new methylene blue or Sternheimer-Malbin stain may assist in identification of cells, casts, and bacteria.
      c. Nonstained specimens should be examined under reduced light. The latter may be accomplished by lowering the condenser and closing the diaphragm.
   3. Always interpret findings in association with the specific gravity.
      a. Urine specific gravity serves as an index of the relative concentrations of water and constituents of the sediment.
      b. Hypotonic urine (i.e., urine of low specific gravity) may cause lysis of cells.
   4. In health, urine may contain small numbers of epithelial cells, RBC, WBC, and casts. Approximate limits between normal and abnormal have been established in human medicine, but are not available in veterinary medicine.
   5. Urine sediment may contain any one or more of the following:
      a. Organized sediment.
         (1) RBC.
         (2) WBC.
         (3) Epithelial cells.
         (4) Casts.
         (5) Bacteria.
         (6) Parasite ova.
         (7) Yeast and fungi.
         (8) Spermatozoa.
      b. Non-organized sediment.
         (1) Crystals and amorphous material.
   6. Hematuria.
      a. An occasional RBC per high power field (HPF) is normal.
      b. Hematuria may be gross or microscopic.
         (1) Gross hematuria or large numbers of RBC in a microscopic field always indicate hemorrhage, inflammation, necrosis, trauma, or neoplasia somewhere along the urinary tract.
      c. Gross hematuria (generalities only. See Chapter 4, Physical Examination of the Urinary System).
         (1) When hematuria is most prominent at the beginning of urination

or when it occurs without urination, it may be associated with a lesion of the uterus, vagina, prostate, penis, or urethra.
- (2) When hematuria is most prominent at the end of urination, it may suggest a lesion of the urinary bladder because RBC tend to settle to the bottom of the bladder.
- (3) If hematuria is uniform throughout the sample, it may suggest a lesion of the bladder, kidneys, or ureters.

d. Causes of hematuria include:
   (1) Violent exercise.
   (2) Iatrogenic trauma.
      (a) Palpation of the bladder or kidneys.
      (b) Catheterization of the bladder.
   (3) Trauma.
   (4) Urinary calculi in any location.
   (5) Infection of any portion of the urinary system.
   (6) Benign or malignant neoplasms of any portion of the urinary system.
   (7) Chronic passive congestion due to any cause.
   (8) Renal infarcts due to any cause.
   (9) Systemic diseases with hemorrhagic tendencies.
      (a) Thrombocytopenia.
      (b) Warfarin poisoning.
      (c) Leptospirosis.
      (d) Systemic lupus erythematosus.
   (10) Drugs such as sulfonamides.
   (11) Parasites.
      (a) *Dictophyma renale.*
      (b) *Capillaria plica.*
      (c) Microfilaria of *Dirofilaria immitis.*

e. Extra-urinary causes of hematuria include:
   (1) Inflammation or tumors of the genital tract.
   (2) Estrum.
   (3) Trauma to the genital tract.

7. Hemoglobinuria.
   a. Hemoglobinuria occurs as a result of an increased plasma concentration of hemoglobin.
   b. If it is caused by hemolysis of red cells in low specific gravity or alkaline urine, it will be accompanied by ghost RBC in urine sediment.
   c. Gross hemoglobinuria should be suspected if the urine remains wine red after centrifugation.
   d. Causes of hemoglobinuria include:
      (1) Any cause of intravascular hemolysis.
         (a) Transfusion reactions.
         (b) Hemolytic anemia (dependent upon severity).
            [1] Autoimmune hemolytic anemia.
            [2] Babesiasis.
            [3] Hemolytic disease of newborn.
            [4] Snake venom.
            [5] Toxic agents.
            [6] Others.

52 DIAGNOSIS OF URINARY DISEASES

8. Pyuria.
   a. An occasional WBC per HPF may occur in normal patients.
   b. Large numbers of WBC indicate inflammation or necrosis anywhere along the urinary tract.
   c. The possibility that WBC have occurred as the result of passage of urine through the genital tract must be considered in noncatheterized samples of urine.
   d. The presence of WBC is a more reliable indicator of urinary disease if the urine sample is obtained by catheterization utilizing proper technique.
9. Epithelial cells.
   a. Three types of epithelial cells may be observed.
      (1) Squamous cells:
         (a) From the genital tract.
         (b) Common in noncatheterized samples.
      (2) Transitional cells:
         (a) From the urinary tract.
         (b) An occasional cell is normal.
         (c) Increased numbers of transitional epithelial cells often occur in association with inflammation or neoplasia.
      (3) Renal cells:
         (a) From the renal tubules.
         (b) An occasional cell is normal.
   b. Accurate data regarding the number of epithelial cells which may normally be present in the urine of dogs and cats is not available.
   c. Large numbers of cells may suggest disease, but there are more reliable signs upon which to establish such a conclusion.
   d. Tumor cells may be diagnostic, especially those arising from malignant epithelial neoplasms such as transitional cell carcinomas of the urinary bladder.

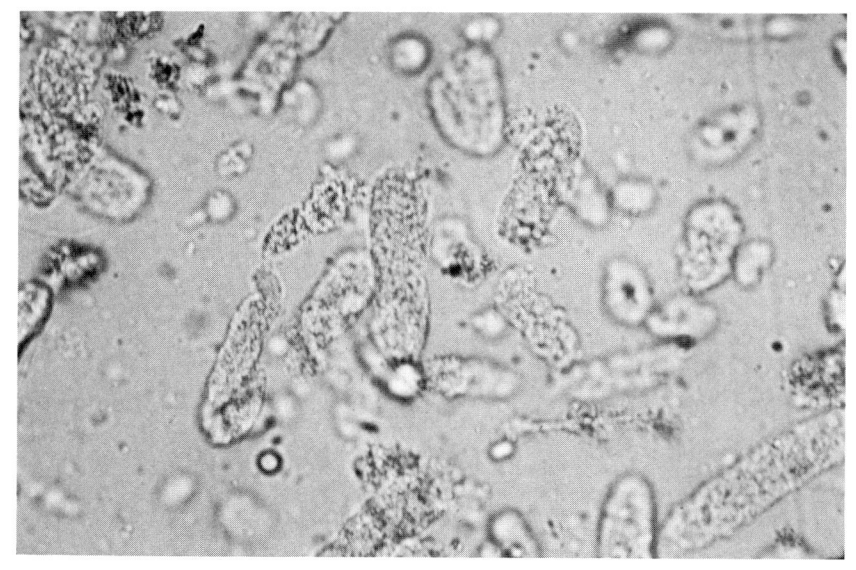

Figure 6–1. Photomicrograph of canine urine sediment containing numerous granular casts. ×450. (Courtesy of Dr. Victor Perman, College of Veterinary Medicine. University of Minnesota.)

LABORATORY FINDINGS IN DISEASES OF THE URINARY SYSTEM

10. Casts.
    a. A few casts are often observed in normal animals and appear to have no diagnostic or prognostic significance.
        (1) Two to four casts per low power field (LPF) is a rough approximation of the borderline between normal and abnormal. Always consider the number of casts per LPF in association with specific gravity.
        (2) The presence of casts in urine indicates some pathologic change in the renal tubules, but this change may be minor and transitory.
    b. Casts in significant numbers always indicate renal disease.
        (1) Casts are tubular molds composed primarily of mucoprotein (Tamm-Horsfall mucoprotein) and some protein (Fig. 6-1).
        (2) Casts are formed in the loops of Henle, distal convoluted tubules, and collecting ducts. Urine reaches maximum concentration and acidity here, and favors precipitation of protein and mucoprotein. In the dog and cat, it has been demonstrated that mucoprotein is secreted in the loops of Henle, distal convoluted tubules, and collecting ducts, but not in the proximal tubules and glomeruli.
        (3) Any lesion in the tubule which is present at the time the cast is formed may be reflected in the composition of the cast. Therefore, casts are classified according to the material which they contain.
        (4) The number and morphologic characteristics of casts are generally of little specific diagnostic significance.
        (5) The number of casts is not a reliable index of the mildness or severity of disease. For example, casts are often absent in progressive generalized chronic nephritis.
    c. The following are different types of casts which may be seen:
        (1) Hyaline casts.
        (2) Epithelial casts.
        (3) Granular casts.
        (4) Waxy casts.
        (5) Renal failure (broad) casts.
        (6) Fatty casts.
        (7) RBC casts.
        (8) WBC casts.
        (9) Bile-stained casts.
        (10) Mixed casts.
    d. Hyaline casts are:
        (1) Composed of mucoprotein and protein and are commonly seen in association with proteinuria.
        (2) Often observed in association with transient conditions (fever, chronic passive congestion), but may occur in association with generalized and irreversible renal disease (chronic nephritis, amyloidosis).
        (3) Not a reliable index of the severity of the underlying lesion.
    e. Epithelial casts are:
        (1) Formed as a result of desquamation of tubular cells which have not disintegrated.
        (2) Similar in significance to granular casts.
    f. Granular casts.
        (1) The granules are derived from disintegrated tubular cells which are embedded in a mucoprotein-protein matrix (Fig. 6-1).

(2) Large numbers are usually associated with renal disease causing necrosis of tubular epithelial cells, including:
    (a) Nephritis due to any cause.
    (b) Nephrotoxins.
    (c) Infarcts due to any cause.

g. Waxy casts:
    (1) Are formed from long-standing granular casts.
    (2) Indicate the presence of a chronic tubular lesion.
    (3) Are uncommonly associated with renal amyloidosis.

h. Renal failure casts (broad casts):
    (1) Are similar to, but larger than, granular casts.
    (2) Originate in collecting ducts and indicate loss or obstruction of more than one nephron.
    (3) They may also be formed in dilated tubules of the nephron.

i. Fatty casts occur in association with degenerative tubular diseases such as diabetes mellitus.

j. RBC casts occur in association with hemorrhage into renal tubules.

k. WBC casts occur in association with inflammation of renal tubules.

l. Bile-stained casts. Any cast may be pigmented with bile when large quantities of bilirubin are excreted by the kidneys.

m. Mixed casts. Casts may be of mixed composition.

11. Bacteria.
    a. Normally urine is sterile until it reaches the neck of the bladder. The urethra of dogs normally contains a resident population of bacteria which are greatest in number at the distal end of the urethra.
    b. Great significance should not be placed on the presence of bacteria in noncatheterized urine samples because such samples may be contaminated with bacteria from the distal urethra, genital tract, or collecting vial (see IV, Bacterial culture of urine).
    c. Great significance should not be placed on the presence of bacteria in urine samples allowed to incubate at room temperature prior to analysis as the bacteria may have proliferated following collection.
    d. Large numbers of bacteria which are observed in catheterized, midstream, or urine samples obtained by cystocentesis, suggest bacterial infection somewhere along the urinary tract, especially when associated with other signals of inflammation such as WBC, RBC, and protein (see Chapter 5, Collection of Urine).
    e. Bacteria observed with a microscope in a noncentrifuged sample of urine suggest a concentration in excess of 1 million bacteria per ml. of urine. New methylene blue or Gram stains may facilitate detection of bacteria.
    f. Bacterial culture and antibiotic sensitivity should be evaluated prior to treatment of patients with bacterial diseases of the urinary system.

12. Yeast and fungi usually represent contaminants.

13. Metazoan parasite ova which may be detected in urine include:
    a. *Dioctophyma renale.*
    b. *Capillaria plica.*
    c. *Capillaria felis-cati.*
    d. The microfilaria of *Dirofilaria immitis* may be occasionally observed in the urine as a result of hematuria.

14. Spermatozoa are a normal finding in the urine of male dogs.

15. Lipiduria.
    a. In cats, lipiduria may occur as a result of physiological breakdown of lipid-laden cells of the renal tubules, and is usually of no clinical significance.
    b. In dogs, the significance of lipiduria is questionable, but it is probably similar to lipiduria in cats. Lipiduria has been observed in association with nephrotic syndromes in dogs (see Chapter 27, Nephrotic Syndrome).
16. Nonorganized urinary sediment.
    a. Crystals and amorphous material seen in the urine sediment provide little diagnostic information about diseases of the urinary system.
    b. The types of crystals seen depend on:
        (1) Urine pH.
        (2) Solubility of the crystalloid.
        (3) Concentration of the crystalloid in urine.
    c. Crystals seen in alkaline urine include:
        (1) Triple phosphates (ammonium and magnesium).
        (2) Amorphous phosphates.
        (3) Calcium carbonate.
        (4) Ammonium urate.
    d. Crystals seen in acid urine include:
        (1) Urate crystals.
        (2) Cystine crystals (uncommon).
        (3) Calcium oxalate.
        (4) Hippuric acid.
    e. The presence of certain types of crystals may be of diagnostic value.
        (1) Large numbers of cystine crystals may occur in association with cystinuria.
        (2) Oxalate crystals may occur in the urine of dogs or cats poisoned with ethylene glycol.

IV. Bacterial culture of urine

  A. *If the patient has been receiving antibacterial therapy, urine should not be cultured for bacteria until therapy has been withdrawn for a period of three to five days.* Antibiotics may suppress the *in vitro* growth of pathogens and lead to erroneous results.
  B. *Urine specimens for bacterial culture may be obtained by:*
    1. Collection of a midstream sample during spontaneous micturition.
    2. Collection of a midstream sample during manual compression of the bladder.
    3. Catheterization of the urinary bladder.
    4. Cystocentesis.
  C. *Collection of urine specimens during spontaneous micturition, by manual compression of the bladder, or by catheterization*
    1. Normal canine urine is sterile until it reaches the neck of the bladder. The same is true for human beings and is presumably true for cats.
      a. The urethra of dogs normally contains a resident population of bacteria which are greatest in number at the distal end of the urethra.
      b. Many of the bacteria in the urethra are nonpathogenic.

56   DIAGNOSIS OF URINARY DISEASES

    2. The use of any of these techniques does not guarantee collection of a urine sample free of urethral bacteria.
       a. By not collecting the first portion of a urine sample, the likelihood of contamination with urethral bacteria is reduced.
       b. The technique of quantitative bacterial culture (i.e., determination of the number of bacteria per unit volume of urine) may permit differentiation between urethral contamination and urinary infection with bacteria. Urinary infection is typically associated with significantly greater numbers of bacteria per unit volume of urine than contamination of urine with bacteria from the urethra. A commercial laboratory kit* is available that permits isolation of common bacterial pathogens, quantitation of bacterial growth, and determination of bacterial sensitivity to antibiotics.
       c. If qualitative bacterial culture of urine collected by one of these techniques is sterile, it may be assumed that bacterial infection due to common bacterial pathogens is not present.
         (1) If bacterial growth occurs, differentiation between urethral contamination and urinary infection cannot always be predicted.
         (2) Correlation of bacteriology data with information obtained from the history, physical examination, and urinalysis will be of benefit in interpretation of results (see Interpretation of urinalysis, in this chapter).

D. *Cystocentesis*
    1. The problem of urethral contamination of urine samples may be eliminated by obtaining urine directly from the bladder with a needle and syringe.
    2. See Chapter 5, Collection of Urine.

E. *Biopsy samples obtained from the kidney during percutaneous needle biopsy with a punch biopsy instrument or a fine needle** may be used for bacterial culture.*

F. *Laboratory technique*
    1. The success of bacterial culture of urine is dependent on good laboratory technique.
    2. Urine should be transported to the laboratory in a sterile container.***
    3. Urine should be cultured as soon as possible following collection. If a delay is unavoidable, refrigeration of the sample may still permit satisfactory results after a delay of several hours.
    4. Consult textbooks of veterinary bacteriology and specific references for specific information about bacterial culture media, laboratory technique, and interpretation of results.

V. Serum electrolytes

A. *Although evaluation of serum or plasma concentrations of electrolytes is helpful, the serum concentration of an electrolyte is not a reliable index of its total body concentration.*

---

*Uro-Bacti-Lab, Bacti-Lab, Mountain View, California 94040.
**Franzen Thin Biopsy Needle, United States Catheter and Instrument Corp., Glens Falls, New York 12801
***Culturette, Medi/Flex Division, Medical Supply Company, Rockford, Illinois 61101.

1. The serum concentration of an electrolyte only indicates the ratio of that electrolyte to water.
2. There are significant differences between intracellular and extracellular electrolyte composition.
3. The serum or plasma concentration of any electrolyte may fluctuate rapidly due to changes in intracellular or extracellular composition. Any change in the concentration of solutes in cells or extracellular fluid will result in redistribution of water between body fluid compartments in order to restore and maintain osmotic equilibrium.

B. *Sodium*

In dogs and cats with generalized polyuric renal disease, the kidneys eventually lose the ability to effectively conserve sodium and, generally, a sodium deficit exists. Serum levels of sodium may be normal despite the deficit in total body sodium because the loss of sodium through the kidneys is accompanied by a loss of water (isotonic contraction of body fluid). For this reason drugs containing sodium are often used as a part of the regimen of therapy of polyuric renal failure (see Chapter 31, Treatment of Renal Failure).

C. *Chloride*

The body concentration of chloride tends to parallel that of sodium in patients with renal failure. Reabsorption of chloride by normal kidneys is thought to be a passive process (i.e., no energy-requiring transport systems are necessary). Dogs with advanced renal failure generally tend to have varying degrees of chloride deficit.

D. *Potassium*
1. Normally potassium is removed from tubular fluid by active reabsorption in the proximal tubules, and is secreted into the tubular fluid by distal tubular cells. Normally, the amount of potassium secreted is approximately equal to potassium intake, and potassium balance is maintained.
2. In patients with renal failure associated with oliguria or anuria, potassium is retained in the body. The effect of hyperkalemia on the heart is thought to be one of the major factors which contribute to the death of patients with irreversible oliguric or anuric renal failure.
3. Provided patients with renal failure can maintain an adequate urine volume, the serum concentration of potassium tends to remain within normal limits. The ability of a reduced number of functioning nephrons to maintain a relatively normal serum concentration of potassium is thought to occur as the result of adaptive changes in viable nephrons (see Chapter 12, Pathophysiology of Renal Failure).

E. *Plasma bicarbonate*

In dogs and cats with generalized renal disease, the kidneys lose the ability to effectively conserve bicarbonate. Generally, a bicarbonate deficit exists in the late stages of the disease. Bicarbonate is a significant buffer of hydrogen ions, and for this reason bicarbonate is often used as a part of the regimen of therapy of renal failure (see Chapter 31, Treatment of Renal Failure).

F. *Calcium and phosphorus*
1. The serum concentration of calcium is usually not markedly affected in acute renal failure.

2. In man, rats and dogs, hypercalcemia may induce varying degrees of damage to the nephrons, especially the renal tubules (see Malignant lymphoma, in Chapter 28). The effects of elevated levels of plasma calcium on the kidneys of cats have not been extensively evaluated.
    a. Hyposthenuria is one of the most common clinical signs associated with calcium nephropathy, although it is not invariably present.
    b. Morphologic changes associated with calcium nephropathy include thickening and calcification of tubular basement membranes, cellular necrosis and calcification, and cellular sloughing.
    c. Hypercalciuria associated with severe functional damage to the kidneys is usually associated with an abnormal increase in serum calcium concentration.
    d. Calcium nephropathy of sufficient severity to induce renal failure is not invariably associated with radiographic evidence of renal calcification.
    e. The degree of reversibility of the renal damage caused by calcium deposition is dependent on the degree of permanent damage to nephrons (see Chapter 12, Pathophysiology of Renal Failure).
3. Hyperphosphatemia is a consistent finding in generalized acute renal disease and chronic progressive renal disease of dogs and cats because phosphorus is normally eliminated by the kidneys.
4. Hypocalcemia occurs in association with chronic generalized renal disease. Although the pathogenesis of hypocalcemia has not been clearly defined, the following factors have been incriminated:
    a. Imbalance of the normal calcium-phosphorus ratio in the body with resultant precipitation of calcium salts in various body tissues.
    b. Excretion of abnormal quantities of phosphorus into the intestines with resultant formation of nonabsorbable calcium salts.
    c. Impaired metabolism of vitamin D to its active form, which impairs intestinal absorption of calcium.
5. The hypocalcemia of uremia stimulates the parathyroid glands to secrete parathormone. As a result, calcium is mobilized from the bones in an effort to maintain the concentration of serum calcium within normal limits.
6. The serum concentration of calcium tends to remain within normal limits until the terminal phase of the renal disease has been reached. At that time, the total serum concentration of calcium may decrease to as low as 5 to 8 mg. per 100 ml. Hypocalcemic tetany is not commonly observed in dogs with terminal chronic renal failure, even when they are markedly hypocalcemic, because the associated renal acidosis causes a greater proportion of the total calcium to become ionized. Ionized calcium is the biologically active form of blood calcium.
7. In chronic renal failure, varying degrees of renal osteodystrophy occur secondary to mobilization of calcium from the bones. Microscopic evidence of osteodystrophy and secondary parathyroid hyperplasia can be detected in most dogs and cats with generalized chronic nephritis. In severe cases, renal osteodystrophy may be detected radiographically and is characterized by demineralization of the skeleton, which is especially prominent in the bones of the skull. As a generality, renal osteodystrophy of sufficient severity to cause pathologic fractures, pain, or deformity of bones is uncommonly encountered in association with spontaneously occurring renal diseases of the dog and cat.

VI. Blood pH

Patients with renal failure often have metabolic acidosis. In most cases of generalized renal disease, the urine is maximally acidified. Metabolic acidosis develops because the amount of H$^+$ that can be secreted by tubular cells is reduced. This reduction occurs because of impaired renal tubular production of ammonia (see Applied Physiology of the Urinary System, Chapter 2). The maximal H$^+$ gradient against which the tubular transport mechanism can secrete hydrogen ions corresponds to a pH of about 4.5 to 5.0. The metabolic acidosis associated with renal failure may also be caused by inability of the kidneys to excrete an adequate quantity of the acid breakdown products of digestion and metabolism, and loss of renal capacity to conserve buffer electrolytes such as bicarbonate.

A. *If the buffer systems of the body are able to compensate for the acidosis, the pH of the blood will remain within normal limits.*

When blood pH is in the normal range, the state of compensated acidosis may be recognized by an abnormally low plasma concentration of bicarbonate.

B. *If the buffer systems of the body cannot completely compensate for the metabolic acidosis, the pH of the blood will be below normal.*

A blood pH below 6.8 to 7.0 is usually fatal.

VII. Serum amylase

Because amylase is dependent upon renal excretion for removal from the blood, serum amylase concentrations are usually elevated in uremic dogs and cats. There is no obvious relationship between the degree of amylasemia and the serum concentrations of BUN or creatinine. In man, serum amylase may be determined by either saccharogenic or amyloclastic methods. In dogs, however, only amyloclastic methods should be used. Significant levels of maltase in dog serum contribute to erroneous values for amylase concentration when the latter is determined by saccharogenic methods based on rate of appearance of reducing groups. Amyloclastic methods of amylase assay are based on the rate of disappearance of substrate as indicated by changes in starch-iodine color, viscosity, or turbidity. Thus amyloclastic methods of amylase determination in dogs eliminate the variable caused by the presence of maltase.

VIII. Alkaline phosphatase

Although it has been reported that alkaline phosphatase is normally excreted by the kidneys of cats, the serum concentration of alkaline phosphatase rarely, if ever, becomes elevated in cats with renal failure.

IX. Cholesterol

Hypercholesterolemia is a frequent, but not invariable, finding in dogs with generalized renal disease. Patients with renal disease and an elevated concentration of total cholesterol usually have a normal percentage (60 to 80 per cent) of cholesterol esters. The mechanisms responsible for hypercholesterolemia in dogs with renal disease are obscure. Experimental evidence has been interpreted to suggest that hypoalbuminemia, which may occur secondary to albuminuria, may play a role in the pathogenesis. Clinical and experimental observations have revealed that hypercholesterolemia in dogs often occurs in association with generalized primary or secondary diseases of the glomeruli associated with proteinuria (i.e., renal amyloidosis, glomerulonephritis associated with pyometra, membranous glomerulonephritis, nephrotoxic serum nephritis).

X. **Serum proteins**

　A. *Generalized renal diseases which cause diffuse damage to the glomerular capillary walls are often associated with proteinuria.*

　　The first plasma protein to escape through the glomeruli in significant quantity is albumin (molecular weight = 68,000). Smaller quantities of plasma globulins also escape into the urine, but globulins with higher molecular weights are retained in the blood vascular system. Hypoalbuminemia may occur in association with severe albuminuria. If the loss of plasma albumin is severe enough to cause a large change in colloidal osmotic pressure, a nephrotic syndrome may be initiated (see Chapter 27, Nephrotic Syndrome).

　B. *Infectious diseases may be associated with a mild to moderate increase in serum globulins.*

　　Systemic lupus erythematosus (see systemic lupus erythematosus, in Chapter 28) may be associated with moderate to marked increases in serum globulins, and if the kidneys are involved with glomerulonephritis, a mild to moderate decrease in serum albumin.

　C. *Evaluation of the concentration of total serum protein without regard to albumin and globulin composition may mask hypoalbuminemia in patients with elevated globulin concentrations (as in SLE described above).*

REFERENCES

Bagdade, J. D.: Uremic lipemia. Arch. Int. Med., *126*:875–881, 1970.
Balazs, T., Sekella, R., and Pauls, J. F.: Renal concentration test in beagle dogs. Laboratory Animal Science, *21*:546–548, 1971.
Benjamin, M.M.: Outline of Veterinary Clinical Pathology. 2nd edition. Ames, Iowa, The Iowa State University Press, 1961.
Bricker, N. S., Slatopolsky, E., Reiss, E., and Avioli, L. V.: Calcium, phosphorus and bone in renal disease and transplantation. Arch. Int. Med., *123*:543–553, 1969.
Brody, L. H., Salladay, J. R., and Armbruster, K.: Urinalysis and the urinary sediment. Med. Clin. N. Amer., *55*:243–266, 1971.
Carone, F. A., Epstein, F. H., Beck, D., and Levitin, H.: The effects upon the kidney of transient hypercalcemia induced by parathyroid extract. Amer. J. Path., *36*:77–103, 1960.
Coles, E. H.: Veterinary Clinical Pathology. Philadelphia, Pa., W. B. Saunders Co., 1967.
Coye, R. D., Maude, D. L., Dibble, R. F., and Yoile, C. L.: Experimental Proteinuria: An electrophoretic study of 3 different types in dogs. Arch. Path., *60*:548–555, 1955.
Coye, R. D., Niehoff, R., Rammer, M., and Tanner, J.: Proteinuria associated with experimentally produced abscesses and fever in dogs. Arch. Path., *68*:126–133, 1959.
Doggart, J. R., McCredie, J. A., and Welbourne, R. B.: Urinary amino acids in normal dogs and in those with experimentally induced cirrhosis. Vet. Rec., *70*:279–282, 1958.
Duffy, J. L., Suzuki, Y., and Chung, J.: Acute calcium nephropathy. Arch. Path., *91*:340–350, 1971.
Edwards, O. M.: Urinary creatinine excretion as an index of the completeness of 24 hour urine collection. Lancet, *2*:1165–1166, 1969.
Epstein, F.: Calcium and the kidney. Amer. J. Med., *45*:700–714, 1968.
Epstein, F. H., Beck, D., Carone, F. A., Levitin, H., and Manitus, A.: Changes in renal concentrating ability produced by parathyroid extract. J. Clin. Invest., *38*:1214–1221, 1959.
Farrow, B. R. H., and Penny, R.: Multiple myeloma in the cat. J.A.V.M.A., *158*:606–611, 1971.
Finco, D. R., and Stevens, J. B.: The clinical significance of serum amylase activity in the dog. J.A.V.M.A., *155*:1686–1691, 1969.

Grollman, A.: The role of the kidney in the parathyroid control of the blood calcium as determined by studies on nephrectomized dogs. Endocrinology, 55:166–172, 1954.
Harvey, D. G., and Hoe, C. M.: The use of paper electrophoresis for the routine identification of urinary proteins in the dog. J. Sm. Anim. Pract., 7:431–440, 1966.
Kaneko, J. J., and Cornelius, C. E.: Clinical Biochemistry of Domestic Animals. Vols. I & II. 2nd ed. New York, N.Y., Academic Press, 1971.
Kern, W. H.: Epithelial cells in urine sediments. Am. J. Clin. Path., 56:67–72, 1971.
Laboratory Diagnosis of Kidney Diseases. Edited by F. W. Sunderman and F. W. Sunderman, Jr., Warren H. Green, Inc., St. Louis, Mo., 1970.
Levy, M., Lester, R., and Levinsky, N. G.: Renal excretion of urobilinogen in the dog. J. Clin. Invest., 47:2117–2124, 1968.
Manuel, Y., Revillard, J. P., and Betvel, H.: Proteins in Normal and Pathological Urine. S. Karger, Basel, New York, N.Y., 1970.
McIntyre, M., and Mon, T. W.: Persistence of leucocytes and erythrocytes in refrigerated and alkaline urine. Amer. J. Clin. Path., 43:53–57, 1965.
McQueen, E. G.: Composition of urinary casts. Lancet, 1:397–398, 1966.
Morgan, H. C.: Practitioner's laboratory. Vet. Med./Small Animal Clin., 62:312–317, 416–423, 585–586, 637–640, 737–742, 984–988, 1182–1191, 1967.
Morgan, H. C.: Practitioner's laboratory, Vet. Med./Small Animal Clin., 63:112–119, 356–361, 1968.
Naets, J. P.: Erythropoiesis in nephrectomized dogs. Nature, 181:1134–1135, 1958.
Osbaldiston, G. W.: The kidney. Its function and evaluation in health and disease. In Clinical Biochemistry of Domestic Animals. Vol. 2. 2nd ed. Edited by J. J. Kaneko and C. E. Cornelius. New York, N.Y., Academic Press, 1971.
Osbaldiston, G. W., and Stowe, E. C.: Diagnostic bacteriology—identification of aerobic pathogens. Vet. Med./Sm. Animal Clin., 66:998–1006, 1971.
Osborne, C. A.: Urologic Logic—Diagnosis of renal disease. J.A.V.M.A., 157:1656–1666, 1970.
Perman, V., and Stevens, J. B.: Clinical evaluation of the acinar pancreas of the dog. J.A.V.M.A., 155: 2053–2058, 1969.
Pollak, V. E., and Arbel, C.: The Distribution of Tamm Horsfall mucoprotein (Uromucoid) in the human nephron. Nephron, 6:667–672, 1969.
Richards, M. A., and Hoe, C. M.: A long term study of renal disease in the dog. Vet. Rec., 80:640–646, 1967.
Schalm, O. W.: Veterinary Hematology. 2nd edition. Philadelphia, Pa., Lea and Febiger, 1965.
Schalm, O. W.: Clinical significance of plasma protein concentration. J.A.V.M.A., 157:1672–1675, 1970.
Schecter, R. D.: The significance of bacteria in feline cystitis and urolithiasis. J.A.V.M.A., 156:1567–1573, 1970.
Schenk, E. A., Schwartz, R. H., and Lewis, R. A.: Tamm-Horsfall mucoprotein. I. Localization in the kidney. Lab. Invest., 25:92–95, 1971.
Silk, M., Sigman, E., and Silk, M.: Serum enzymes after acute experimental renal infarction. Invest. Urol., 9:154–155, 1971.
Terry, R., Hawkins, D. R., Church, E. H., and Whipple, G. H.: Proteinuria related to hyperproteinemia in dogs following plasma given parenterally: A renal threshold for plasma proteins. J. Exper. Med., 87:561–573, 1948.
Textbook of Veterinary Clinical Pathology. Edited by W. Medway, J. E. Prier, and J. S. Wilkinson. Baltimore, Md., The Williams and Wilkins Co., 1969.
Thysell, H.: A Comparison between Albustix, Hema-Combistix, Labstix, the Sulphosalicylic-Acid Test, Heller's Nitric-Acid Test, and a biuret method. Acta Med. Scand., 185:401–407, 1969.
Vaughn, E. D., and Wyker, A. W.: Effect of osmolality on the evaluation of microscopic hematuria. J. Urol., 105:709–711, 1971.
Walker, D. M.: Free amino acids in the blood and urine of the bitch. Vet. Rec., 70:923–924, 1958.
Wallach, S., and Carter, A. C.: Metabolic and renal effects of acute hypercalcemia in dogs. Amer. J. Physiol., 200:359–366, 1961.
Worden, A. N., Waterhouse, C. E., and Sellwood, E. H. B.: Studies on the composition of normal cat urine. J. Sm. Anim Pract., 1:11–23, 1960.
Yano, H., Sonoda, T., Ohkawa, T., Takeuchi, M., Miyagawa, M., Kinoshita, K., Kusunoki, T.: An electron microscopic study on the kidney in experimentally induced hyperparathyroidism. Urol. Int., 20: 319–335, 1965.
Zabor, L.: Preservation of urine sediments on slides. Amer. J. Med. Technol., 36:544–545, 1970.

Chapter 7
TESTS OF RENAL FUNCTION

I. Perspective of renal function tests

A. *Laboratory tests are helpful, but not infallible, and their value is directly proportional to the clinician's ability to interpret them.*

In addition to biological variation, the results of laboratory tests are influenced by methods and techniques of analysis. While some tests have minimal variation due to these factors, the variation associated with others is great. Like any other factor being evaluated in patients with renal disease, the results of renal function tests must be evaluated in combination with available clinical, radiographic, biopsy, and other laboratory findings if they are to be meaningful. Because an incorrect diagnosis may be established, erroneous conclusions established on the basis of misinterpretation of laboratory findings are often of worse consequence than inability to establish a diagnosis due to lack of laboratory data.

B. *The purpose of renal function tests is to help determine the location and extent of renal functional impairment, and thereby provide additional information with which to establish a meaningful diagnosis and prognosis.*

1. As is the situation with the history and physical examination, however, functional abnormalities indicated by renal function tests lack specificity because they are similar in a wide variety of renal diseases. Functional abnormalities encountered in patients with progressive renal failure are similar regardless of the nature of the underlying disease (see Chapter 12, Pathophysiology of Renal Failure).
2. Single determinations of most renal function tests indicate the functional competence of the kidneys at the time the tests are performed. They do not indicate:
   a. The specific cause of the disease.
   b. The acuteness or chronicity of the underlying renal lesions.
   c. The degree of reversibility or irreversibility of the lesions.
   d. The likelihood of regaining renal function adequate to permit patient recovery.
3. To perform a test of renal function once is analogous to obtaining body temperature once. In either situation, the clinician cannot determine whether the abnormality is remaining static, increasing, or decreasing in severity.
4. Because single determinations of renal function tests are of limited diagnostic and prognostic value, renal function should be re-evaluated at appropriate intervals in order to establish the trend of abnormal renal function. Detection of remission or exacerbation of abnormal renal function

by serially performed function tests often provides a reliable index with which to establish a prognosis or determine efficacy of treatment.

C. *Precise measurements of renal function require quantitative estimates of glomerular filtration rate, renal plasma flow, and maximal tubular excretory capacity.*

Because of limits imposed by time and economics, clinicians are forced to use qualitative and semiquantitative measurements of renal function. Unfortunately the latter tests are relatively crude, are often influenced by nonrenal variables, and only provide rough approximations of the functional capabilities of the kidneys. For this reason, and because of functional reserve capacity and adaptive processes characteristic of kidneys, the results of renal function tests may be normal in the presence of extensive renal histopathologic changes. Once abnormalities in renal function are severe enough to allow detection by conventional laboratory methods, there is a rough correlation between the degree of functional impairment detected by renal function tests and the severity, but not the type (i.e., specific cause), of the underlying renal disease. Generally, the results of renal function tests are related to the amount of renal parenchyma that is nonfunctional at the time the test is performed.

II. Renal function tests

A. *Urine specific gravity*
   1. The ability of patients to excrete urine with a specific gravity above or below the specific gravity of glomerular filtrate is dependent on an intact system for secretion of antidiuretic hormone (ADH) and a sufficient quantity of functional nephrons.
   2. The ability to concentrate urine (S.G. = 1.025 or greater) indicates functional competence of the distal tubules and collecting ducts, since it is in these areas that water absorption or excretion is controlled by ADH.
   3. Once the specific gravity becomes fixed at that of glomerular filtrate (1.008 to 1.012), however, it is more an indicator of nephron function than tubular function since, in addition to generalized tubular disease, fixation of specific gravity may occur as a result of factors not specifically related to intrinsic tubular damage. These factors include:
      a. Obligatory solute diuresis affecting viable nephrons.
      b. Destruction of the renal countercurrent mechanism.
      c. Rapid flow of an abnormally large volume of filtrate through viable nephrons.
   4. Diminution in the capacity to concentrate or dilute urine is a consistent finding in acute or chronic renal disease in which a sufficient quantity of functional parenchyma has been damaged. Because the kidneys have tremendous reserve capacity, impairment of the kidneys' ability to concentrate or dilute urine is usually not detectable until at least two thirds of the total functional parenchyma has been incapacitated.
   5. Detection of a specific gravity similar to that of glomerular filtrate in a randomly obtained sample of urine is not reliable evidence of generalized renal disease. Since the ability of normal kidneys to alter specific gravity overlaps the specific gravity of glomerular filtrate, such an assumption can only be made if the specific gravity of urine remains at this "fixed" level after a suitable period of water deprivation, or if the patient is clinically

dehydrated or uremic at the time the isosthenuric sample of urine is collected.
   a. If the kidneys are unable to conserve water in the presence of endogenous ADH, the obvious conclusion is that the nephrons are unable to concentrate urine.
   b. In patients with primary uremia, inability to concentrate or dilute urine is related, at least in part, to obligatory osmotic diuresis and loss of the countercurrent interstitial osmotic gradient.
   c. See Urinalysis, in Chapter 6, for additional details.
6. Detection of a specific gravity greater than approximately 1.025 in association with uremia is often a favorable prognostic sign, since it indicates that a sufficient quantity of nephrons are present to concentrate urine, and that the uremia may be prerenal in origin. An elevated urine specific gravity associated with prerenal uremia reflects a compensatory response by the body to combat low renal perfusion pressure and blood volume by secreting ADH to conserve water filtered through glomeruli.
7. Detection of urine specific gravity below that of glomerular filtrate (1.001 to 1.006) is reliable evidence of functional nephrons since metabolic work is required to remove solute from glomerular filtrate.
8. Because evaluation of urine specific gravity only reflects the functional competence of the kidneys at the time the urine is formed and collected, urine specific gravity should be re-evaluated at appropriate intervals when being used as an aid to establishment of a diagnosis and prognosis.
9. Once the ability of the kidneys to concentrate or dilute urine has been permanently destroyed, repeated evaluation of specific gravity will not be of aid in evaluation of progressive deterioration of renal function. Therefore serial evaluation of urine specific gravity is of greatest aid in detecting functional changes earlier during the course of progressive generalized renal diseases. Following fixation of specific gravity at 1.008 to 1.012, further deterioration is best monitored by evaluation of tubular excretion (PSP test), glomerular filtration rate (endogenous creatinine clearance), or the concentrations of blood urea nitrogen and serum creatinine.
10. Serial evaluation of urine specific gravity may also be of value in monitoring functional recovery associated with reversible renal diseases.

B. *Osmolality*
1. Osmotic pressure is one of the colligative properties of solutions.
   a. It is dependent on the number of particles of solute per unit volume of solvent.
   b. It is independent of the chemical nature, size, molecular weight, and electrical charge of solutes.
   c. Most osmotic activity in body fluids is due to electrolytes, because they are the predominant form of solute present in the body.
      (1) Sodium, chloride, and bicarbonate account for approximately 90 per cent of the osmotic activity of extracellular fluid.
      (2) Nonelectrolytes such as urea, proteins, and glucose account for the remainder of the osmotic activity.
2. In clinical medicine, the osmotic concentration of solutions is not measured in terms of osmotic pressure, but rather in terms of another colligative property, freezing point depression.
   a. Freezing point depression of solutions is measured with an instrument called a freezing point osmometer.

(1) Pure water freezes at 0°C.
(2) As the number of free particles of solute increase in the solvent, the freezing point becomes progressively lower. The lower the freezing point, the higher the osmotic concentration.
b. The unit of osmotic concentration is the osmole.
(1) One osmole of an ideal solute in one Kg. of water will have a freezing point of $-1.86°C$, as compared to pure water.
(2) Since the osmole represents a large mass of solute, the milliosmole has been devised for clinical use.
(a) One milliosmole (mOsm) = 0.001 osmole.
(b) The use of milliosmoles eliminates the necessity to use fractions when evaluating osmolality of biological fluids.
(c) Osmolality is expressed as mOsm. per Kg. of solution.
(3) Following determination of the freezing point of a sample, the osmolality is determined with the aid of conversion tables.
c. Osmolarity is sometimes used instead of osmolality and may be defined as the osmole content per liter of solution. The difference between osmolarity and osmolality readings is usually small.
3. The osmotic concentration of plasma, interstitial fluid, transcellular fluid, and intracellular fluid is approximately 300 mOsm. per Kg. of water. There is no significant difference between serum and plasma osmolality since fibrinogen does not exert a significant osmotic effect.
4. Normally, the osmotic concentration of urine is variable, being dependent on the fluid and electrolyte balance of the body, and the nitrogen content of the diet.
a. In dogs and cats, urine osmolality may be as low as approximately 50 mOsm. per Kg. in states of extreme diuresis.
b. In dogs, urine osmolality may be as high as 2000 to 2400 mOsm. per Kg. in states of physiologic oliguria.
c. In normally hydrated dogs and cats, urine osmolality is usually 500 to 1200 mOsm. per Kg.
5. The ratio of urine osmolality (U_{osm}) to plasma osmolality (P_{osm}) is a good index of one renal function.
a. A ratio of U/P_{osm} above one indicates that the kidneys are capable of concentrating urine above that of plasma. Following a 24 hour water deprivation period, the normal canine U/P_{osm} is 3 or higher.
b. A U/P_{osm} ratio of 1 indicates that water and solute are being excreted in a state which is iso-osmotic with plasma.
c. A U/P_{osm} ratio below 1 indicates that the kidneys are capable of absorbing solute in excess of water.
d. See Urine concentration test in this chapter.
6. Osmolality versus specific gravity.
a. Urine S.G. is a measure of the density of urine as compared to pure water, while urine osmolality is a measure of the number of osmotic particles per unit of solvent.
(1) The relationship between specific gravity and total solute is only approximate.
(a) Urine specific gravity may be significantly altered by protein, glucose, and other abnormal solutes since specific gravity is dependent on molecular size and weight of solutes, as well as on the number of molecules of solute.

(b) Equal numbers of molecules of urea, sodium chloride, albumin, globulin, fibrinogen, and glucose all have a different quantitative effect on specific gravity.
  (c) Urine specific gravity may be altered by temperature.
 b. Specific gravity provides only a rough approximation of the solute concentration of urine.
 c. Because of the high degree of individual biologic variability seen when specific gravity or osmolality of serial urine samples obtained from the same patient are compared, the accuracy gained by the use of osmolality tends to be minimized.
 d. Because of the high cost of osmometers, their use in clinical medicine is, in most instances, impractical.
 e. In clinical medicine, determination of urine S.G. with an instrument* which measures the refractive index of urine is very satisfactory.
  (1) The refractive index of urine is dependent on the quantity of dissolved substances it contains.
  (2) Substances such as protein will increase the specific gravity determined with refractometers.
  (3) Refractometers are superior to urinometers.
   (a) Refractometers which are temperature compensated (60 to 100°F.) may be purchased.
   (b) Determination of S.G. with a refractometer can be accomplished with a fraction of a milliliter of urine.
   (c) Refractometers are technically easy to use.
   (d) Reproducibility of results obtained with refractometers is better than that obtained with urinometers.
  (4) While more expensive than urinometers, refractometers can be purchased for a fraction of the cost of freezing point osmometers.

C. *Urine concentration test (water deprivation test)*
 1. Basis for the test
  a. When patients are deprived of fluids for a suitable period of time (approximately 24 hours), endogenous antidiuretic hormone is released from the posterior pituitary gland as a compensatory response to hydropenia.
  b. Antidiuretic hormone enhances fluid reabsorption by the distal tubules and collecting ducts by increasing tubular cell permeability to water. In normal patients, this mechanism permits excretion of urine of high specific gravity, high osmolality, and low volume.
 2. Procedure.
  a. Deprive the patient of water. Food may be given provided it is not high in moisture content. Fasting is not recommended since the excretion of urea influences the ability of the kidneys to concentrate urine. The concentration of urine depends not only on the degree of hydropenia, but also on the prevailing rate of solute excretion.
  b. Accurately weigh the patient. This weight will serve as a baseline with which to determine future water loss from the body. The weight of the food consumed and feces eliminated should be approximated, especially in small patients.

---

*T/C Refractometer, Americal Optical Corporation, Scientific Instrument Division, Buffalo, N.Y. 14215.

c. Approximately 12 hours after starting the period of water deprivation, remove and discard all urine from the bladder. This step will eliminate errors induced by mixture of dilute urine contained in the urinary bladder with urine formed under conditions of water deprivation.
d. Allow a sufficient period for urine to collect in the bladder. Collect a sample of urine and determine its specific gravity.
   (1) If the specific gravity of the urine exceeds 1.025, it may be concluded that the nephrons are capable of concentrating urine. Discontinue the test.
   (2) If the urine specific gravity is below 1.025, continue the test for an additional 12 or more hours.
e. At the end of 24 hours, repeat steps c and d.
   (1) If at the end of 24 hours urine specific gravity is greater than 1.025, discontinue the test.
   (2) If at the end of 24 hours urine specific gravity is not greater than approximately 1.025, evaluate the physical status of the patient, the concentration of BUN or serum creatinine, and the patient's body weight. If the patient has lost more than 5 per cent of its body weight, or if the concentration of BUN or serum creatinine is abnormally elevated, discontinue the test. If not, continue the test for an additional six to 12 hours and repeat the above.
f. The period of time chosen for water deprivation is arbitrary. The test should be continued until it is determined that the patient can or cannot concentrate urine. In the majority of cases this can be accomplished in 24 hours.
3. Intepretation of results.
   a. A patient with normal ability to concentrate urine should excrete urine with a specific gravity of approximately 1.025 or higher.
   b. In one experimental study, the results of water deprivation tests (16 to 23 hours of water deprivation) in healthy beagle dogs were interpreted to indicate that urine specific gravity values of greater than 1.039 implied normal renal concentrating ability.
   c. If the urine has a specific gravity of less than 1.025 after the patient has been deprived of water for an appropriate period of time, any of the following conclusions may apply:
      (1) The kidneys have impaired ability to concentrate urine because of generalized renal disease.
      (2) Production or release of antidiuretic hormone may be impaired as a result of diabetes insipidus. In diabetes insipidus, the specific gravity of urine is typically below that of glomerular filtrate (1.001 to 1.006) because the nephrons retain the ability to reabsorb solute in excess of water.
      (3) The nephrons may have impaired ability to respond to antidiuretic hormone as a result of renal diabetes insipidus. In this disease, the renal tubules are refractory to the pharmacologic action of antidiuretic hormone although other parameters of renal function may be normal.
      (4) A technical error characterized by mixture of dilute and concentrated urine may have occurred.
4. Contraindications for the test.
   a. Patients with uremia, regardless of cause, should not be subjected to

the test. Not only may conclusions about nephron concentrating ability be established on the basis of randomly obtained urine samples combined with physical examination and laboratory data, but also deprivation of water may precipitate a uremic crisis and cause death.
   b. Clinically dehydrated patients should not be subjected to water deprivation since there is already maximal stimulation for the release of antidiuretic hormone.
   c. Patients with polyuria should be weighed several times during the course of water deprivation. The test should be discontinued in any patient that has lost 5 per cent of its body weight due to loss of fluids.

D. *Exogenous antidiuretic hormone concentration test (Pitressin concentration test)*
   1. Basis for the test.
      a. By injecting exogenous antidiuretic hormone into a patient, the permeability of normal distal tubules and collecting ducts to water is increased. Water will be absorbed despite the patient's state of hydration.
      b. Provided a sufficient quantity of ADH is administered, normal kidneys will excrete urine with a concentration above that of glomerular filtrate.
   2. Indications.
      a. Administration of exogenous antidiuretic hormone to aid in evaluation of the kidneys' ability to concentrate urine should be considered for patients that cannot tolerate water deprivation because:
         (1) They are debilitated.
         (2) The findings of the history and physical examination suggest that water deprivation may precipitate a uremic crisis.
      b. Provided the patient can tolerate water deprivation without undue risk, the latter procedure is preferred to exogenous administration of vasopressin since the results are more reliable.
      c. When concentration of urine does not occur following water deprivation, the exogenous antidiuretic hormone test should be utilized to determine if concentration of urine occurs. Failure to concentrate urine following water deprivation, but adequate concentration of urine during the exogenous antidiuretic hormone test is indicative of diabetes insipidus.
   3. Procedure.
      a. A precise dosage schedule and urine collection schedule have not been established for clinical use of a single injection of aqueous or repositol antidiuretic hormone (vasopressin) in dogs and cats. The following recommendations are general guidelines which have been established on the basis of empirical use of the test on clinical patients (dogs).
      b. Aqueous vasopressin test.
         (1) Inject subcutaneously ¼ unit of aqueous vasopressin* per Kg. of body weight up to a maximum of 5 units.
         (2) Withhold food and fluids during the test period.
         (3) Empty the bladder 30 minutes after injecting the vasopressin so that urine formed prior to the action of ADH will not invalidate the results by mixing with urine formed under the influence of ADH.
         (4) Collect urine samples at 30, 60, 90, and 120 minute intervals following administration of ADH. Determine the specific gravity of each sample.

---
*Pitressin, Parke, Davis and Co., Detroit, Michigan 48232.

c. Repositol vasopressin test.
   (1) Inject intramuscularly 3 to 5 units of vasopressin tannate in oil.*
   (2) Withhold food and fluids during the test period.
   (3) Empty the bladder 3 hours after injecting the vasopressin in order to eliminate residual dilute urine.
   (4) Collect urine samples at 3, 6, and 9 hours following administration of ADH. Determine the specific gravity of each sample.
4. Interpretation of results.
   a. A patient with normal ability to concentrate urine should excrete urine with a specific gravity higher than that of glomerular filtrate. Although precise response values for normal dogs have not been established, it is suggested that a value of 1.020 to 1.025 or higher represents a normal response.
   b. Experimental studies in normal dogs have revealed that urine osmolalities achieved following parenteral administration of pitressin were less than those achieved following water deprivation. Although the reason for this discrepancy has not been established, it has been hypothesized that it may be related to one or both of the following:
      (1) Dilute urine present in the excretory pathway may have mixed with concentrated urine formed after administration of ADH. The error caused by dilution would be of greatest significance at low rates of urine flow.
      (2) Substances with antidiuretic activity other than ADH may be present in hydropenic patients.
   c. If the urine has a specific gravity of less than 1.020 following completion of the test, any of the following conclusions may apply:
      (1) The kidneys may have impaired ability to concentrate urine because of generalized renal disease.
      (2) The nephrons may have impaired ability to respond to antidiuretic hormone as a result of renal diabetes insipidus.
      (3) A technical error characterized by a mixture of dilute and concentrated urine may have occurred.
5. Contraindications for the test.
   a. Vasopressin should be used with caution in any patient in which expansion of fluid volume may be hazardous. This precaution is only significant when continued oral intake of fluid is allowed during the interval of action of the vasopressin. Generally, aqueous vasopressin will have an effect for a few hours, and repositol vasopressin may have an effect for 48 to 72 hours.
   b. Patients with uremia, regardless of cause, should not be subjected to the test.
   c. Vasopressin causes contraction of smooth muscle and therefore should be used with caution in pregnant animals.

E. *Urine dilution test*
1. Basis for the test:
   a. The ability of the kidneys to perform metabolic work can be evaluated by the degree to which they can dilute glomerular filtrate.
   b. When a patient is challenged with a relatively large oral dose of water,

---
*Pitressin tannate in oil, Parke, Davis and Co., Detroit, Michigan 48232.

the kidneys are forced to absorb solute against a relatively large concentration gradient. Metabolic work is required to dilute as well as to concentrate glomerular filtrate.
2. Indications.
   a. The water dilution test is discussed to emphasize the fact that urine of low specific gravity does not always indicate the presence of renal disease.
   b. This test is not recommended as a routine test for evaluation of renal function.
      (1) The urine concentration test provides a similar measurement of the ability of the kidneys to perform metabolic work.
      (2) Persistent impairment of urine dilution occurs somewhat later in the course of generalized renal disease than does loss of the ability to concentrate urine.
      (3) Because a large volume of water is given orally, vomiting may be induced.
      (4) The test may aggravate cardiovascular dysfunction in patients with generalized circulatory disease.
      (5) Patients with impaired renal function may develop hydroplasmia because they are unable to excrete the water load.
3. Procedure.
   a. Evaluation of this procedure in normal or diseased dogs and cats has not been reported.
   b. The procedure recommended for human patients is as follows:
      (1) Withhold food for approximately 12 hours.
      (2) Empty the urinary bladder.
      (3) Administer 20 ml. of water per Kg. of body weight per os over a one-half hour period.
      (4) Collect urine samples at hourly intervals for the next four hours and determine specific gravity.
4. Interpretation of results (man).
   a. With normal renal function, most of the fluid should be eliminated within the four-hour test period.
   b. The specific gravity of one of the specimens will usually be below 1.003 if renal function is normal.
   c. In patients with impaired renal function, smaller amounts of urine will be eliminated and the specific gravity will be higher than 1.003. In some patients, values as high as 1.010 may occur.

F. *Phenolsulphonphthalein (PSP) excretion test*
   1. Basis for the test.
      a. Following parenteral injection into the body, PSP dye is predominantly bound to plasma proteins at a ratio dependent on the concentration of PSP in plasma. With the usual clinical test dose of PSP (6 mg.), a low plasma concentration is obtained, and only about 15 to 20 per cent of the dye is in free form which can be filtered by glomeruli.
      b. PSP dye is primarily excreted into urine by the proximal tubules. A small amount (5 per cent) is excreted by glomerular filtration.
      c. A small amount of dye is excreted by the biliary tract, but the dye is rapidly reabsorbed from the intestinal lumen.

d. Because it is predominantly excreted by proximal tubules, urinary excretion of PSP dye has been advocated by some as a test of proximal tubular function.
e. The dose of dye (6 mg.) commonly used in clinical trials results in a total plasma concentration of PSP far below the tubular capacity to excrete the dye.
   (1) The maximum tubular capacity (T_m) for excretion of PSP is about 50 times greater than that required for excretion of the 6 mg. dose.
   (2) If renal plasma flow per unit of time were to remain constant, there would have to be extensive destruction of tubules to result in diminished excretion of dye following administration of the 6 mg. test dose.
   (3) The limiting factor in renal excretion of PSP is the rate of delivery of the dye to the tubules rather than tubular integrity. For this reason, the 6 mg. PSP excretion test most accurately reflects renal plasma flow rather than tubular excretion, although both are involved.
f. Determination of urinary excretion of larger doses (100 mg. per sq. meter of body surface area) of PSP dye may provide a better index of tubular function, although plasma T_m levels are probably still not achieved by this dose.
g. Following intravenous injection of 6 mg. of PSP dye, it begins to appear in urine in approximately three minutes in the dog. Seventy-five per cent of the dose will be excreted in urine one hour following administration.
   (1) Excretion of PSP dye by the kidney provides the most significant results soon after its injection.
   (2) Even damaged kidneys may eventually remove the majority of dye from plasma if given enough time to do so.
   (3) For these reasons, a relatively short test period (20 minutes) in which only a fraction of the total dose of dye is removed is recommended.

2. Indications.
   a. Although precise figures have not been determined, it is thought that excretion of PSP dye will reflect abnormal renal function earlier in the course of generalized progressive renal diseases than will evaluation of BUN concentration or serum creatinine concentration.
   b. Evaluation of the progression of generalized renal diseases in which "fixation" of urine specific gravity has already occurred may be monitored by excretion of PSP dye. A state may be reached, however, when evaluation of PSP excretion will not reflect further deterioration of renal function.

3. Dosage.
   a. In an experimental study of excretion of PSP dye in normal dogs, use of a standard dosage (6 mg.) regardless of body size was compared with dosage calculated on the basis of square meters of body surface area (100 mg. per square meter of body surface area).
   b. In both procedures, the PSP was administered intravenously and a 20 minute test period was used.
   c. There was no significant correlation between body weight and the percentage of the 6.0 mg. dose excreted in urine in 20 minutes.

d. It was concluded that administration of a dose of PSP calculated on the basis of body surface area resulted in nearly the same percentage of urinary excretion of dye as when a standard 6.0 mg. dose was used, although the standard deviation with dosage calculated on the basis of body surface area was smaller.
4. Procedure.
   a. Empty the bladder by catheterization or by allowing the patient to micturate.
      (1) Since test results are calculated on the basis of the total quantity of dye excreted in urine, and not on urine volume, it is not necessary to have the bladder completely empty.
      (2) The bladder must not be allowed to contain a large volume of residual urine since the latter will interfere with attempts to remove all of the dye excreted during a 20 minute test period.
   b. Inject 6 mg. of PSP dye* intravenously and note the exact time of injection.
      (1) Only the intravenous route of injection should be used.
      (2) The subcutaneous route of injection should be avoided since it complicates interpretation of results by adding the variable of absorption of dye from the subcutaneous tissue.
   c. If the patient has not yet been catheterized, insert a catheter into the bladder approximately 10 minutes following injection of the dye. In order to remove all urine from the bladder, the tip of the catheter should be positioned so that it is just beyond the junction of the neck of the bladder with the urethra (see Chapter 5, Collection of Urine).
   d. Gently aspirate the contents of the bladder with a syringe; collect all the urine in a flask.
      (1) In order to minimize collection error, rinse the bladder with 10 to 15 ml. of sterilized physiologic saline three or more times. Aspirate the saline rinse each time and add it to the urine in the collection flask.
      (2) The injection and recovery of 10 to 15 ml. of air following the final saline rinse often improves dye collection. The latter may be repeated several times.
      (3) These maneuvers will facilitate removal of residual PSP dye from the bladder.
   e. Complete the procedure exactly 20 minutes following the time of injection of the dye.
5. Methodology to determine quantity of dye excreted.
   a. Dilute all urine and dye collected from the bladder to 400 ml. in a 1 liter graduated cylinder or other suitable liter container.
   b. Add 10 ml. of 10% sodium hydroxide and mix. PSP dye has an intense pink color in an alkaline solution.
      (1) If the color is deep pink, add a sufficient quantity of water to bring the total volume to 1 liter.
      (2) If the color is light pink, add a sufficient quantity of water to bring the total volume to 500 ml. Divide the final results by two.
      (3) If the solution is turbid, filter it through quantitative filter paper before proceeding.

---
*Phenolsulfonphthalein Injection U.S.P., Scientific Products, Evanston, Illinois 60201.

c. To determine the quantity of dye excreted in urine perform either of the following:
  (1) Transfer an aliquot of the urine-dye mixture to a cuvette and determine optical density in a spectrophotometer set at a wavelength of 550 millimicrons.
  (2) Visually compare the color of the unknown to the color standards in a PSP comparator block.*
d. Interferences.
  (1) Sulfobromophthalein dye used in liver function studies may appear in urine and cause interference in readings of PSP. For this reason it is best not to perform both of these tests on the same day.
  (2) Hemoglobin and bilirubin have also been reported to cause interference in evaluation of PSP.

6. Interpretation of results.
  a. In an experimental study of urinary excretion of PSP dye in normal dogs during a 20 minute test period, it was observed that:
    (1) An average of 43.8 ± 11.1 per cent of the dye (range = 26 to 64%) was excreted following administration of a 6 mg. dose.
    (2) An average of 42.1 ± 7.7 per cent of the dye (range = 31 to 60%) was excreted following administration of 100 mg. of the dye per square meter of body surface.
  b. With the 6.0 mg. dose, 67 per cent of normal dogs can be expected to excrete 33 to 55 per cent of the dye in 20 minutes; 95 per cent of normal dogs can be expected to excrete 21 to 66 per cent of the dye in 20 minutes.
  c. With the 100 mg. per square meter dose, 67 per cent of normal dogs can be expected to excrete 34 to 52 per cent of the dye in 20 minutes; 95 per cent of normal dogs can be expected to excrete 28 to 56 per cent of the dye in 20 minutes.
  d. Abnormal decrease in urinary excretion of PSP dye may occur as a result of:
    (1) Poor renal perfusion due to any cause, including:
      (a) Generalized renal disease.
      (b) Dehydration.
      (c) Congestive heart failure.
      (d) Hypoadrenalcorticism.
    (2) Generalized destruction of proximal tubules due to any cause.
    (3) Both of the above.
    (4) A technical error in collection of dye from the bladder.

G. *Blood urea nitrogen (BUN)*
  1. Basis of the test.
    a. Urea is a nonprotein nitrogen substance that is formed during protein catabolism.
    b. The main site of urea formation is the liver. Following hepatectomy, there is a progressive decline in the concentration of urea in blood and urine.
    c. Urea is a small molecule (MW = 60) that is distributed throughout total body water and is equal in concentration in the intracellular and extra-

---

*PSP comparator block, Lamotte Chemical Products Company, Chestertown, Maryland 21620.

cellular fluid. Thus its concentration is the same in whole blood, plasma, and serum.
  d. Urea is not utilized or excreted to any significant degree by organs other than the kidneys.
     (1) In disease and health, the rate of excretion of urea is related to the rate of its production in the body.
     (2) Urea is excreted by glomerular filtration, although approximately 25 to 40 per cent of the amount filtered is reabsorbed during its passage through tubules. High rates of urine flow diminish tubular reabsorption of urea, while low rates of urine flow enhance tubular reabsorption of urea.
     (3) The relationship between BUN and glomerular filtration rate (GFR) is such that, provided urea production is relatively constant, their product remains constant (GFR × BUN = constant). Thus measurement of the concentration of BUN provides a crude index of GFR.
2. Factors influencing BUN concentration. The concentration of BUN may be affected by:
  a. The rate of its production.
     (1) Exogenous sources such as high protein diets cause a mild elevation of the concentration of BUN.
        (a) The effect of diet on the concentration of BUN must be kept in perspective.
           [1] Evaluation of normal dogs revealed that the concentration of BUN may increase to 40 mg. per 100 ml. following ingestion of normal diets.
           [2] In cases where the significance of a mildly elevated BUN concentration (35 to 45 mg. per 100 ml.) cannot be determined because of the variable of diet, withhold food from the patient for 12 to 18 hours and re-evaluate BUN concentration.
     (2) Endogenous sources such as rapid catabolism of body tissue (trauma, fever, infection) or gastrointestinal hemorrhage cause a significant elevation in the concentration of BUN.
     (3) Drugs that increase protein catabolism (corticosteroids, thyroid preparations) or decrease protein anabolism (tetracyclines) may cause an increase in the concentration of BUN.
  b. Body fluid balance.
     (1) As a result of a decrease in the percentage of water in plasma, dehydration will be associated with a minor increase in the concentration of BUN.
     (2) Dehydration may cause prerenal uremia as a result of decreased renal perfusion and glomerular filtration (see below).
  c. The rate of its excretion.
     (1) Any abnormality (prerenal, primary renal, or postrenal) which decreases GFR will cause an increase in the concentration of BUN (see Chapter 12, Pathophysiology of Renal Failure).
     (2) Although the concentration of BUN rises during progressive reduction in GFR, the increase is gradual at first and is hidden within the so-called normal concentration of BUN (10 to 30 mg. per 100 ml.). Abnormal elevations in the concentration of BUN which occur as a result of impairment of renal function are not detectable until

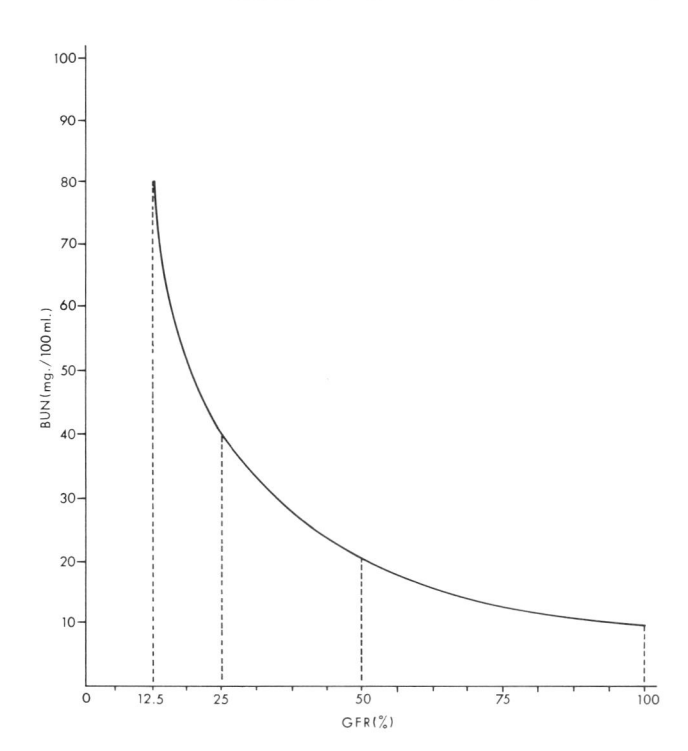

Figure 7-1. Relationship of BUN to GFR.

approximately 70 to 75 per cent or more of the nephrons of both kidneys become nonfunctional. Although an oversimplification, it is easy to understand this phenomenon by considering that each time GFR is reduced by one half, the concentration of BUN doubles (Fig. 7-1).

(3) Early stages of progressive renal diseases are usually accompanied by only minor changes in the concentration of BUN even though there has been destruction of a relatively large quantity of renal parenchyma. As the disease progresses, however, eventually a stage is reached where destruction of a relatively small number of nephrons is accompanied by a large change in concentration of BUN.

3. Methodology.
   a. Many techniques are available for determining the concentration of BUN.
   b. Plasma urea nitrogen (PUN), serum urea nitrogen (SUN), or blood urea nitrogen may be used because urea is freely diffusable in RBC.
   c. Values for BUN vary slightly with different methods of determination. Concentrations between 10 and 30 mg. per 100 ml. are usually considered to be normal.
   d. Avoid use of ammonium-containing anticoagulants in samples to be used for BUN determination.
   e. Consult standard textbooks of veterinary clinical pathology for specific details about methodology.
4. Interpretation of results.
   a. When the concentration of BUN exceeds 35 to 45 mg. per 100 ml., GFR is diminished.

b. Abnormal BUN concentration known to be caused by abnormal renal excretion may be caused by prerenal, primary renal, or postrenal uremia. Every effort should be made to determine the underlying cause of uremia in order to establish a meaningful prognosis and to select appropriate treatment.
c. There is only a rough correlation between the degree of elevation of BUN and the severity of renal functional impairment.
 (1) This may be related, at least in part, to the duration of the renal disease. Progressive renal diseases that destroy renal parenchyma at a relatively slow rate allow remaining viable nephrons to undergo structural and functional compensation. Thus more renal parenchyma may be destroyed in chronic renal diseases before functional abnormalities become detectable than in acute renal diseases.
 (2) Time must elapse for a sufficient quantity of urea to accumulate to be considered abnormal. Acute renal shutdown will not be associated with an abnormal increase in the concentration of BUN during very early stages of the disease.
d. Single determinations of BUN concentration, regardless of value obtained, do not provide a reliable index of the reversibility or irreversibility of the underlying damage.
 (1) Serial determinations of BUN provide a more reliable index of prognosis.
 (2) Progressive increase in the concentration of BUN despite appropriate therapy is justification for a guarded to poor prognosis.
5. Clinical use of BUN.
 a. Advantages. While many factors tend to limit the usefulness of BUN as an index of renal function, the test is of great clinical value provided it is properly interpreted.
  (1) It allows the presence of renal failure to be established.
  (2) If performed serially, it provides a good index of response to therapy of uremia.
  (3) If performed serially and interpreted in association with other clinical, laboratory, and biopsy findings, it provides information which is useful in establishing a prognosis.
  (4) Determination of BUN concentration is technically easy and economical.
 b. Disadvantages.
  (1) The test lacks specificity because:
   (a) Several nonrenal factors may alter the concentration of BUN while renal function remains unchanged.
   (b) Abnormal BUN concentrations may occur in prerenal, primary renal, and postrenal uremia.
  (2) The concentration of BUN may be within the normal range despite a reduction in GFR by more than 60 to 65 per cent. It is not a good test of renal function in early stages of renal disease.

H. Creatinine

1. Basis of the test.
 a. Creatinine is a nonprotein nitrogen substance that is formed during metabolism of muscle creatine and phosphocreatine. Creatinine is not reutilized by the body and therefore is excreted in urine.
 b. The quantity of creatinine produced and excreted depends on skeletal

TESTS OF RENAL FUNCTION

muscle mass and renal excretion. In normal individuals, creatinine concentration tends to remain constant from day to day.
  c. Creatinine is excreted by glomerular filtration. In dogs, significant quantities of creatinine are neither excreted nor reabsorbed by the tubules. Provided production is constant, the measurement of creatinine concentration provides a crude index of glomerular filtration rate (GFR × creatinine = constant).
2. Factors influencing creatinine concentration. The concentration of creatinine may be affected by:
  a. The rate of its production.
    (1) Daily production of creatinine from muscle metabolism is relatively constant.
    (2) Although creatinine excretion is proportional to lean muscle mass, its production is not readily influenced by catabolic factors that affect urea formation (e.g., fever, infection, corticosteroids, and others).
    (3) Creatinine concentration is not significantly influenced by diet.
  b. Body fluid balance.
    (1) As a result of a decrease in the percentage of water in plasma, dehydration will cause a minor increase in the concentration of creatinine.
    (2) Dehydration may cause prerenal uremia as a result of decreased renal perfusion and glomerular filtration (see below).
  c. The rate of its excretion.
    (1) Any abnormality (prerenal, primary renal, or postrenal) which decreases GFR will cause an increase in the serum concentration of creatinine.
    (2) Abnormal elevations in the concentration of creatinine which occur as a result of impairment of renal function are not detectable until approximately 70 to 75 per cent or more of the nephrons of both kidneys become nonfunctional.
    (3) See discussion of rate of BUN excretion in Blood urea nitrogen in this chapter.
3. Methodology.
  a. Creatinine concentrations between 1 and 2 mg. per 100 ml. are usually considered to be normal.
  b. Several techniques have been advocated for determining the concentration of creatinine.
    (1) The alkaline picrate method (Jaffe) of creatinine determination measures non-creatinine chromogens present in plasma as well as creatinine. Thus this method gives erroneously high creatinine values.
    (2) The use of Lloyd's reagent (Fuller's earth) has been reported to allow measurement of "true" creatinine by removing noncreatinine chromogens.
  c. Consult standard textbooks of veterinary clinical pathology and specific references for details about methodology.
4. Interpretation of results.
  a. When the concentration of creatinine exceeds 2.0 mg. per 100 ml., GFR is reduced.
  b. Elevation in creatinine concentration may be caused by prerenal, pri-

mary renal, or postrenal uremia. Every effort should be made to determine the underlying cause of uremia in order to establish a meaningful prognosis and to select appropriate treatment.
- c. There is only a rough correlation between the degree of elevation of creatinine and the severity of renal functional impairment (see II,G,4, discussion of interpretation of results, under Blood urea nitrogen).
- d. Single determinations of creatinine concentration, regardless of value obtained, do not provide a reliable index of the reversibility or irreversibility of the underlying damage.
    - (1) Serial determinations of creatinine provide a more reliable index of prognosis.
    - (2) Progressive increase in the serum concentration of creatinine despite appropriate therapy is justification for a guarded to poor prognosis.
- e. Because it is affected by fewer nonrenal variables and because it tends to become elevated later in the course of many generalized renal diseases, creatinine has the reputation for being a more specific index of the severity of renal damage and a more reliable index of prognosis than BUN. Unfortunately the latter generality has been overemphasized. The assumption that recovery cannot occur if creatinine levels exceed 5 mg. per 100 ml. is erroneous. Although a marked elevation in serum creatinine concentration does indicate severe functional or organic impairment of nephron function, it is not of significantly greater value than BUN concentration in indicating the degree of reversibility or irreversibility of the underlying disease process, since it does not permit establishment of a specific diagnosis.

5. Clinical use of creatinine.
    - a. Advantages.
        - (1) Creatinine has all the advantages listed for BUN, except that the technical aspects of creatinine determination are not as simple as those available for BUN determination.
        - (2) Creatinine is affected by fewer nonrenal variables than BUN.
    - b. Disadvantages.
        - (1) Some techniques for determination of creatinine concentration provide falsely high values since they also measure noncreatinine chromogens.
        - (2) Like BUN, its value is limited in early renal failure when marked reduction of GFR may be associated with little change in creatinine concentration.

I. Nonprotein nitrogen (NPN)
1. Nonprotein nitrogen substances include all nitrogenous constituents of blood except protein (i.e., urea, uric acid, creatine, creatinine, amino acids, polypeptides).
2. Determination of NPN is not commonly used as a clinical test of renal function since a technically easy method of determination is not available.
3. Determination of NPN concentration provides essentially the same information as BUN or creatinine determinations, but provides no advantages over either. There is no logical reason to use this test if either BUN or creatinine determinations are available.

J. *Excretory urography*
 1. Excretory urograms provide crude qualitative, not quantitative, evaluation of the renal function of each kidney.
 2. Excretory urograms should not be used as a substitute for renal function tests.
    a. The following variables affect the degree of visualization provided by contrast material.
       (1) Type, dosage, and route of administration of the contrast material.
       (2) Injection time.
       (3) Radiographic technique.
       (4) Degree of patient hydration.
       (5) Factors influencing renal blood flow.
       (6) Functional capacity of the kidneys.
    b. The excretion of contrast material gives no indication of the number of nephrons taking part in the process, and thus gives no reliable information as to the quantity of functioning nephrons present.
    c. Good contrast density of the urinary tract is not always associated with normal renal function, and poor contrast density is not always associated with reduced renal function.

K. *Renal clearance and glomerular filtration rate*
 1. The following is a discussion of the concepts related to quantitative evaluation of various aspects of renal function. With the exception of determination of glomerular filtration rate by endogenous creatinine clearance, no attempt has been made to provide specific details about methods by which quantitative renal function tests are performed. Textbooks of veterinary clinical pathology and specific references should be consulted for information related to performing quantitative renal function tests.
 2. Clearance concept.
    a. Renal clearance is a term used as a quantitative description of the rate at which the kidney excretes various substances in relation to their concentration in plasma.
       (1) Clearance denotes the amount of plasma that is completely cleared of a substance in a unit of time.
       (2) The volume is only theoretical or "virtual" if the substance is not completely removed from plasma in a single circulation through the kidney.
    b. If U_c is the concentration (mg.) of a substance in each milliliter of urine (U), and V is the rate of urine formation in ml. per minute, $U_c V$ equals the rate of excretion of the substance in mg. per minute.
       (1) The amount of the substance excreted equals the amount filtered by glomeruli plus the net amount transferred by the tubules.
       (2) The amount of a substance in the urine per unit of time must have been provided by clearing exactly the number of milliliters of plasma which contained this amount of substance.
       (3) Plasma clearance is equal to the concentration of the substance in urine (U_c) times urine flow per unit of time (V) divided by the plasma concentration (P_c) of the substance. Clearance $= \dfrac{U_c V}{P_c}$.
          (a) Clearance is equal to glomerular filtration rate (GFR) provided

there is no net tubular secretion or reabsorption of the substance.
- (b) Clearance exceeds GFR if there is net tubular excretion.
- (c) Clearance is less than GFR if there is net tubular reabsorption.
3. Glomerular filtration rate can be determined by measuring the excretion and plasma concentration of a substance which is freely filtered through glomeruli and neither secreted nor reabsorbed by tubules.
   a. The quantity of such a substance in the urine per unit of time is provided by filtering exactly that volume of plasma which contains an identical amount of substance.
      (1) Glomerular filtration rate (GFR) is equal to the concentration (c) of the substance in urine (U) times the urine volume (V) per unit of time, divided by the arterial plasma concentration of the substance (P_c).

$$GFR = \frac{U_c V}{P_c}$$

   (2) If the body does not metabolize or store a significant quantity of the substance, the concentration of the substance in peripheral venous plasma may be substituted for the concentration of the substance in peripheral arterial plasma.
   b. Substances used to determine GFR include:
      (1) Inulin.
         (a) Inulin is a polymer of fructose that is found in dahlia tubers.
         (b) The molecular weight of inulin is 5200.
         (c) Inulin clearance is used as the reference method for GFR because:
            [1] It is freely filtered by glomeruli.
            [2] It is not reabsorbed or secreted by renal tubules.
            [3] It is not metabolized in the body.
            [4] It is not stored in kidneys.
            [5] It is not toxic.
            [6] It is not protein bound.
            [7] It has no effect on glomerular filtration rate.
            [8] It can be measured in plasma and urine.
         (d) Because determination of GFR with inulin is very time consuming, the technique is rarely used in clinical practice.
      (2) Creatinine.
         (a) In dogs, creatinine clearance is frequently used to determine GFR.
            [1] Creatinine is freely filtered by glomeruli, and significant quantities of creatinine are neither reabsorbed nor secreted by the tubules.
            [2] Exogenous creatinine clearance.
               [a] A loading dose of creatinine is administered intravenously to increase plasma concentration of creatinine.
               [b] Exogenous creatinine is infused at a constant rate to maintain the plasma concentration constant.
               [c] After exogenous creatinine has equilibrated with body fluids, an accurately timed urine specimen is collected.
               [d] A venous plasma sample is collected approximately halfway through the timed urine collection.

[e] GFR is calculated by utilizing the preceding formula.
[3] Endogenous creatinine clearance.
  [a] This procedure is based on the principles used for exogenous creatinine clearance except that exogenous creatinine is not administered. The endogenous plasma concentration of creatinine is substituted for exogenous creatinine since the plasma concentration of creatinine remains relatively stable during the test period.
  [b] Procedure.
    [1'] Catheterize the bladder and remove residual urine. In order to permit aspiration of all urine from the urinary bladder, the tip of the catheter should be positioned so that it is just beyond the junction of the neck of the bladder with the urethra (see Chapter 5, Collection of Urine).
    [2'] Rinse the bladder several times with sterilized physiologic saline. With the aid of an air flush, remove all the residual solution. Discard the rinse solution.
    [3'] Begin timing urine formation immediately following the rinsing procedure.
    [4'] Collect a serum sample approximately halfway through the test period and save it for creatinine determination.
    [5'] Gently aspirate the contents of the bladder with a syringe; collect all the urine in a flask. Rinse the bladder several times with sterilized physiologic saline solution. Aspirate the saline rinse each time and add it to the urine collection flask. During the last minute of collection, rinse the bladder once or twice with saline, and once or twice with air in order to insure complete collection of fluid.
    [6'] Complete the collection 15 or 20 minutes following the rinsing procedure. The time allotted for the procedure is not critical, but it must be accurately determined.
    [7'] The creatinine concentration of urine should be determined by the alkaline picrate method.
    [8'] Plasma creatinine should be determined by the alkaline picrate method after adsorption of creatinine on Lloyd's reagent.
    [9'] Calculate GFR by utilizing the preceding formula.
    [10'] The most reliable data are obtained by repeating the procedure two or more times and using the average of the results.
c. Indications.
  (1) If properly performed, determination of GFR will permit a more precise evaluation of renal function than can be obtained by evaluating urine specific gravity, urine osmolality, BUN or creatinine concentration, or urinary excretion of PSP dye.
  (2) Abnormalities of renal function may be detected earlier during

the course of generalized renal disease by evaluation of glomerular filtration rate than by evaluation of urinalysis or the concentration of BUN or creatinine.
  d. Interpretation of results.
    (1) When glomerular filtration rate is reduced, it may be concluded that a prerenal, primary renal, or postrenal abnormality is altering renal function.
    (2) Reduced glomerular filtration rate may be caused by technical errors in urine collection or determination of plasma creatinine concentration.
      (a) The alkaline picrate method of creatinine determination measures non-creatinine chromogens in the plasma as well as creatinine.
      (b) Since these non-creatinine chromogens are virtually absent from the urine of the dog, endogenous creatinine clearance calculated from values obtained by this method gives erroneously low values.
      (c) The use of Lloyd's reagent to adsorb creatinine prior to its analysis in plasma is reported to allow measurement of "true" creatinine, and thus gives values that accurately reflect GFR.
    (3) Reported normal values for endogenous creatinine clearance in the dog.
      (a) 2.98 ± 0.96 ml. per minute per Kg. of body weight.
      (b) 60 ± 22 ml. per minute per square meter of body surface area.

L. *Simultaneous determination of PSP excretion and endogenous creatinine clearance*
  1. A laboratory method has been described that converts PSP to a colorless form, and thus allows analysis of biological fluids for both PSP and creatinine. This procedure has been used to simultaneously determine urinary PSP excretion and endogenous creatinine clearance in dogs.
  2. Indications.
    a. The procurement of samples for simultaneous determination of endogenous creatinine clearance and PSP excretion in the dog requires two additional procedures that are not required when the PSP test is performed alone.
      (1) A sample of blood must be obtained prior to injection of PSP dye.
      (2) The urinary bladder must be empty and thoroughly rinsed immediately prior to injection of PSP, as well as at the end of the collection period.
    b. Since these procedures do not greatly complicate the test, the feasibility of performing both tests simultaneously approaches the feasibility of collecting urine for the PSP excretion test.
    c. Utilization of endogenous creatinine clearance for estimation of GFR, and administration of a large dose of PSP for estimating proximal tubular function could provide valuable information concerning glomerulotubular balance during early stages of renal disease.
  3. Procedure.
    a. Collect a sample of blood for determination of the concentration of serum or plasma creatinine.
    b. Catheterize the bladder and remove residual urine (see PSP excretion test in this chapter).

c. After the bladder has been thoroughly rinsed several times with sterile saline, immediately administer 6.0 mg. of PSP dye intravenously.
d. Collect all urine during the next 20 minute period (see PSP excretion test in this chapter).
e. Analyze an aliquot of urine for creatinine by first boiling the sample with zinc dust. The latter will convert the PSP to a colorless form. Creatinine concentration may then be determined by the alkaline picrate method.
f. Analyze the remainder of the urine for PSP content (see PSP excretion test in this chapter).
g. Determine the plasma or serum creatinine concentration by the alkaline picrate method after adsorption of creatinine on Lloyd's reagent.
h. GFR may be calculated using the clearance formula.

REFERENCES

Anderson, R. S., and Edney, A. T. B.: Protein intake and blood urea in the dog. Vet. Rec., *84*:343–349, 1969.
Asheim, A., Helander, C. G., and Persson, F.: Studies on renal function in dogs. Extraction values for PAH obtained by percutaneous catheterization and clearance studies on single kidneys. Acta Physiol. Scand., *44*:103–117, 1958.
Asheim, A., Persson, F., and Persson, S.: Renal clearance in dogs with regard to variations according to age and sex. Acta Physiol. Scand., *51*:150–162, 1961.
Balint, P.: Parameters of renal function of the anesthetized and unanesthetized dog. Acta Physiol. Acad. Sci. Hung., *31*:99–106, 1967.
Balint, P., and Visy, M.: "True creatinine" and "pseudocreatinine" in blood plasma of the dog. Acta Physiol. Hung., *28*:265–272, 1965.
Benjamin, M. M.: Outline of Veterinary Clinical Pathology. 2nd ed. Ames, Iowa, The Iowa State University Press, 1961.
Bold, A. M., Menzies, I. S., and Walker, G.: Assessment of the Azostix Strip Test. J. Clin. Path., *23*:85–89, 1970.
Bovee, K. C.: Urine osmolarity as a definite indicator of renal concentrating capacity. J.A.V.M.A., *155*:30–35, 1969.
Bradford, J. R.: The results following partial nephrectomy and the influence of the kidney on metabolism. J. Physiol., *25*:415–496, 1898.
Bricker, N. S., Dewey, R. R., Lubowitz, H., Stokes, J., and Kirkensgaard, T.: Observations on the concentrating and diluting mechanisms of the diseased kidney. J. Clin. Invest., *38*:516–523, 1959.
Brobst, D. F.: Plasma Phenolsulfonphthalein Determination as a Measure of Renal Function in Dogs. Gaines Veterinary Symposium. Gaines Dog Research Center, White Plains, N. Y., 1967.
Carlson, G. P., and Kaneko, J. J.: Simultaneous estimation of renal function in dogs using sodium sulfanilate and sodium iodohippurate 131. J.A.V.M.A., *158*:1229–1234, 1971.
Carlson, G. P., and Kaneko, J. J.: Sulfanilate clearance in clinical renal disease in the dog. J.A.V.M.A., *158*:1235–1239, 1971.
Coles, E. H.: Veterinary Clinical Pathology. Philadelphia, Pa., W. B. Saunders Co., 1967.
Eggleton, M. G., and Habib, Y. A.: Excretion of para-aminohippurate by the kidney of the cat. J. Physiol., *110*:458–467, 1950.
Elser, R. C., and Savorg, J.: Comparison of manual, automated, and "kit" methods for measurement of glucose and urea in plasma. Am. J. Clin. Path., *54*:820–827, 1970.
Ewald, B. H.: Renal function in normal beagles. Amer. J. Vet. Res., *28*:741–749, 1967.
Finco, D. R.: Simultaneous determination of phenolsulfonphthalein excretion and endogenous creatinine clearance in the normal dog. J.A.V.M.A., *159*:336–340, 1971.
Harvey, D. G.: Some biochemical aspects of urology in the dog. J. Sm. Anim. Pract., *8*:599–604, 1967.
Harvey, D. G., and Hoe, C. M.: A simple clearance test for the assessment of renal function in dogs. J. Sm. Anim. Pract., *7*:361–373, 1966.
Harvey, D. G., and Richards, M. A.: A comparison of two methods used for determination of blood urea nitrogen in the dog. Vet. Rec., *77*:450–452, 1965.
Hayman, J. M., Shumway, N. P., Dumke, R., and Miller, M.: Experimental hyposthenuria. J. Clin. Invest., *18*:195–212, 1939.
Heetderks, D. R.: Localization of PSP excretion by stop flow analysis. J. Urol., *92*:221–223, 1964.
Hoe, C. M., and O'Shea, J. D.: The correlation of biochemistry and histopathology in kidney disease in the dog. Vet. Rec., *77*:210–218, 1965.

Holliday, M. A., and Egan, T. J.: Renal function in man, dog, and rat. Nature, *193*:748–750, 1962.
Houck, C. R.: Statistical analysis of filtration rate and effective renal plasma flow related to weight and surface area in dogs. Amer. J. Physiol., *153*:169–175, 1948.
Isaacson, L. C.: Urine osmolality and specific gravity. Lancet, *1*:72–73, 1959.
Kaneko, J. J., and Cornelius, C. E.: Clinical Biochemistry of Domestic Animals. Vol. I & II. 2nd ed. New York, N. Y., Academic Press, 1971.
Lacher, D. L.: The use of the osmometer in the clinical laboratory. Amer. J. Med. Tech., *37*:240–246, 1971.
Low, D. G., Bergman, E. N., Hiatt, C. W., and Gleiser, C. A.: Experimental canine leptospirosis. II. Renal function studies. J. Infect. Dis., *98*:260–265, 1956.
Matter, B. J., and Smith, W. O.: Use and interpretation of renal function tests. Okla. State Med. Assoc., *62*:146–152, 1969.
Morgan, H. C.: Practitioner's laboratory. Vet. Med./S.A.C., *62*:312–317, 416–423, 585–586, 637–640, 737–742, 984–988, 1182–1191, 1967.
Morgan, H. C.: Practitioner's laboratory. Vet. Med./S.A.C., *63*:112–119, 356–361, 1968.
Myers, L. J., and Pierce, K. R.: Determination of blood urea nitrogen concentration in canine blood. An evaluation of two paper-strip test methods. Southw. Vet., *24*:183–187, 1971.
Noel, P. R. B., and Walker, A. D.: Comparison of four dog diets (including nitrogen balance study). J. Sm. Anim. Pract., *11*:3–16, 1970.
O'Connell, J. M. B., Romeo, J. A., and Mudge, G. H.: Renal tubular secretion of creatinine in the dog. Amer. J. Physiol., *203*:985–990, 1962.
Oester, A., Olesson, S., and Madsen, P. O.: Determination of glomerular filtration rate: Old and new methods. A comparative study in dogs. Invest. Urol., *6*:315–321, 1968.
Osbaldiston, G. W.: The kidney: Its function and evaluation in health and disease. *In* Clinical Biochemistry of Domestic Animals. Vol. 2. 2nd edition. Edited by J. J. Kaneko and C. E. Cornelius. New York, N. Y., Academic Press, 1971.
Osbaldiston, G. W., and Fuhrman, W.: The clearance of creatinine, inulin, para-aminohippurate, and phenolsulphonphthalein in the cat. Canad. J. Comp. Med., *34*:138–141, 1970.
Osborne, C. A.: Urologic logic—diagnosis of renal disease. J.A.V.M.A., *157*:1656–1666, 1970.
Richards, M. A., and Hoe, C. M.: A long term study of renal disease in the dog. Vet. Rec., *80*:640–646, 1967.
Roscoe, M. H.: Plasma chromogen and the endogenous creatinine clearance. J. Clin. Path., *11*:173–176, 1958.
Smith, H. W.: The Kidney. Structure and Function in Health and Disease. New York, N. Y., Oxford University Press, 1951.
Street, A. E.: Blood urea elevation after feeding. Toxicol. Appl. Pharmacol., *13*:363–371, 1968.
Swanson, R. E., and Hakim, A. A.: Stop flow analysis of creatinine excretion in the dog. Amer. J. Physiol., *203*:980–984, 1962.
Textbook of Veterinary Clinical Pathology. Edited by Medway, W., J. E. Prier, and J. S. Wilkinson. Baltimore, Md., The Williams and Wilkins Co., 1969.
Van Pilsum, J. F.: Determination of creatinine and related guanidinium compounds. *In* Methods of Biochemical Analysis. Edited by D. Glick. New York, N. Y., Interscience Publications Inc., 1959.
West, C. D., Traeger, J., and Kaplan, S. A.: A comparison of the relative effectiveness of hydropenia and of Pitressin in producing a concentrated urine. J. Clin. Invest., *34*:887–898, 1955.
Wolf, A. V., and Pillay, V. K. G.: Renal concentration tests, osmotic pressure, specific gravity, and electrical conductivity compared. Amer. J. Med., *46*:837–843, 1969.

Chapter 8
RADIOGRAPHIC EVALUATION OF THE URINARY SYSTEM

I. Pre-radiographic considerations

   A. *Familiarity with the anatomy of the urinary system is essential for proper interpretation of radiographs (see Chapter 1, Applied Anatomy of the Urinary System).*

   B. *Adequate radiographic equipment, proper positioning, correct exposure factors, proper developing technique, and correct interpretation are essential if information gained from radiography of the urinary system is to be consistently meaningful (see standard texts on veterinary radiology).*

   C. *Radiography of the urinary system should not be used as a substitute for careful clinical evaluation of the patient by history, physical examination, and pertinent laboratory procedures.*

   1. Abdominal palpation is an especially important prerequisite to radiographic examination of the urinary system because it:
      a. Often allows localization of the disease process.
      b. Facilitates more meaningful interpretation of radiographic findings.
      c. May facilitate the decision as to whether additional radiographs or special radiographic techniques are likely to be of value in establishing a diagnosis.
   2. Radiographic findings may confirm, deny, or correct diagnostic probabilities formulated on the basis of history, physical examination, and laboratory procedures.

II. Radiographic estimation of kidney size of dogs

   A. *Value of estimating kidney size*
   1. Renal disease, depending on its etiology and stage of progression, may result in changes in kidney size.
      a. Increase in kidney size may occur as a result of:
         (1) Any acute renal disease.
         (2) Hydronephrosis or pyonephrosis.
         (3) Neoplasia.
      b. Decrease in kidney size may occur as a result of:
         (1) Any cause of end-stage kidney.
         (2) Renal hypoplasia.
   2. Estimation of kidney size may aid in the diagnosis and prognosis of renal disease.

a. Knowledge of kidney size, considered together with history, physical examination, and laboratory aids, may allow the clinician to narrow the list of diagnostic possibilities or to make a specific diagnosis.
b. Prognosis of renal disease is based on the reversibility or irreversibility of renal disease (see Chapter 12, Pathophysiology of Renal Failure).
  (1) Chronic generalized renal diseases are generally irreversible; small, contracted kidneys are present in the end-stage of chronic renal diseases.
  (2) Acute renal diseases have the potential for being reversible; increase in kidney size may be, but is not invariably, present in acute renal disease.

B. *Results of studies to evaluate the reliability of estimating kidney size by radiographic techniques*
  1. Adequacy of visualization of the kidneys.
    a. Without the use of contrast media, the right kidney can rarely be visualized well enough to permit measurement; the left kidney can be adequately visualized about 50 per cent of the time.
    b. Intravenous nephrography and aortography almost invariably allow adequate visualization of normal dog kidneys. Because of its technical ease, intravenous nephrography is the technique of choice.
  2. Relationship of actual renal size to measurements of kidneys obtained from radiographs.
    a. Kidney size is best estimated by measurement of kidney dimensions in three planes; however, measurement of kidneys visualized on radiographs is limited to two planes.
    b. Experimental studies in dogs have revealed that kidney length provided a better correlation with kidney weight than did kidney area or kidney length cubed. Kidney length should be used to estimate kidney size from radiographs.
  3. Reliability of radiographic measurements.
    a. Due to geometry of radiographic procedures, measurements obtained from radiographs represent a magnification of the actual dimensions of an anatomic structure.
    b. The degree of magnification induced by radiography is dependent primarily on the distance between the structure and the film; however, magnification is also affected by the distance between the X-ray tube and the structure.
    c. The exact position of the kidneys with respect to the film and X-ray tube cannot be determined under the usual conditions of radiography. Variables such as body size, body condition, stage of respiration, and patient position on the table all affect the spatial relationship of the kidneys to the X-ray tube and film.
    d. Comparison of kidney length to an adjacent anatomic structure, such as a lumbar vertebra, has been used in effort to avoid errors in interpretation due to magnification. Studies comparing kidney and vertebrae lengths determined at necropsy to the same measurements obtained from radiographs indicate that in normal dogs, kidneys are magnified to a slightly greater degree than are vertebrae.
    e. Comparison of kidney-vertebra length ratios obtained by radiography of several dogs indicates that the relationship between the necropsy

and radiographic measurements is not constant. Some dogs have marked differences between the necropsy and radiography ratios, whereas the same measurements obtained in other dogs are in close agreement.
   f. Necropsy measurements indicate that considerable variation in kidney length and weight occurs in dogs of the same size.
4. Method of determination of the kidney-vertebra length ratio.
   a. Perform intravenous urography by techniques described in this section.
   b. With the dog in ventrodorsal recumbency, expose the film ten seconds after completion of injection of radiopaque material.
   c. Measure maximum kidney length (extreme cranial pole to extreme caudal pole).
   d. Measure the length of the second lumbar vertebra. Do not include intervertebral spaces in the measurement.
   e. Divide kidney length by vertebra length.
5. Interpretation of results.
   a. Results of measurements obtained from intravenous nephrograms of 27 normal dogs indicate that the kidney-vertebra-length ratio is 3.03 ± 0.25. Tube-film distance was 101.6 cm.
   b. These data suggest that 95 per cent of normal dogs will have a kidney-vertebra-length ratio between approximately 2.5 and 3.5. Values outside this range suggest abnormal kidney size.
   c. In view of the many variables associated with the technique, it should be emphasized that results of these measurements should be correlated with history, physical examination, and laboratory aids in the evaluation of the patient.
   d. Values within the normal range do not eliminate the possibility of renal disease. Depending on the etiology and duration of the disease, kidney size can be within normal limits with generalized renal disease.
   e. Significant differences between right and left kidney size may provide valuable information. Knowledge of the normal range for kidney-vertebra-length ratios may aid in establishing which kidney is abnormal.
   f. If kidneys are not obviously abnormal in size, significant information may still be obtained by reexamining kidney size at various time intervals, and comparing results obtained at different times.

III. Patient Preparation

Proper preparation of the patient is an essential prerequisite to optimal roentgenographic visualization of lesions of the urinary system.

   A. Because alterations which may be detected radiographically are often subtle, it is essential that the intestines contain no fecal material or gas at the time films are exposed.
   1. Food should be withheld for 24 hours prior to elective radiography.
      a. Even after a 24 hour fast, the intestines often contain enough ingesta to interfere with interpretation of radiographs.
      b. A mild irritant cathartic such as castor oil given at the start of the fast is often helpful.

88   DIAGNOSIS OF URINARY DISEASES

2. Warm water enemas may be given if fecal material can be palpated in the intestines or if feces are visualized on survey films.
   a. Since enemas are often associated with introduction of air into the lower intestinal tract, they should be administered several hours prior to elective radiography. Five to 10 units of vasopressin* may be administered parenterally one-half to one hour prior to radiography to eliminate intestinal gas. The latter may hinder contrast cystographic techniques since the smooth muscle of the urinary bladder may also be stimulated to contract.
   b. If water has been restricted in preparation for intravenous urography, enemas should be avoided if possible as they tend to rehydrate the patient. A Fleet** enema may be used if necessary.

B. *If ascitic fluid is present, it should be removed and evaluated prior to radiography.*

IV. Survey films

A. *Organs of the urinary system may not be well visualized on survey radiographs.*

Radiographic visualization of organs of the urinary system is dependent upon the contrast between them and surrounding tissues. The outline of the

---

*Pitressin, Parke, Davis and Company, Detroit, Michigan 48232.
**Sodium phosphate and sodium biphosphate. Eaton Laboratories, Norwich, New York 13815.

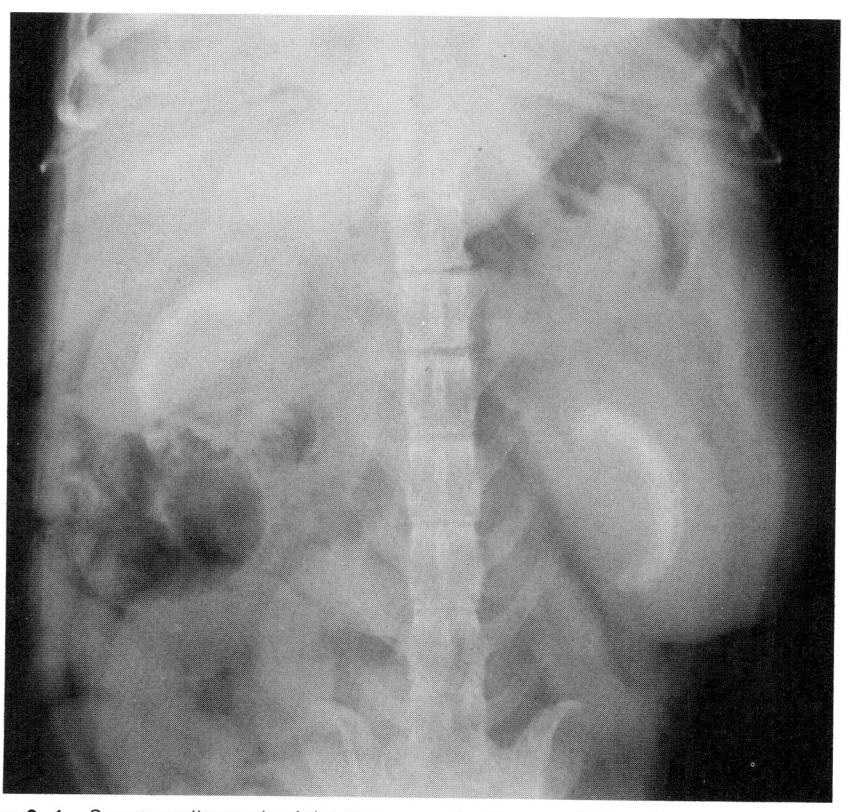

Figure 8–1. Survey radiograph of the abdomen of a 10-year-old female cocker spaniel dog. There is extensive calcification in the corticomedullary portions of both kidneys. The serum concentrations of calcium and phosphorus were normal. The specific cause of the renal calcification was not determined.

RADIOGRAPHIC EVALUATION OF THE URINARY SYSTEM 89

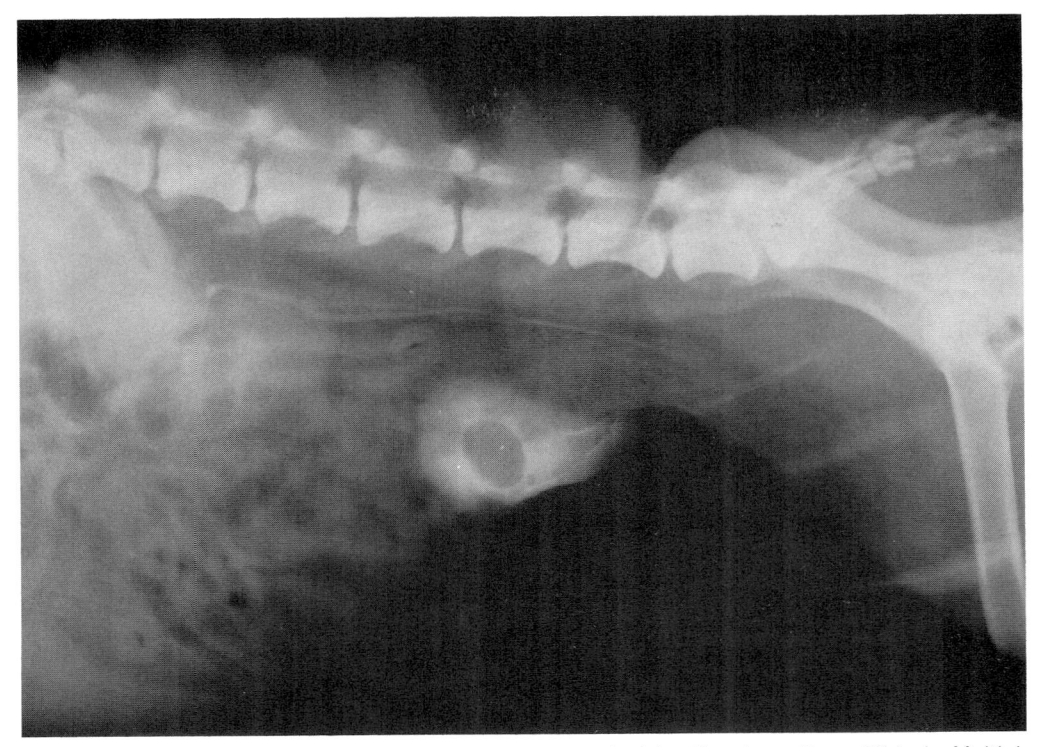

Figure 8–2. Intravenous urogram of a 14-year-old male dalmatian dog with urolithiasis. Multiple radiolucent uroliths are present in the urinary bladder. Analysis of the stones revealed that they were composed predominantly of ammonium urates. (Courtesy of Dr. G. F. Hanlon, College of Veterinary Medicine, University of Minnesota.)

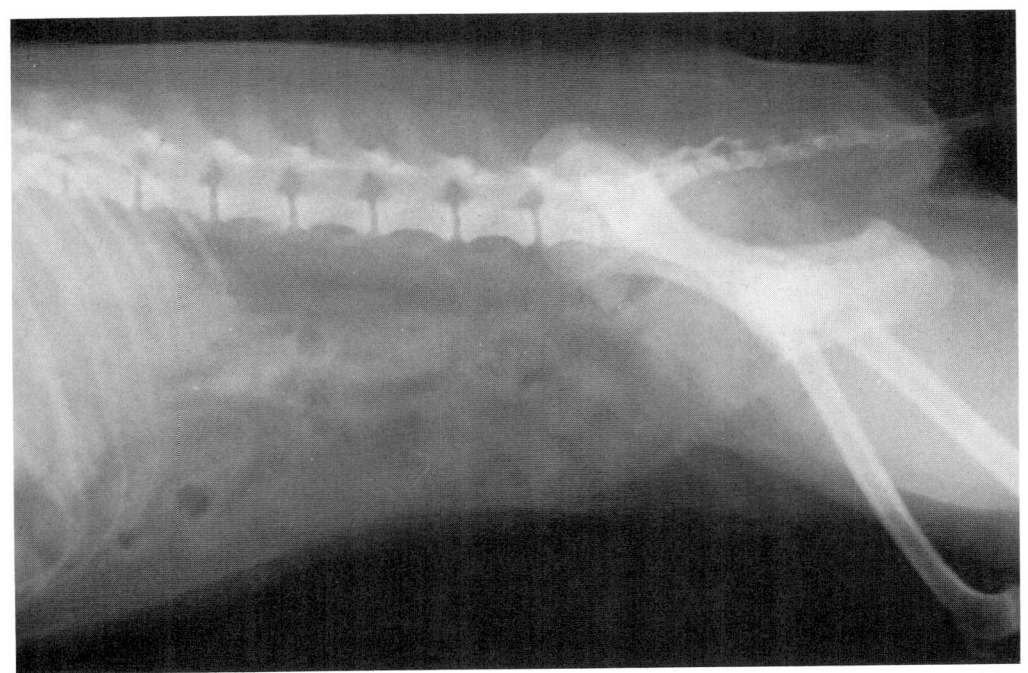

Figure 8–3. Survey radiograph of the abdomen of a 2-year-old female pomeranian dog with a urethral calculus. Visualization of the calculus has been obscured by the bony pelvis.

90 DIAGNOSIS OF URINARY DISEASES

kidneys and urinary bladder may be visualized if a sufficient quantity of adipose tissue surrounds them, because the radiographic density of fat is different than that of adjacent tissues.

B. *Good quality radiographs combined with careful interpretation may reveal abnormalities without the use of special techniques (Fig. 8–1).*
   1. Changes in size, shape, and position may be detected; however, organs of the urinary system may be severely damaged and yet maintain normal size and shape when visualized radiographically.
   2. Radiopaque calculi may be detected.
      a. Visibility depends on composition and size of calculi.
         (1) Calcium, phosphate, and oxalate containing calculi are usually radiopaque.
         (2) Calculi composed of uric acid, xanthine, or matrix concretions may not be visible on scout films, but may be detected as radiolucent structures by positive contrast radiography (Fig. 8–2).

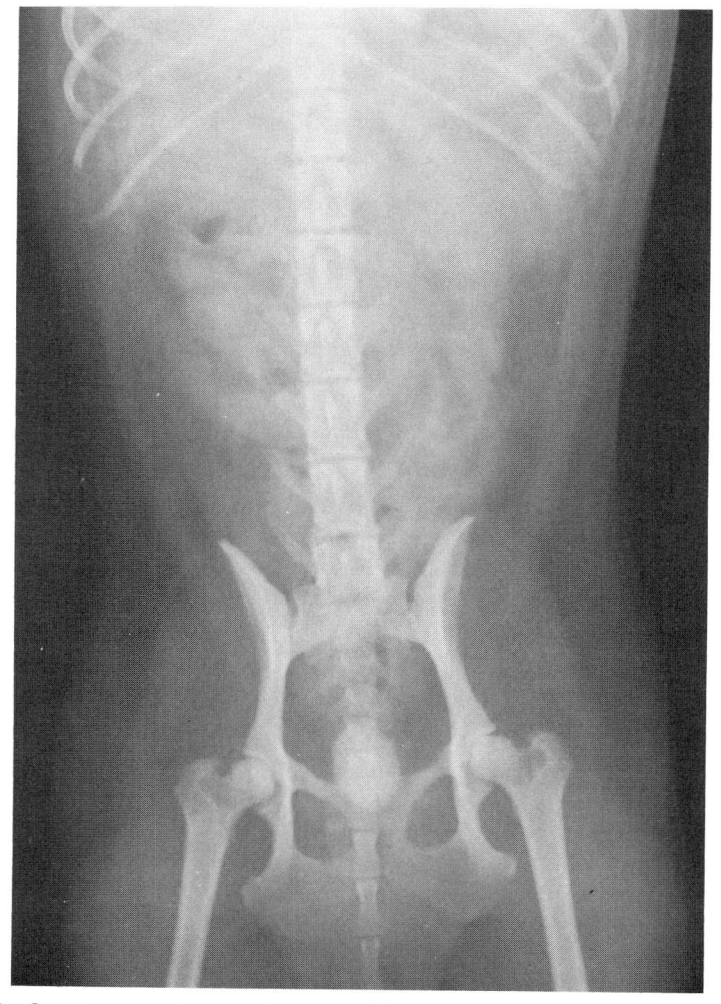

Figure 8–4. Survey ventrodorsal radiograph of the abdomen of the dog described in Figure 8–3. A solitary calculus is present in the proximal urethra.

b. Calculi found in one part of the urinary tract dictate examination of other portions of the system for the presence of calculi.
c. Always expose at least two views (ventrodorsal and lateral). Oblique views may be of value. Interposition of skeletal bone between calculi and film is a common cause of failure to visualize calculi (Figs. 8–3 and 8–4).
3. Chronic generalized nephrocalcinosis may be detected.

V. Contrast radiography of the urinary system

A. *Contrast radiography is often indicated as a diagnostic aid because of poor visualization of organs of the urinary system on survey films.*

B. *Positive contrast agents (diagnostic opaques)*
1. Organic iodinated compounds.
    a. Tri-iodinated (excreted mainly by glomerular filtration).
        (1) Conray, or Conray-400 (Mallinckrodt Chemical Works). Intravenous urography and drip infusion urography.
        (2) Hypaque sodium, 50% (Winthrop Laboratories). Intravenous urography.
        (3) Hypaque sodium, 20% (Winthrop Laboratories). Retrograde urography.
        (4) Hypaque-M, 75% and 90% (Winthrop Laboratories). Nephrography and nephrotomography.
        (5) Renografin, 30%, 60%, and 76% (E. R. Squibb and Sons). Intravenous urography and retrograde urography.
        (7) Retrografin (E. R. Squibb and Sons). Retrograde urography in the presence of infection.
        (7) Renovist (E. R. Squibb and Sons). Intravenous Urography.
        (8) Miakon sodium, 50% (Mallinckrodt Chemical Works). Intravenous urography.
        (9) Urokon, 30%, 50%, 70% (Mallinckrodt Chemical Works).
            (a) Intravenous urography, nephrotomography.
            (b) Secreted by proximal convuluted tubules at low concentrations but primarily by glomerular filtration at high concentrations.
    b. Di-iodinated (excreted by glomerular filtration and secreted by proximal convoluted tubules).
        (1) Diodrast 35%, Diodrast concentrated, Diodrast Compound (Winthrop Laboratories). Intravenous and retrograde urography.
        (2) Neo-Iopax 50%, 75% (Schering Corporation). Intravenous urography, retrograde urography, and intravenous nephrography.
2. The quality of intravenous urograms often varies more from patient to patient than between different diagnostic opaques.
3. Tri-iodinated compounds are most commonly used because they are well tolerated and provide excellent contrast.
4. Although serious reactions, including sensitivity reactions (angioneurotic edema, anaphylactic shock), cardiopulmonary reactions (hypotension, apnea, pulmonary edema, cardiac arrest), and convulsions, have been reported in human patients following injection of organic iodide compounds, they are apparently rarely encountered in dogs and cats.
    a. On occasion, vomition and urticaria have been reported in dogs following administration of organic iodinated compounds.
    b. Although injection of small pretest doses of diagnostic opaques is of no proven value, manufacturers commonly recommend intravenous

injection of a small dose of the diagnostic opaque in question prior to administration of the calculated dose as an effort to determine whether or not unfavorable reactions are likely to occur.

C. *Negative contrast agents*
  1. Radiolucent substances provide contrast with the walls of organs of the urinary tract and thus facilitate better visualization.
      a. Air is satisfactory for routine use in dogs and cats. There have been no documented instances of complications associated with the use of air as a negative contrast agent in veterinary medicine.
      b. Carbon dioxide and nitrous oxide. The high solubility coefficient of these gases in blood prevents embolism in instances of inadvertent intravascular injections.
      c. Negative contrast agents are used in pneumocystography, double contrast cystography, and pneumoperitoneum (Fig. 8–5).

D. *Excretory urography (intravenous urography, descending urography)*
  1. The capacity of the kidneys to excrete circulating organic iodinated compounds in concentrations sufficiently high to cause the urine to become radiopaque is the basis for the excretory urogram.

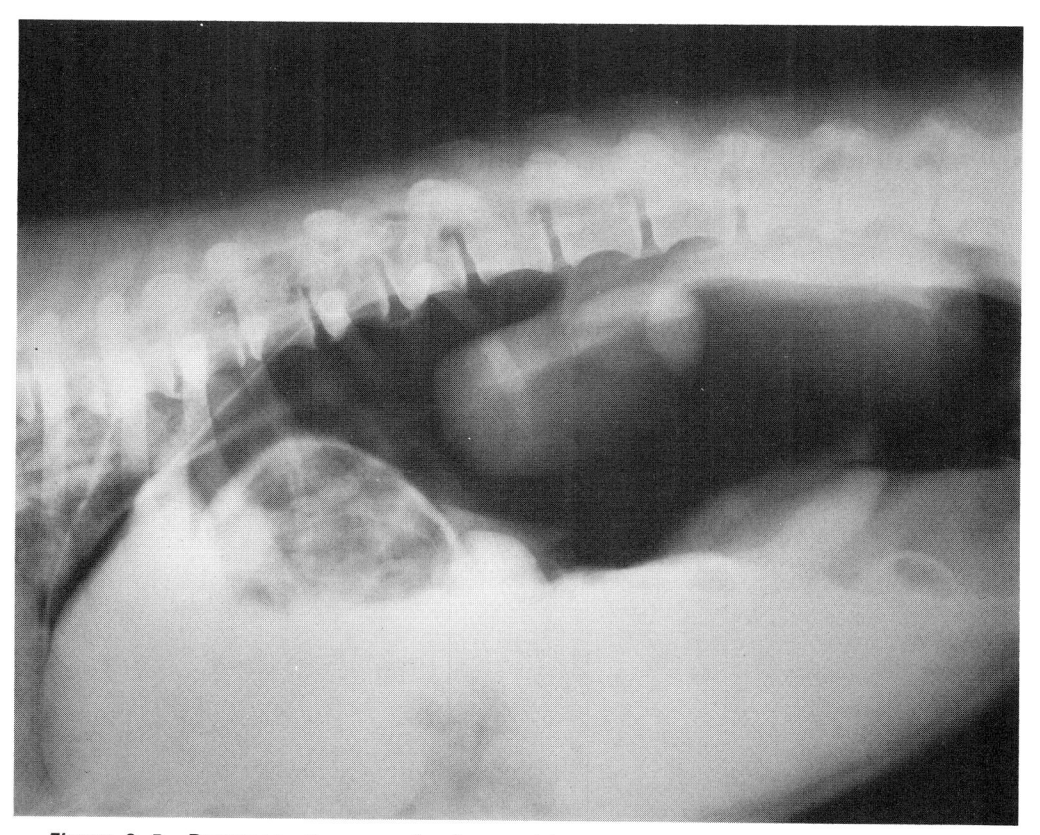

Figure 8–5. Pneumoperitoneum of a 9-year-old male bassett hound. Following induction of pneumoperitoneum with nitrous oxide gas, a lateral radiograph of the abdomen was exposed with the dog in the standing position. The negative contrast provided by nitrous oxide permits visualization of both kidneys.

2. It facilitates evaluation of the excretory pattern of the urinary system.
    a. Excretory urography is the only practical method of radiographic visualization of the renal pelves and ureters of dogs and cats.
    b. It may indicate whether a renal or ureteral lesion is bilateral or unilateral, and, if unilateral, the side affected. This information is especially important if surgical correction or biopsy is contemplated.
3. Excretory urograms provide crude qualitative (not quantitative) evaluation of the renal function of each kidney. Such information is of significance if a nephrectomy is contemplated. Urography should *not* be used as a substitute for renal function tests (see Chapter 7, Tests of Renal Function, and Urinalysis, in Chapter 6).
4. The use of excretory urography is indicated in the diagnosis of:
    a. Primary or metastatic neoplasms of the kidneys or ureters.
    b. Hydronephrosis, whether unilateral or bilateral.
    c. Partial or complete obstructive uropathy due to any cause.
    d. Congenital anomalies of the kidneys and ureters, including:
        (1) Unilateral renal aplasia.
        (2) Unilateral or bilateral hypoplasia.
        (3) Double pelves.
        (4) Horseshoe kidneys.
        (5) Ectopic kidneys.
        (6) Cystic kidneys.
        (7) Ectopic ureters.
    e. Radiolucent calculi.
    f. Rupture of kidney or ureters due to any cause.
    g. Excretory cystography is especially useful in small dogs and cats when catheterization of the urinary bladder is difficult or impossible. It may be of value in the diagnosis of:
        (1) Primary or metastatic neoplasms.
        (2) Patent urachus.
        (3) Congenital or acquired diverticula.
        (4) Radiolucent calculi.
        (5) Abnormal locations of the bladder, including:
            (a) Perineal, inguinal, or ventral abdominal hernias.
            (b) Displacement of the urinary bladder by an enlarged prostate or abdominal mass.
        (6) Rupture of the urinary bladder accompanied by urethral obstruction which prevents catheterization.
        (7) Polypoid and emphysematous cystitis.
5. Limitations.
    a. Excretory urograms do not indicate whether the underlying lesion is reversible or irreversible.
    b. They do not indicate the reserve capacity of the kidneys.
    c. Early or focal lesions may not be visualized.
    d. Satisfactory films may be hard to obtain if severe renal insufficiency is present. At least two factors are responsible:
        (1) The total quantity of dye excreted during the test period is decreased as a result of a decrease in renal function.
        (2) The remaining functional nephrons excrete a greater than normal quantity of filtered water, which causes dilution of contrast material.

e. Excretory urography does not provide any quantitative information about renal function.
   (1) The following variables affect the degree of visualization provided by contrast material:
       (a) Type, dosage, and route of administration of the contrast material.
       (b) Injection time.
       (c) Radiographic technique.
       (d) State of hydration of the patient.
       (e) Factors influencing renal blood flow.
       (f) Functional capacity of the kidneys.
   (2) The excretion of contrast material gives no indication of the number of nephrons taking part in the process, and thus gives no reliable information as to the quantity of functioning nephrons present.
   (3) Varying degrees of visualization of the urinary tract may occur in patients with unilateral or bilateral impairment of renal function.
   (4) Good contrast density of the urinary tract is not always associated with normal renal function and poor contrast density is not always associated with reduced renal function.
6. Nonvisualization of one kidney may occur as a result of one or more of the following:
   a. The absence of one kidney.
   b. Severe destruction of the nephron population of the involved kidney.
   c. Obstruction of the renal artery.
   d. Marked or total obstruction to urine flow.
   e. A high rate of solute and water excretion by the involved kidney.
7. Technique.
   a. Withhold food for 24 hours and give a laxative.
   b. The amount of water in which the excreted contrast material is contained is of great significance.
      (1) The final concentration of radiopaque dye in urine is dependent on tubular concentration mechanisms, and the latter is related to the patient's body water balance. The larger the quantity of water excreted, the lower the concentration of the contrast material in the urine.
      (2) Withhold fluid for 12 to 15 hours in patients that can tolerate partial dehydration.
      (3) Withholding fluid for as little as four hours may improve contrast to some degree.
      (4) Vasopressin may be administered to patients unable to tolerate the stress of water deprivation.
      (5) Warm water enemas should be avoided as they promote rehydration.
      (6) Withholding water is absolutely contraindicated in patients with renal insufficiency because:
          (a) It will not be effective in increasing the concentration of the contrast agent due to impaired ability of the kidneys to concentrate and dilute urine.
          (b) It may precipitate a uremic crisis.
   c. Sedation or anesthesia may be needed, depending on the attitude of the patient.

RADIOGRAPHIC EVALUATION OF THE URINARY SYSTEM 95

(1) Avoid hypotension in patients with renal insufficiency.
(2) Manual restraint often suffices.
d. Always take survey radiographs prior to administration of contrast material.
  (1) Patient preparation may be evaluated.
  (2) Exposure factors may be evaluated.
  (3) Survey radiographs may provide the diagnosis.
  (4) Contrast material may obscure existing lesions.
  (5) Survey radiographs of the thorax should be taken if malignant neoplasia is suspected.
e. Medias and dosages.
  (1) Tri-iodinated water-soluble organic compounds provide good contrast and are well tolerated.
  (2) Hypaque 50%. Inject 0.5 to 1 cc. per lb. of body weight intravenously. Usually not more than 30 to 50 cc. of the contrast media is necessary for dogs with adequate renal function (see High dose urography, in this chapter).
f. Abdominal compression.
  (1) Abdominal compression devices are designed to compress the ureters and thus increase the filling of the renal pelves and ureters with contrast material.
    (a) Normal peristaltic movements of the ureters may prevent distention of the ureters and renal pelves with urine.
    (b) Incomplete filling makes interpretation difficult.
  (2) Diagnostic radiographs of many diseases may be obtained without compression devices, especially if an adequate dose of radiopaque dye is administered.
  (3) Apply the compression device before the injection of contrast media and leave it in place for the 5 and 10 minute exposures.
  (4) To visualize the ureters, expose the film immediately after removal of the compression device.
  (5) Compression devices should be placed just in front of the pubis.
    (a) Standard compression bands are available from manufacturers of radiographic equipment.
    (b) Other compression devices that may be used include:
      [1] Blocks of balsa wood.
      [2] Blocks of cellulose sponge.
      [3] Muslin, gauze, or cotton bands with a wad of cotton placed over each ureter.
  (6) Disadvantages. Abdominal compression tends to cause displacement and distortion of the ureters and other abdominal organs, but such artefacts should not be present on films exposed prior to and after application of abdominal compression devices.
  (7) See high dose urography.
g. Exposure.
  (1) Exposure technique is dependent on diagnostic possibilities and the segment of the urinary system that is to be visualized.
  (2) Center the tube over the area of interest.
    (a) Kidneys and ureters are usually best visualized on ventrodorsal views.
    (b) The bladder is usually best visualized on lateral and oblique views.

(c) Take at least two views in planes which are at right angles to each other in order to determine the exact position and extent of lesions.
(3) Patients with normal renal function. When renal function is normal or only moderately decreased, contrast visualization is usually excellent.
  (a) Kidneys begin to excrete contrast material almost immediately and are usually visible after injection of the contrast media has been completed.
  (b) Develop films after each exposure and allow the radiographic findings to serve as a guide for subsequent exposure times.
  (c) Five minutes following injection, the kidneys, renal pelves, and ureters are usually visible, and some dye is present in the urinary bladder.
  (d) Ten minutes following injection, the kidneys, ureters, and urinary bladder are usually visible.
  (e) Fifteen minutes following injection, the kidneys, ureters, and urinary bladder are usually visible.
  (f) The urinary bladder is usually best visualized on 25 to 30 minute exposures.
  (g) Need for additional exposures is dependent on the lesions present.
  (h) In patients with impaired renal function, visualization of the urinary tract may be obtained by delayed exposures at one, two, or three hours following injection of the dye (see High dose urography, below).
h. High dose urography.
  (1) Intravenous urography should not be performed in patients with renal insufficiency unless it is probable that information of diagnostic value is likely to be obtained.
  (2) There are no published data defining the degree of renal insufficiency incompatible with satisfactory urographic examination.
  (3) Available data do not provide information which suggests that excretory urography of patients with renal insufficiency is associated with increased risk.
  (4) If excretory urography by conventional methods proves to be inconclusive, or if the patient is uremic, high dose urography should be considered. The efficacy of this technique is related to the fact that contrast mediums act as osmotic diuretics, and therefore augment filling of the collecting system with radiopaque material.
  (5) Technique.
    (a) Take standard survey radiographs after preparing the patient.
    (b) Administer 50% Hypaque. Conray or Conray-400 may be used instead of Hypaque. Although the exact dosage which will provide satisfactory radiographs is variable, the following dosages are provided as guide lines.
      [1] Inject 2 to 3 cc. of Hypaque per lb. of body weight for patients under 40 lbs.
      [2] Inject 1.5 to 2 cc. of Hypaque per lb. of body weight for patients above 40 lbs.

RADIOGRAPHIC EVALUATION OF THE URINARY SYSTEM 97

[3] The contrast material should be injected intravenously with a syringe.

[4] When large volumes are used, they may be administered with a reservoir container and an 18-gauge needle without restriction to flow (drip infusion urography), but more rapid injection with a syringe is preferable. Drip infusion urography provides no advantage over high dose urography in which an identical dose of contrast medium is injected. The higher plasma concentration of radiopaque dye associated with injection techniques provides a denser nephrogram than a slow infusion.

(c) Expose films at 10, 20, and 30 minutes (or longer if necessary) following completion of administration of the contrast media.

(6) This technique may be especially useful in veterinary medicine since retrograde pyelography is not feasible in the majority of patients.

(7) The use of high dose urography in patients with normal renal function is usually associated with better filling of the excretory pathway of the urinary system. It may be used in place of abdominal compression bands to enhance visualization of the renal pelves and ureters. In the latter instance, use standard exposure times.

E. *Nephrography*
   1. Nephrography refers to the temporary increase in the radiopacity of the kidneys following intravenous injection of contrast material.
   2. Exposure.
      a. Films should be exposed approximately 10 to 20 seconds following completion of administration of contrast medium (Hypaque-M 90%).
      b. Injection of contrast media should be completed in approximately 30 seconds.
      c. High dose urography may be considered.
   3. Indications.
      a. Nephrograms often reveal abnormalities in size, shape, and contour of the kidneys.
      b. They may be used to facilitate measurement of kidneys.
      c. They may facilitate localization of renal cysts and neoplasms.

F. *Retrograde pyelography and ureterography*
   1. This technique is not practical in the majority of dogs and cats with the equipment currently available. The technique may be performed with the aid of a cystoscope in female dogs of sufficient body size (see Chapter 10, Cystoscopy).
   2. The technique is useful in the diagnosis of ectopic ureters which enter the urethra or vagina of female dogs (see Ectopic ureters, in Chapter 35).

G. *Pneumocystography*
   1. Medias available for pneumocystography are radiolucent substances which provide contrast with the radiopaque wall of the urinary bladder.
      a. Air is satisfactory for routine use.
      b. Carbon dioxide or nitrous oxide may be used.

2. Technique.
   a. Prepare the patient as previously outlined.
   b. Remove all of the urine from the bladder by catheterization.
      (1) Aseptic technique is essential.
      (2) Avoid metal female catheters as they often traumatize the bladder mucosa. Use flexible fiber catheters.
      (3) It may be necessary to flush the bladder with sterile saline to remove blood clots.
   c. Obtain survey radiographs and evaluate them.
   d. Inject air through a catheter into the bladder utilizing a three-way valve and syringe.
      (1) The volume of air that should be placed in the bladder is variable and depends on the size of the patient and the lesions present. The quantity must be determined on the basis of clinical judgment.
      (2) As a generality, air should be injected until a rebound on the syringe plunger is felt, or until air escapes through the urethra around the periphery of the catheter. Once sufficient intravesical pressure has been reached to stimulate contraction of the wall of the urinary bladder, most of the air instilled into the bladder may be expelled. In the latter instance, a smaller volume of air should be replaced.
      (3) In order to develop a consistent technique, and one which facilitates reproduction of results, maximum intravesical pressure should be maintained throughout the study. If air escapes around the catheter during positioning of the patient, additional air should be replaced before further films are exposed.
   e. Expose at least two views (ventrodorsal and lateral).
      (1) Right lateral, left lateral, ventrodorsal, dorsoventral, and oblique views have been recommended by some investigators because lesions visible in one view may not be visible on others, or may vary in appearance.
   f. Pneumocystography may be combined with pneumoperitoneum.
3. Indications include:
   a. Radiopaque calculi too small to be palpated per abdomen, or to be visualized on survey films.
   b. Primary or metastatic neoplasia of the urinary bladder.
   c. Rupture of the urinary bladder due to any cause. Watch for the presence of air which has escaped from the bladder into the peritoneal cavity. Intraperitoneal fluid will also be present in the majority of cases.
      (1) The patient should be positioned for standing-lateral exposure. In such a position air will accumulate under the vertebrae. Alternatively, the patient may be positioned in lateral recumbency. In such a position, air will accumulate under the uppermost portion of the abdominal wall.
      (2) Fluoroscopy may be used. Gas bubbles may be observed escaping into the peritoneal cavity immediately following injection of air into the bladder via a catheter.
   d. Abnormal locations of the urinary bladder, including:
      (1) Perineal, inguinal, and ventral abdominal hernias.
      (2) Displacement of urinary bladder by the prostate gland or abdominal masses.

RADIOGRAPHIC EVALUATION OF THE URINARY SYSTEM 99

   e. Cystitis in which predisposing causes such as calculi or neoplasms are suspected.
- H. *Positive contrast cystography*
    1. Mediums available:
        a. Water soluble organic iodinated material.
        b. Sterile barium sulfate (see Double contrast cystography, in this chapter).
    2. Technique.
        a. Prepare the patient as previously described.
        b. Remove all urine from the bladder by catheterization (see Pneumocystography, in this chapter).
        c. Blood clots and air bubbles may produce identifiable shadows, and may obscure visualization of lesions. In patients with gross hematuria, the presence of blood clots should be suspected, and the bladder should be rinsed prior to injection of contrast medium.
        d. Expose survey radiographs and evaluate them.
        e. Dilute aqueous organic iodinated material to a 2.5% to 5% concentra-

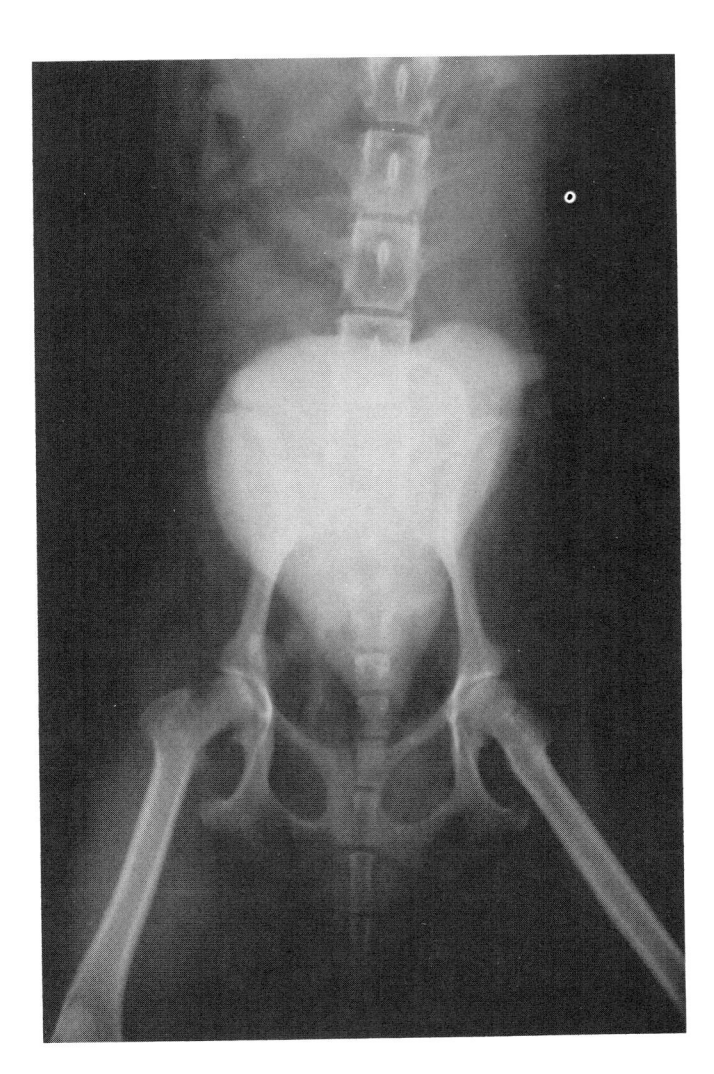

Figure 8-6. Positive contrast cystogram of the urinary bladder of a 3-year-old female mixed breed dog. A diverticulum is present in the wall of the urinary bladder. A solitary radiopaque cystolith is also present, but its presence has been partially obscured by radiopaque contrast material.

tion with sterilized water or saline. Small lesions may be obscured by administration of highly concentrated radiopaque materials into the bladder.
   f. Expose a minimum of 2 views (lateral and ventrodorsal).
   g. Additional contrast may be obtained by combining this technique with pneumoperitoneum.
   h. Indications include detection of:
      (1) Radiolucent calculi.
      (2) Ulceration of the mucosa of the urinary bladder.
      (3) Diverticula of the urinary bladder wall (Fig. 8–6).
      (4) See Indications for pneumocystography, in this chapter.

I. *Double contrast cystography*
   1. In this technique a negative contrast medium and a positive contrast medium are used in combination.
   2. Mediums available.
      a. A finely ground emulsion of barium sulfate is the positive contrast medium of choice. The mucosal coating quality of barium mixtures has been reported to be enhanced by using products with barium particles of small and uniform size.
         (1) A sterilized suspension of micropulverized barium sulfate* in water is commercially available in England, but has not been approved for commercial sale in the United States or Canada.
         (2) A barium emulsion made by thoroughly mixing 6 ounces of barium sulfate, sterilized by dry heat in an oven, with 100 ml. of sterile saline has been successfully used in man.
         (3) Barium preparations**,† which have been sterilized and diluted with sterile water to a concentration of 15 to 30 per cent have been successfully used in dogs. Preparations with a high viscosity have been unsatisfactory because of difficulty in injecting them into and removing them from the urinary bladder with a catheter.
      b. Barium is pharmacologically inert and adheres to the surface of abnormalities in the bladder mucosa.
      c. Water soluble organic iodinated contrast agents are not recommended for use in double contrast cystography because of their poor ability to adhere to defects in the bladder mucosa.
      d. Metallic tantalum has been successfully used for double contrast cystography in normal dogs. Tantalum is biologically inert, radiopaque, and adheres to the bladder mucosa.
      e. Room air provides a satisfactory negative contrast agent.
   3. Technique.
      a. Prepare the patient as previously outlined.
      b. Remove all residual urine from the bladder by catheterization. The diameter of the catheter should be as large as is consistent with atraumatic technique, to facilitate instillation and recovery of urine and contrast medium from the urinary bladder.
      c. Expose and evaluate survey films.

---

*Steripaque, Nicholas Laboratories Limited, P.O. Box 17, 225 Bath Road, Slough, Bucks, England SL1 4AU.
**Redi-Flow, Flow Pharmaceuticals, Inc., Mountain View, California 94040.
†Barosperse, Mallinckrodt Pharmaceuticals, St. Louis, Missouri 63160.

d. Utilizing a large capacity syringe, a sufficient quantity (50 to 300 ml.) of barium sulfate should be instilled into the urinary bladder to mildly distend its mucosal surface. In this fashion, the entire mucosal surface comes in contact with barium sulfate. The volume of barium instilled should not be great enough to increase intravesical pressure to such a degree that the wall of the urinary bladder is stimulated to contract. The latter should be avoided since barium expelled from the urinary tract will contaminate the patient's skin and hair and the x-ray unit, and thus may interfere with the quality of subsequent radiographs.
e. An alternative method is to inject a smaller quantity of barium sulfate into the urinary bladder, and then slowly rotate the patient 360 degrees in a horizontal plane. Rotation enhances coating of all portions of the bladder mucosa with barium.
f. Barium which fails to adhere to defects in the bladder mucosa should then be aspirated with the aid of a catheter and syringe. An effort should be made to remove as much barium as possible since excessive barium allowed to remain in the bladder will gravitate to the dependent portion of the bladder and may obscure visualization of small lesions in this area. In addition, air bubbles trapped in barium may induce artefacts which mimic the appearance of lesions.
g. Inject an appropriate quantity of air (see Pneumocystography, in this chapter).
h. Following injection of air and barium into the urinary bladder, exposure of the bladder in at least 2 planes which are at right angles to each other should be made. Exposure factors determined on the basis of evaluation of survey radiographs should be used.
i. Following exposure of the x-ray films, it is usually unnecessary to remove air or barium from the bladder since most patients will expel them spontaneously. If desirable, residual barium may be removed by lavage with several hundred milliliters of sterilized water or saline.
j. Double contrast cystography may be combined with pneumoperitoneum in order to enhance evaluation of bladder wall thickness, and to detect lesions outside the lumen of the urinary bladder.
k. Stereoscopic pair radiography may be combined with double contrast cystography to improve three dimensional visualization of space occupying lesions in the urinary bladder.
4. Interpretation.
a. The use of double contrast cystograms in dogs with normal urinary bladders has revealed that a significant quantity of barium sulfate does not adhere to the mucosa of the urinary bladder.
b. Space occupying lesions with a roughened surface are readily coated with barium and are easy to visualize since they are silhouetted against the air in the bladder (Figs. 8-7 and 8-8).
c. Barium clings to defects in the bladder mucosa caused by ulcerations or diverticulae.
d. Radiolucent calculi or blood clots may be coated with barium, but tend to shift to the most dependent portion of the bladder when the position of the patient is changed.
e. As is the situation with other contrast cystographic techniques, double contrast cystography may be ineffective in demonstrating small lesions in the bladder.

102   DIAGNOSIS OF URINARY DISEASES

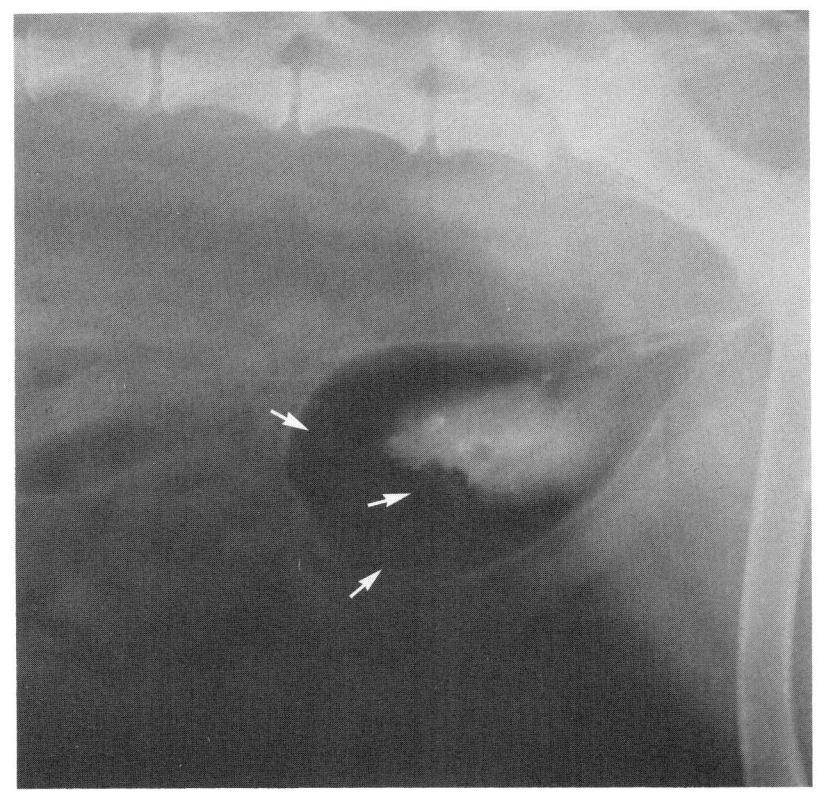

Figure 8–7. Double contrast cystogram of a 5-year-old female mixed breed dog with chronic hematuria. Multiple space-occupying lesions have been coated with barium sulfate and are silhouetted against a background of air (arrows). (J.A.V.M.A., *159*:1400–1404, 1971.)

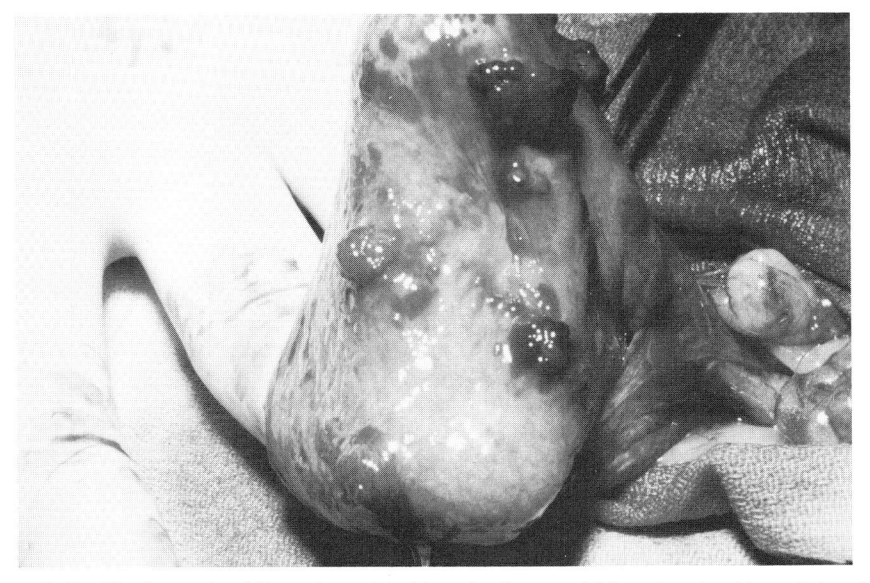

Figure 8–8. Photograph of the urinary bladder of a 5-year-old female mixed breed dog. Multiple polypoid lesions are protruding from the mucosal surface of the bladder. The polyps were removed with the aid of electrocautery. A diagnosis of polypoid cystitis was established by microscopic examination of a surgical biopsy specimen. (J.A.V.M.A., *159*:1400–1404, 1971.)

5. Indications.
    a. The indications for double contrast cystography are similar to those for pneumocystography and positive contrast cystography.
    b. Double contrast cystography has all of the advantages of either positive contrast cystography or pneumocystography and requires a minimum of extra material and time.
    c. Double contrast cystography is superior to other contrast cystographic techniques because better contrast is provided by using two contrast agents of different densities.
    d. Double contrast cystography is particularly useful in detection of:
        (1) Space occupying lesions.
        (2) Ulcerations.
        (3) Diverticulae of the urinary bladder.
    e. This technique increases the probability of detecting lesions when only two views of the urinary bladder are exposed and evaluated.
6. Complications.
    a. Provided aseptic technique is used, double contrast cystography should not be associated with complications.
    b. Air embolism following pneumocystography has not been documented in the veterinary literature.
    c. Although exceedingly rare, a small friable calculus composed of barium sulfate was found in a diverticulum of the urinary bladder of a human being.

J. *Fractional superimposition cystography*
   1. Definition. Fractional superimposition cystography is a technique characterized by superimposition of the radiographic images of serially diluted cystograms obtained by distending the bladder to varying degrees.
   2. Technique. Only the equipment and materials required for conventional positive contrast cystography are required.
       a. Prepare the patient as previously described. Anesthesia may facilitate patient positioning.
       b. Remove all the urine from the bladder by catheterization.
       c. Expose and evaluate survey films.
       d. Introduce 10 to 30 ml. of 50% Hypaque into the urinary bladder. The exact dose is dependent on the size of the patient and the lesions present.
       e. With the patient in lateral recumbency, and without moving either the animal or the cassette:
           (1) Expose the film at 50% of the calculated MAS time at the end of expiration.
           (2) Introduce 10 to 30 ml. of sterilized saline into the bladder and again expose the same film at 50% of the calculated MAS time at the end of expiration.
           (3) Introduce 10 to 30 ml. of sterile saline into the bladder and expose the same film at 33% of the calculated MAS time at the end of expiration.
           (4) Introduce 10 to 30 ml. of sterile saline into the bladder and again expose the same film at 33% of the calculated MAS time at the end of expiration.
           (5) Care must be used not to move the patient while performing the above technique.

104 DIAGNOSIS OF URINARY DISEASES

    f. Remove all of the contrast medium and saline from the urinary bladder by catheterization and repeat as above with the patient in dorsal recumbency.

    g. The exposure time should not be divided into four equal parts because the overall end result would be an underexposed film. A shorter exposure time is used for the last two exposures of the film because of the dilution of the contrast material and resultant decrease in radiodensity.

3. Indications.
    a. Fractional superimposition cystographs may be helpful in evaluation of the location and depth of infiltration of neoplasms in the wall of the urinary bladder.
    b. This technique may facilitate evaluation of the functional capacity of the urinary bladder when severe cystitis is present.
    c. Comments.
        (1) Superimposition cystographs facilitate comparison and evaluation of the distensibility and mobility of various segments of the bladder wall.

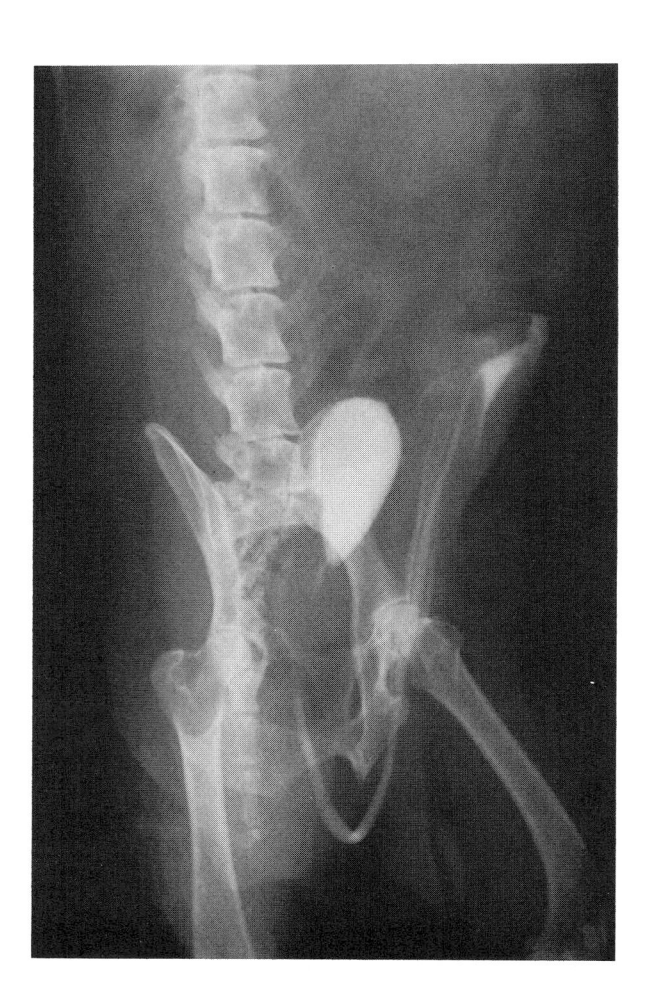

Figure 8-9. Positive contrast urethrogram of a 13-year-old male cocker spaniel. The contrast material was prepared by mixing 1 part aqueous radiopaque medium with 3 parts aqueous sterilized lubricant. Although the prostatic urethra was compressed by hyperplastic enlargement of the prostate gland, the dog had only mild dysuria.

(2) A lack of distensibility of a segment of the bladder wall is suggested by:
    (a) Increased asymmetry during fractional distention of the bladder.
    (b) Disturbance in the layering (halos) of contrast material above the fixed segment of the bladder wall.
(3) Either infiltrating neoplasms, acute or chronic inflammatory disease, or postsurgical scar tissue may cause fixation of the bladder wall.
(4) Patients with impaired innervation of the urinary bladder are not amenable to examination by superimposition cystography because of altered contractility of the bladder wall.

K. *Urethrography*
  1. Technique.
     a. Mix one part of radiopaque material (50% Hypaque) with three to four parts of sterilized aqueous lubricant. Use care not to introduce air bubbles into the mixture during the mixing process.
     b. Inject the radiopaque mixture into the urethra with a fiber catheter or teat cannula.
     c. Expose films in at least two views which are at right angles to each other.
     d. If desirable, the mixture may be removed by lavage with sterile water or saline.
  2. Indications include:
     a. Congenital or acquired stenosis of the urethra (Fig. 8-9).
     b. Neoplasia.
     c. Diverticulae.
     d. Urethrorectal fistula.
     e. Periurethral abscess.

REFERENCES

Benness, G. T.: An evaluation of antidiuretic hormone in intravenous urography. Sniff urography. Clin. Radiol., *21*:157–162, 1970.

Blank, N. K.: Experimental double contrast cystography with tantalum dust. Invest. Radiol., 5:250–253, July-Aug., 1970.

Borthwick, R., and Robbie, B.: Urography in the dog by an intravenous transfusion technique. J. Sm. Anim. Pract., *10*:465–470, 1969.

Dove-Smith, P.: The dose of contrast medium in intravenous urography: A physiologic assessment. Amer. J. Roentgenol., *108*:691–697, 1970.

Doyle, F. H.: Cystography in bladder tumors. A technique using steripaque and carbon dioxide. Brit. J. Radiol., *34*:205–215, 1961.

Edling, N. P. G., Edvall, C. A., and Helander, C. G.: Correlation of urography and tests of renal function. Acta Radiol., *54*:433–438, 1960.

Finco, D. R., Stiles, N. S., Kneller, S. K., Lewis, R. E., and Barrett, R. B.: Radiologic estimation of kidney size of the dog. J.A.V.M.A., *159*:995–1000, 1971.

Griffith, D. P.: A simple, inexpensive technique for photographing roentgenograms. J. Urol., *104*:751–752, 1970.

Helander, C. G., Asheim, A., and Odman, P.: A percutaneous method for catheterization of the renal vein in dogs. Acta Physiol. Scand., *43*:228–232, 1958.

Hoffman, W. W., and Grayhack, J. T.: The limitations of the intravenous pyelogram as a test of renal function. Surg. Gynec. & Obst., *110*:503–508, 1960.

Johansson, S.: Variation in the size of the kidney during nephroangiography in anesthetized dogs. Clin. Radiol., *20*:308–314, 1969.

Lang, E. K.: Superimposition cystography. J. Indiana Med. Assn., *60*:1372–1373, 1967.

Lindell, S. E., and Olin, T.: Catheterization of the renal arteries in dogs and cats. Acta Physiol. Scand., 73:39–40, 1957.
McClennan, B. L., and Becker, J. A.: Excretory urography. Choice of contrast media—experimental. Radiology, 100:585–590, 1971.
Osborne, C. A., and Jessen, C. R.: Double contrast cystography in the dog. J.A.V.M.A., 159:1400–1404, 1971.
Osborne, C. A., Yoho, B. C., Low, D. G., and Wall, B. E.: Radiographic evaluation of the canine urinary system. J. Amer. Hosp. Assoc., 5:136–149, 1969.
Pochaczevsky, R., and Grabstald, H.: Double contrast barium cystography utilizing carbon dioxide. Amer. J. Roentgenol., 92:365–374, 1964.
Porter, G. A.: Sequential effect of angiographic contrast agent on canine renal and systemic hemodynamics. Amer. Heart J., 81:80–92, 1971.
Rhodes, W. H.: Pneumocystography in the dog. J. Amer. Vet. Rad. Soc., 8:45–53, 1967.
Sadi, A., Malali, A. M., and Saad, F.: Histological features of glomeruli and tubules after the injection of an iodinated contrast medium through puncture of the left ventricle for renal angiography. Urol. Int., 11:193–201, 1961.
Schultz, M. L.: Acute changes in renal size in normal and hypertensive dogs. J. Urol., 104:629–634, 1970.
Tennille, N. B., and Thornton, G. W.: Intravenous urography studies in the unanesthetized dog. Vet. Med., 53:29–40, 1958.
Yulis, G. P., Morrin, P. A. F., Mackie, F. W., and Bruie, A. W.: Intravenous urography in the presence of uremia. Surg. Gynec. & Obstet., 120:810–816, 1965.

Chapter 9
PERCUTANEOUS RENAL BIOPSY

I. Indications

A. *Percutaneous renal biopsy in the dog and cat has proved to be a valuable aid to clinical evaluation of patients with primary renal failure because of the need for diagnostic specificity, and the fact that morphologic alterations constitute the principal criteria for classifying most renal diseases.*

Renal biopsies are indicated to confirm, support, or eliminate diagnostic possibilities formulated on the basis of history, physical examination, radiographic evaluation, and laboratory data.

1. The detection of specific renal disease before there is serious impairment of renal function is often difficult because:
    a. The onset of many renal diseases is insidious.
    b. Clinical signs which one can detect by history and physical examination usually are not sufficiently specific to permit a diagnosis other than renal dysfunction. They do not provide consistently reliable information upon which to predict the potential reversibility or irreversibility of the underlying disease.
    c. Functional abnormalities that are detected by laboratory procedures are similar in a wide variety of renal disorders.
2. Representative biopsy samples are more likely to be obtained in generalized renal diseases, as listed below, than in focal renal disease.
    a. Amyloidosis.
    b. Acute generalized nephritis.
    c. Chronic generalized nephritis.
    d. Renal cortical hypoplasia.
    e. Generalized neoplasia.
    f. Generalized pyelonephritis.

B. *To aid in the choice of treatment*
1. Evaluation of biopsy specimens may indicate whether underlying lesions are potentially reversible or irreversible.
    a. It is often difficult to distinguish between potentially reversible and irreversible renal disease in the dog and cat on the basis of clinical findings and laboratory data.
        (1) Potentially reversible lesions are justification for vigorous therapy.
        (2) Generalized progressive irreversible lesions may not warrant such effort and expense.
2. Microscopic evaluation of a biopsy specimen may result in establishment of a specific histopathologic diagnosis which differs from the clinical

impression, necessitating revision of regimen of the therapy considered prior to biopsy.

3. Biopsy findings may serve as a baseline which may be used to determine response to therapy.

C. *To aid in prognosis*

Establishment of a specific morphologic diagnosis facilitates prediction of the biological behavior of the disease.

II. Pre-biopsy considerations

A. *Renal biopsy should not be used as a substitute for careful clinical evaluation by history, physical examination and laboratory procedures.*

B. *Because hemorrhage is the most serious potential complication to renal biopsy, the hemostatic capabilities of the patient should be evaluated, and any hemorrhagic tendency should be corrected prior to biopsy.*

If a hemorrhagic tendency cannot be corrected, percutaneous needle biopsy of the kidney should not be performed.

III. Equipment

A. *A Franklin modified Vim-Silverman biopsy needle* (small size) should be used (Fig. 9–1).*

1. The Franklin modification consists of metal plugs which seal the tips of the cutting prongs. This modification allows the base of the biopsy specimen to be cut from the surrounding tissue. The unmodified Vim-Silverman needle should not be used for renal biopsy, as the open tips of the cutting prongs are often responsible for failure to obtain biopsy samples.
2. Biopsy needles *must* be maintained in excellent condition if good renal biopsy specimens are to be consistently obtained.
3. The clinician should acquire experience in using the biopsy needle by practicing on necropsy specimens.

---

*Available from V. Mueller and Co., 6600 West Touhy Ave., Chicago, Illinois 60648.

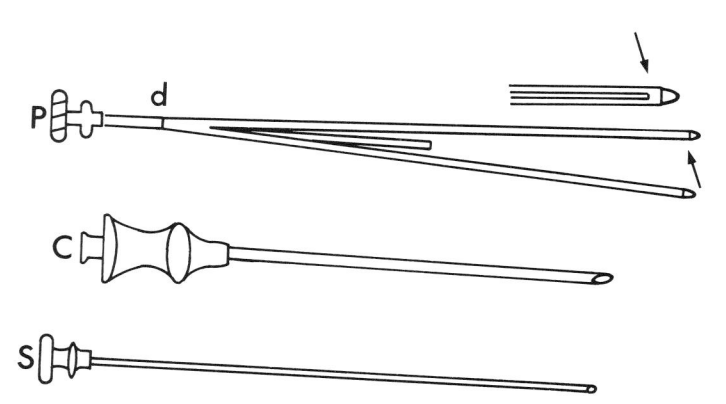

Figure 9–1. Franklin modified Vim-Silverman biopsy needle: *P*, cutting prongs; *d*, change in outside diameter of cutting prongs; *C*, outer cannula; *S*, stylet. The tips of the cutting prongs have been sealed (arrows). (Current Veterinary Therapy, Vol. 4, Philadelphia, W. B. Saunders Co., 1971.)

B. *A surgical pack containing the following items should be prepared.*
   1. Sharp pointed tissue scissors and scalpel.
   2. Hemostats.
   3. Thumb forceps.
   4. Needle holder, suture needles, suture material, gauze sponges.
   5. Drapes, towel forceps, gloves.

C. *Bacterial culturing equipment and appropriate fixtures including 10% buffered formalin*

IV. Choice of biopsy site

Either the right or left kidney may be biopsied.

A. *In dogs to be biopsied by the blind percutaneous technique, the left kidney may be chosen if it can be adequately immobilized by digital palpation per abdomen.*

The right kidney is rarely palpable per abdomen in the dog. In general the blind percutaneous technique should be avoided in dogs because of difficulty in controlling the path of the needle.

B. *Both kidneys can usually be localized and immobilized by digital palpation per abdomen in the cat.*

C. *The right kidney is usually chosen in the dog if the "key-hole" technique is used.*

Its anatomical position is more constant than the left kidney's because the right kidney is more firmly attached to the body wall.

V. Restraint

A. *Morphine sulfate (1 mg. per lb. of body weight) combined with atropine sulfate and a local anesthetic (lidocaine hydrochloride) provides satisfactory restraint and anesthesia for most dogs.*

B. *Meperidine hydrochloride* (5 mg. per lb. of body weight) combined with promazine hydrochloride** (2 mg. per lb. of body weight) prior to local anesthesia with lidocaine hydrochloride is adequate for most cats.*

C. *Ketamine hydrochloride may be used in cats, provided renal function is adequate to excrete the drug.*

Ketamine hydrochloride should be used with great caution, if at all, in uremic cats since the drug is excreted in active form in urine.

D. *General anesthesia with halothane may be used in dogs and cats if the patients are not poor anesthetic risks.*

In the majority of patients, this is the preferred method of anesthesia.

E. *In patients that are profoundly depressed, local anesthesia may suffice.*

Epidural anesthesia may be considered.

VI. Techniques

A. *The technique for the keyhole biopsy procedure is as follows:*
   1. Surgically prepare a wide area over the kidney to be biopsied.
   2. Induce local or general anesthesia.

---
*Demerol Hydrochloride, Winthrop Laboratories, New York, N.Y.
**Sparine, Wyeth Laboratories Inc., Philadelphia, Pa.

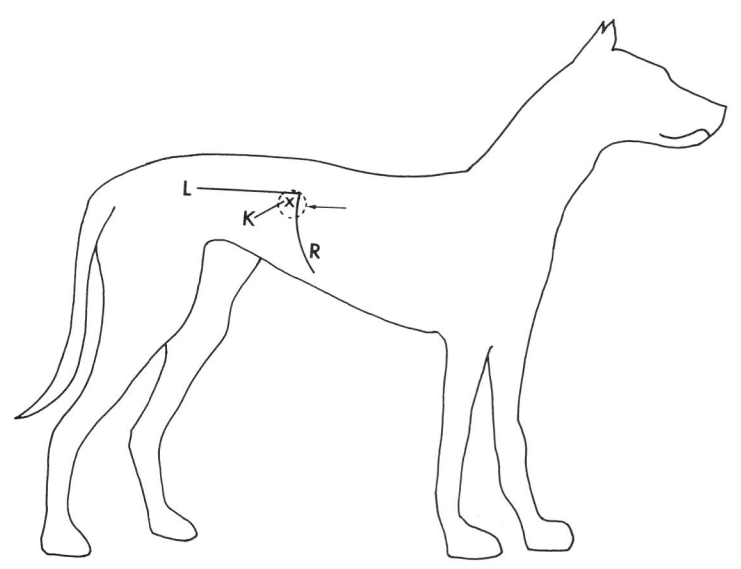

Figure 9–2. Diagram of landmarks for the keyhole technique of percutaneous renal biopsy: L, ventral border of lumbar muscles; R, thirteenth rib; arrow, position of right kidney; K, incision line, which is equidistant between the caudal border of the thirteenth rib and the ventral border of the lumbar muscles; X, point of insertion of biopsy needle over caudal pole of the kidney. (Current Veterinary Therapy, Vol. 4, Philadelphia, W. B. Saunders Co., 1971.)

3. Make an oblique paralumbar skin incision large enough to accommodate an index finger over the caudal pole of the kidney (Fig. 9–2).
    a. The incision should be made caudal to the last rib and just below the ventral border of the lumbar muscles.
    b. The long axis of incision should be equidistant between the last rib and the ventral border of the longissimus muscle mass.
    c. The intercostal artery just caudal to the last rib should be avoided.
4. Bluntly dissect fascia, muscle, and peritoneum with sharp pointed tissue scissors.
5. Insert the index finger through the incision, into the peritoneal cavity, and palpate the kidney and surrounding structures.
    a. Evaluate the size, shape, position, contour, and consistency of the kidney.
    b. Evaluate both kidneys if possible.
    c. Palpate adjacent abdominal viscera, peritoneum, vessels, etc.
6. Introduce the biopsy needle through a separate site in the body wall, cranial to the keyhole site. Insertion of the biopsy needle through the keyhole incision containing the index finger will usually result in inability to properly position the biopsy instrument.
    a. In order to facilitate passage of the needle through the skin, make a small skin incision with a curved scalpel blade.
    b. Guide the biopsy needle into the peritoneal cavity, and then to the kidney, with the index finger.
7. Immobilize the kidney by displacing it against the body wall or other adjacent structures with the index finger.
    a. Position the biopsy needle so that the exact route the cutting prongs will follow can be predetermined.
    b. Direct the long axis of the biopsy needle away from the renal artery,

vein, and renal pelvis, and push the needle just through the renal capsule.
- (1) Proper positioning of the biopsy needle will eliminate the possibility of damage to large vessels and penetration of the renal pelvis.
- (2) Large vessels of the renal medulla should be avoided because the degree of renal damage caused by the biopsy needle is primarily dependent on the size and number of renal vessels damaged. Because the renal vessels of the dog and cat progressively diminish in size from the renal hilus to the capsular surface, significantly less damage will be induced in the renal parenchyma by biopsy tracts confined to the renal cortex. The chance of damaging large vessels progressively increases with depth of penetration into the kidney.
- c. Try to avoid positioning the needle in such a way that the cutting prongs will pass through the renal capsule twice.
- d. *Do not overpenetrate beyond the renal capsule* or the quantity of renal cortex in the biopsy specimen will be inadequate!
8. Replace the stylet with the cutting prongs. Experience has revealed that if the cutting prongs can be inserted to their full depth without meeting resistance, the outer cannula has not penetrated the renal capsule.
9. Rapidly thrust the cutting prongs into the renal tissue. If the cutting prongs are advanced too slowly, the kidney has a tendency to move away from the biopsy instrument, and the size of the biopsy specimen is reduced.
10. An assistant should then grasp the hub of the cutting prongs with an index finger and thumb and firmly hold them in this exact position.
11. Without changing the spatial relationship of the cutting prongs, the outer cannula should be advanced over the blades. Rotation of the outer cannula 5 degrees clockwise and then 5 degrees counterclockwise as it is being advanced over the cutting prongs will help to prevent overpenetration of the outer cannula into the renal parenchyma.
    - a. Care must be used so that the assistant does not exert countertraction on the cutting prongs. If the latter occurs, the length of the biopsy specimen will be reduced, or a biopsy specimen will not be obtained.
    - b. The outer cannula should be advanced just beyond the change in the outside diameter of the nonsplit end of the prongs. This landmark indicates that the outer cannula has forced the cutting prongs into apposition. Further penetration of the outer cannula serves no useful purpose, but causes unnecessary damage to the renal parenchyma. Conservation of functional renal parenchyma is of prime importance to a patient with generalized renal disease. If biopsy needles do not have this landmark, a mark should be placed in the appropriate location on the cutting prongs. This location may easily be determined by inserting the cutting prongs into the outer cannula until the tips of the blades become visible at the end of the outer cannula.
12. Remove the cutting prongs and outer cannula. It is unnecessary to rotate the cutting prongs if the Franklin modified Vim-Silverman needle is used, because the seal at the tips of the cutting prong blades cut the base of the specimen.

13. Carefully remove the biopsy specimen from the biopsy needle.
    a. Place the specimen in an appropriate fixative. Do not damage the sample.
        (1) For routine histologic procedures, the biopsy sample should be fixed in 10% buffered formalin.
        (2) If additional biopsy specimens are not to be taken, the cutting prongs containing the biopsy specimen should be placed in a bottle of fixative. The specimen should be allowed to fix for a short period of time prior to removal from the needle.
        (3) If additional samples are to be taken with the same needle, the biopsy sample may be gently lifted from the cutting prongs with a sterile, pointed, wooden applicator stick.
    b. If a portion of the biopsy specimen is desired for impression smears, it may be divided longitudinally into equal halves with the aid of a hand magnifying lens. In most instances where impression smears are desired, it is usually best to obtain an additional sample. With the exception of biopsy samples obtained from diseased kidneys characterized by highly cellular inflammatory responses or highly cellular neoplasms, cytologic evaluation of impression smears is usually unrewarding.
    c. Biopsy material or blood aspirated from the kidney through the outer cannula may be utilized for culture of bacterial or mycotic agents.
14. The biopsy needle may be repositioned if additional biopsy samples are required.
15. Close the surgical wound in a routine manner.
16. Be sure serious hemorrhage is not present prior to repair of the surgical wound.
    a. Spontaneous hemostasis will usually occur within two to seven minutes following removal of the biopsy needle from the kidney if the procedure has been properly performed.
    b. In the event that significant hemorrhage occurs, digital pressure applied over the biopsy site for a period of minutes is often sufficient to enhance clotting.
    c. In the event that severe uncontrollable hemorrhage continues, oxidized regenerated cellulose* may be placed on the renal capsule over the biopsy site.
    d. If hemorrhage cannot be controlled by these methods, the keyhole incision should be lengthened, and the affected kidney should be exposed and examined. Oxidized regenerated cellulose should be applied over the needle wound in the kidney and sutured to the renal capsule. This emergency procedure will be unnecessary if the biopsy technique is performed correctly.

B. *The technique for percutaneous renal biopsy with manual localization of the kidney per abdomen is as follows:*
  1. Surgically prepare the proposed biopsy site.
  2. Manually localize and immobilize the kidney by digital palpation.
  3. Make a small skin incision over the proposed biopsy site to facilitate entry of the biopsy needle.

---
*Surgicel, Johnson & Johnson, New Brunswick, N.J.

4. Proceed as for the keyhole technique.
5. The correct position of the biopsy needle may be verified by the resistance which the cutting prongs transmit as the renal capsule is encountered. If the cutting prongs can be inserted to full depth without meeting resistance, the outer cannula has not encountered the renal capsule.
6. Although the blind percutaneous technique is satisfactory for percutaneous renal biopsy in cats, it cannot be routinely employed for percutaneous renal biopsy in dogs.
    a. The success of percutaneous renal biopsy techniques in dogs and cats is dependent on adequate localization and immobilization of kidneys, so that representative samples of tissue can be obtained with every biopsy attempt without serious risk to the patient.
    b. Adequate localization and immobilization of normal-sized and abnormally small canine kidneys by digital palpation per abdomen is typically difficult and does not permit precise projection of the path that the cutting prongs will follow as they are thrust into the renal parenchyma.
    c. In cats, the blind percutaneous technique of renal biopsy has been routinely satisfactory because either kidney can usually be localized and immobilized by digital palpation per abdomen with ease.

C. *Biopsy of the kidneys at laparotomy may be indicated when:*
1. Patients have surgically correctable disease processes which are associated with renal failure (e.g., pyometra). Evaluation of a renal biopsy specimen may indicate whether functional impairment of the kidneys is reversible or irreversible.
2. Significant gross alterations of the kidney are detected during an exploratory laparotomy.

D. *Biopsy of the kidneys with a fine needle* is indicated to:*
1. Obtain culture material from kidneys suspected of having disease caused by bacteria.
2. Obtain cells from kidneys suspected of having highly cellular neoplasms (i.e., malignant lymphoma, renal cell carcinoma).
3. Aspirate fluid from pyonephrotic or hydronephrotic kidneys.

VII. Post-Biopsy Care

A. *Closely observe the patient for signs of hemorrhage for 24 hours.*

B. *Provide cage rest.*

C. *Excessive manipulation of the biopsied kidney by digital palpation should be avoided for a short time following completion of the biopsy procedure.*

D. *Whole blood transfusions will usually control most serious bleeding problems in the event they occur.*

E. *Antibiotics are not essential if aseptic technique is maintained (see Chapter 33, Drug Therapy in Renal Failure).*

F. *On rare occasions, nephrectomies have been performed in human patients to arrest uncontrollable hemorrhage from the kidney.*

---

*Franzen Thin Biopsy Needle, United States Catheter and Instrument Corporation, P.O. Box 787, Glens Falls, New York 12801.

114 DIAGNOSIS OF URINARY DISEASES

VIII. Absolute contraindications

  A. *Patients with uncorrected hemorrhagic tendencies*

  B. *Clinicians inexperienced with the use of the biopsy needle and the technique*
   1. Careful attention to the procedural detail is essential if adequate biopsy specimens are to be consistently obtained without serious risk to the patient.
   2. Blind insertion of a biopsy needle on a "hit or miss" basis is never justified.

  C. *Renal abscesses*

  D. *Advanced hydronephrosis or pyonephrosis*

  A 22 to 25 gauge needle and syringe may be used to aspirate a sample of fluid from hydronephrotic or pyonephrotic kidneys.

IX. Post-Biopsy Complications

  A. *The occurrence and frequency of post-biopsy complications are dependent upon:*
   1. The skill of the clinician.
   2. The condition of the patient prior to biopsy.
   3. The degree to which biopsy contraindications are observed.
   4. The technique employed.

  B. *Self-limiting microscopic hematuria usually occurs for one half to three days following biopsy.*

  C. *Transient, self-limiting gross hematuria may be observed in a small percentage of the cases.*

  D. *When severe hemorrhage occurs, it usually is caused by faulty technique.*

  E. *Although uncommon, clotted blood in the renal pelvis caused obstruction to urine flow and secondary hydronephrosis in a cat.*

  Administration of fluids prior to, and immediately following, renal biopsy may prevent blood from clotting in the excretory pathway of the urinary system by inducing diuresis.

  F. *Complications reported in man but not as yet encountered in dogs and cats include:*
   1. Renal arteriovenous fistulas.
   2. Perirenal extravasation of urine.
   3. Injury to adjacent organs.

  G. *Although percutaneous renal biopsy should be regarded as having the potential risk of causing a fatal complication, the risk of fatality should be kept in proper perspective.*

  No fatalities have occurred in approximately 250 consecutive renal biopsies of dogs and cats at the University of Minnesota.

  H. *The possibility of serious post-biopsy complications dictates the clinical use of the procedure only when the information obtained would be of probable benefit to the patient.*

  When the results are likely to establish a specific diagnosis, to determine the type of therapy, or to indicate the prognosis, the indication for renal

PERCUTANEOUS RENAL BIOPSY

biopsy is absolute provided the patient can tolerate the procedure without risk of serious complications.

X. Needle biopsy limitations

A. *Focal distribution of lesions*
1. Inability to consistently detect focal lesions is an inherent limitation of all needle biopsy techniques.
2. The sampling error of needle biopsy must be kept in proper perspective. In general, the success of attempts to detect focal renal lesions by needle biopsy is dependent upon:
   a. The distribution and size of the lesions.
   b. The size of the biopsy specimen.
   c. The number of biopsy samples obtained.
   d. The technique employed (i.e., blind, keyhole, or surgical).
3. The chance of detecting focal renal lesions by needle biopsy in patients with clinical evidence of renal disease is good because focal lesions generally do not cause signs of renal disease until they become widespread in distribution.
4. Detection of focal renal lesions by needle biopsy in patients before there are clinical signs of renal disease is more difficult. By digital palpation of the kidneys during biopsy by the keyhole technique, it may be possible to detect the presence of focal lesions that involve the surface of the kidneys.

B. *Some histopathologic features, such as the presence of amyloid or neoplastic cells, allow establishment of a specific diagnosis, while other changes are not diagnostic and may occur as the result of a variety of different renal diseases (Fig. 9–3).*

C. *Correct interpretations of observations made by histologic examination of renal*

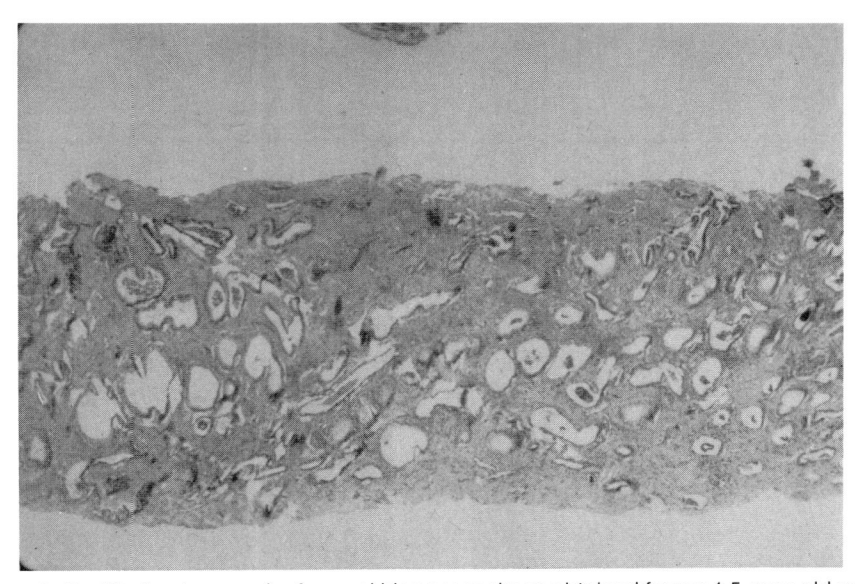

Figure 9–3. Photomicrograph of a renal biopsy specimen obtained from a 1.5-year-old male great dane dog. Microscopic examination of the biopsy sample revealed end-stage kidney disease. The cause of the renal disease could not be established on the basis of light microscopic examination of renal tissue. H&E stain; × 25.

biopsy samples are sometimes difficult to make because of a lack of recognized changes in morphology associated with early stages of specific diseases.

D. *Although various renal diseases have been classified as acute, subacute, and chronic on the basis of morphologic criteria, sharp divisions between various stages of renal diseases often do not exist.*

Depending on the biological behavior of the disease, lesions may undergo resolution, become inactive but irreversible, or they may become progressive and irreversible. In many renal diseases of the dog, the etiology is unknown or cannot be defined on the basis of morphologic alterations. Thus it is not always possible to determine the evolution, reversibility, or probable future behavior of a lesion on the basis of a single biopsy specimen. In many diseases, it is necessary to evaluate serial renal function tests and serial renal biopsies.

E. *Clinical and experimental investigations have revealed that it is often not possible to predict the type and severity of functional abnormalities on the basis of pathologic lesions, and vice versa.*

The degree of reversibility and functional compensation which occurs following injury to the kidneys varies from patient to patient and from disease to disease. Histologic examination alone is not a reliable index of these factors in every instance. Both function and morphology must be evaluated when an attempt is being made to ascertain the ability of the kidneys to repair injury and regain normal function.

XI. Routine processing and staining of biopsy samples

A. *Meaningful evaluation of biopsy samples, especially glomeruli, is dependent on obtaining thin sections of a consistent thickness.*
   1. A tissue thickness of one to six microns has been recommended by various investigators.
   2. Thin sections are favored by most pathologists because they facilitate evaluation of the character of cells, and the degree of cellularity of glomeruli.
   3. If thin sections are desired, excessively long fixation time should be avoided as it may cause the specimen to become brittle, and may prevent satisfactory preparation of thin sections with a microtome. A formalin fixation time of three to four hours is recommended for needle biopsy specimens of kidney.
   4. Regardless of the tissue thickness chosen, it is imperative to have tissue sections consistently cut at the same thickness so that one may become familiar with the morphology of renal structures at that thickness.
      a. Glomeruli can be made to appear hypocellular or hypercellular by varying the thickness of tissue sections.
      b. Thickened basement membranes may be mimicked by thick sections.
      c. These artefacts may be erroneously interpreted as lesions.

B. *Special stains may be of great value.*

C. *Diagnostic probabilities should be discussed with a pathologist prior to biopsy so that special fixatives or stains can be provided when indicated.*

XII. Biopsy sample artefacts

Renal biopsy samples obtained with a Franklin modified Vim-Silverman biopsy needle may contain artefacts induced by the biopsy needle.

A. The edges of the biopsy sample will be compressed to a varying degree.

Lateral movement of the cutting prongs at the time they are in the tissue will induce tissue compression.

B. Intraluminal desquamation of tubular epithelial cells will occur to some degree in all biopsy samples and is usually most prominent in the medulla.

REFERENCES

Lavastida, M. T., Musil, G., and Hulet, W. H.: A disposable needle for percutaneous renal biopsy. Clin. Pediat., 7:170–173, 1968.

Muehrcke, R. C., Mandal, A. K., Gotoff, S. P., Isaccs, E. W., and Violini, F. I.: The clinical value of electron microscopy in renal disease. Arch. Int. Med., 124:170–176, 1969.

Osborne, C. A.: Clinical evaluation of needle biopsy of the kidney and its complications in the dog and cat. J.A.V.M.A., 158:1213–1228, 1971.

Osborne, C. A.: Modified Franklin-Silverman biopsy needle. J. Urol., 107:358–359, Mar., 1972.

Osborne, C. A., and Low, D. G.: Size, adequacy and artifacts of canine renal biopsy samples. Amer. J. Vet. Res., 32:1865–1871, Nov., 1971.

Osborne, C. A., and Low, D. G.: Iatrogenic lesions in serial renal biopsy samples. J. Urol., 106:805–809, Dec., 1971.

Osborne, C. A., Low, D. G., and Jessen, C. R.: Renal parenchymal response to needle biopsy. Invest. Urol., In Press, May, 1972.

Osborne, C. A., Finco, D. R., Low, D. G., and Perman, V.: Percutaneous renal biopsy in the dog and cat. J.A.V.M.A., 151:1474–1480, 1967.

Pirani, C. L., and Salinas-Madrigal, L.: Evaluation of percutaneous renal biopsies. *In* Pathology Annual 1968. Edited by S. C. Sommers. New York, N. Y., Appleton, Century, Crofts, 1968.

Sweet, I. E., Davidson, A. J., and Hayslett, J. P.: Complication of needle biopsy of the kidney in the dog. Radiology, 92:849–854, 1969.

Chapter 10
CYSTOSCOPY

I. **Definition.** Cystoscopy is the technique in which an endoscope is used to visually examine the lower urinary tract.

II. **Equipment**
   A. *A variety of endoscopes have been designed for examination of the human urinary bladder and urethra.*
      1. Cystoscopes and panendoscopes are most commonly used.
         a. A cystoscope permits visualization of structures which are at right angles to the long axis of the instrument.
         b. A panendoscope permits visualization of structures which are directly in front and at oblique angles to the long axis of the instrument. Consequently it can be used as both a cystoscope and a urethroscope.
         c. By interchanging telescopes, some endoscopes can be used as cystoscopes and panendoscopes.
      2. The basic components of cystoscopes and panendoscopes include:
         a. An outer hollow shaft with an obturator.
         b. A telescope which fits inside the outer shaft.
            (1) Telescopes have a variety of different lens systems.
            (2) Alteration of the lens systems permits visualization of structures at various angles in relation to the endoscope.
            (3) The most common types of lens systems are:
               (a) Direct.
               (b) Forward.
               (c) Foroblique.
               (d) Right angle.
               (e) Retrograde.
      3. Accessory components for cystoscopes and panendoscopes include:
         a. Instruments to crush calculi (lithotrites).
         b. Instruments for tissue biopsy.
         c. Instruments which permit electrocautery.
         d. Instruments which aid in catheterization of the ureters.

   B. *Instruments* which have been successfully used in dogs include:*
      1. Wappler cystoscope.
      2. Ravich convertible cystoscope.
      3. Brown-Buerger cystoscope.
      4. McCarthy panendoscope (pediatric size).

---

*American Cystoscope Makers Inc., Pelham Manor, N.Y. 10803.

III. Indications

  A. *Diagnostic indications for cystoscopy include:*
  1. Direct visualization of the mucosa of the urethra or bladder with the objective of detecting ulcers, neoplasms, diverticulae, etc.
  2. Detection of uroliths.
  3. Transurethral biopsy of lesions.
  4. Visualization of ureteral orifices and ureteral expulsion of urine.
  5. Ureteral catheterization for:
     a. Retrograde pyelography.
     b. Renal function studies of individual kidneys.

  B. *Therapeutic indications for cystoscopy include:*
  1. Transurethral treatment of bladder lesions.
     a. Transurethral surgery may be performed with a resectoscope.
     b. Fulguration.
     c. Removal of calculi with a lithotrite.
  2. Dilation of urethral strictures.

IV. Cystoscopy in dogs

  A. *Females*
  1. Medium-size and large dogs may be evaluated with human cystoscopes.
  2. Although general anesthesia may be used, female dogs have been cystoscoped without pharmacologic restraint.
  3. If large instruments are used, it may be necessary to dilate the urethral lumen with sounds prior to cystoscopy.

  B. *Males*
  1. The anatomy of the canine male urethra does not permit the use of human cystoscopes.
  2. Human cystoscopes may be used in medium-size and large male dogs following urethrotomy or urethrostomy. The incision in the urethra should be placed in the area of the ischial arch of the bony pelvis.
  3. Flexible fiberoptic ureteroscopes may be passed into the bladder of male dogs in a manner similar to that described for catheterization (see Chapter 5, Collection of Urine). The value of ureteroscopes is limited since it is difficult to properly irrigate the bladder during cystoscopy. In addition, specialized instruments for biopsy or surgery cannot be used in conjunction with a ureteroscope.

  C. *Technique*
  1. Restrain the patient and thoroughly cleanse periurethral skin.
  2. If necessary, dilate the urethra with an appropriate sound.
  3. Insert a lubricated, sterilized cystoscope into the bladder via the urethra.
  4. Replace the obturator with a telescope.
  5. Irrigate the bladder with sterilized physiologic saline or a commercially prepared genitourinary irrigating solution.
     a. Instill just enough solution to permit adequate visualization.
     b. Do not overdistend the bladder with irrigant solution as this commonly causes petechial hemorrhages in the mucosa.

6. Various portions of the bladder or urethra may be visualized by manipulating the instrument.
    a. A right angle telescope provides best visualization of the ureteral orifices.
    b. A foroblique telescope provides best visualization of the urethra.
7. The ureters may be catheterized with 4 to 6 F. ureteral catheters.

D. *Consult standard textbooks of human urology and specific references for additional details about cystoscopy.*

REFERENCES

Barringer, B. B.: Cystoscopic examination of female dogs. J. Urol., *57*:185–189, 1947.
Bauer, K. M.: Cystoscopic Diagnosis. Philadelphia, Pa., Lea and Febiger, 1969.
Ensor, R. D., Boyarsky, S., and Glenn, J. F.: Cystoscopy and ureteral catheterization in the dog. J.A.V.M.A., *149*:1067–1072, 1966.
Takagi, T., Go, T., Takayasu, H., and Aso, Y.: Fiberoptic pyeloureteroscope. Surgery, *70*:661–666, 1971.
Tanagho, E. A., and Lyon, R. P.: Urethral dilatation versus internal urethrotomy. J. Urol., *105*:242–244, 1971.
Thompson, I. M., and Baker, J. J.: The histologic effects of dilation and internal urethrotomy on the canine urethra. J. Urol., *103*:168–173, 1970.
Vermooten, V.: Cystoscopy in male and female dogs. J. Lab. Clin. Med., *15*:650–657, 1930.

Chapter 11
SUMMARY OF DIAGNOSTIC ASPECTS OF URINARY DISEASE

I. **History and physical examination**

   A. *An accurate history aids the clinician in reducing innumerable diagnostic possibilities to diagnostic probabilities.*

   B. *The results of a physical examination may not be sufficiently specific to allow one to make a definitive diagnosis, but they often allow one to formulate tentative diagnoses comprised of diagnostic probabilities.*

   C. *Once the presence of urinary abnormalities is suspected on the basis of the history and physical examination, appropriate laboratory, radiographic, or biopsy information should be obtained to confirm the presence of urinary dysfunction, to determine whether the cause is related to extraurinary or primary disturbances of urinary function, and to determine whether the disease is reversible or irreversible.*

II. **Urinalyses**

   A. *Significant numbers of RBC, WBC, and protein known to originate from the urinary tract indicate the presence of inflammatory disease.*

   B. *Persistent hematuria in the absence of an inflammatory response that is known to originate from the urinary tract is suggestive of trauma or neoplasia.*

   C. *Persistent and severe proteinuria not associated with hematuria and pyuria indicates the presence of generalized glomerular disease.*

   D. *The presence of significant numbers of casts localizes the disease process to the kidneys, and, depending on their type, may indicate significant damage to distal tubules and collecting ducts.*

III. **Hemograms**

Evaluation of hemograms (PCV, Hb, blood smears) facilitates evaluation of erythropoietin stimulating factor produced by the kidneys. Evaluation of WBC (total count and differential count) may provide information about severe inflammatory processes of the urinary system. Severe inflammatory processes are more likely to cause leucocytosis when they are renal rather than bladder in origin.

IV. **Renal function tests**

   A. *Generally, renal function studies are of little assistance in establishing the etiology of renal disease since function tests indicate the degree and type of abnormal function, but not the underlying cause.*

122 DIAGNOSIS OF URINARY DISEASES

B. *In view of the multiplicity of renal functions and the fact that various renal functions may vary independently of each other, it is evident that no single test is adequate for complete evaluation of the overall functional capacity of the kidneys.*

Meaningful evaluation of renal function is best obtained by serial evaluation of a combination of selected tests. Appropriate selection of the tests must be based on the problem at hand.

C. *Urine specific gravity or osmolality*
1. The ability of the kidneys to excrete urine with a specific gravity or osmolality above or below that of glomerular filtrate provides information relative to the functional competence of the distal tubules and collecting ducts since it is in these areas that water absorption or excretion is governed by antidiuretic hormone. Interpretation may require periods of controlled water intake (urine concentration test), or administration of exogenous antidiuretic hormone (vasopressin concentration test).
2. Once urine specific gravity becomes fixed at that of glomerular filtrate (1.008 to 1.012), it is not a reliable index of intrinsic tubular damage since, in addition to generalized tubular disease, fixation of specific gravity may occur as a result of factors not specifically related to intrinsic tubular damage.
3. Impaired ability to concentrate or dilute urine as detected by evaluation of specific gravity is usually not detectable until approximately two thirds of the total functional capacity has been incapacitated.

D. *Blood urea nitrogen or creatinine concentration*
1. Evaluation of the serum concentration of BUN or creatinine provides a crude index of glomerular filtration rate.
2. Abnormal elevation of the concentration of these substances which occurs as a result of impaired renal function is not detectable until approximately 70 to 75 per cent of the nephrons of both kidneys become nonfunctional.

E. *Endogenous creatinine clearance*

Evaluation of glomerular filtration rate by endogenous creatinine clearance may allow functional abnormalities to be detected earlier during the course of renal diseases than is possible by evaluation of urine specific gravity, BUN, or creatinine concentration.

F. *Urinary excretion of PSP dye*
1. Determination of urinary excretion of a low dose (6 mg.) of PSP dye is primarily an index of renal blood flow.
2. Determination of urinary excretion of larger doses (100 mg. per square meter of surface area) of PSP dye may be used as an index of proximal tubular function.

V. Serum electrolytes

A. *With few exceptions (pseudo-hyperparathyroidism), evaluation of the concentration of serum or plasma electrolytes is not of significant diagnostic value with respect to primary diseases of the kidneys.*

B. *Knowledge of the types and degrees of electrolyte abnormalities often provides information of prognostic and therapeutic significance, however, and may provide information which supports or denies tentative diagnoses.*

VI. Serum and urine enzymes

Enzyme tests which are of significant diagnostic value in urinary disease have not been developed for clinical use in dogs and cats. Lack of specificity, false positive and false negative results, and large fluctuations in normal concentration have been major disadvantages associated with enzyme tests.

VII. Radiology

A. *In general, conventional radiographic techniques localize disease processes to various segments of the urinary system.*
  1. They may provide information of sufficient preciseness to establish a specific diagnosis, especially when related to diseases of the ureters, urinary bladder, and urethra. Some examples include:
     a. Uroliths.
     b. Rents in the excretory pathway which permit the escape of urine (and radiopaque media).
     c. Abnormal locations of organs of the urinary system.
     d. Ectopic ureters.
  2. In several instances, however, radiographs do not provide information of sufficient preciseness to establish a specific diagnosis; this is especially applicable to diseases of the kidneys.

B. *Excretory urograms may be used as a crude qualitative index of renal function.*

C. *Although determination of kidney size by radiography will not provide an etiologic diagnosis, it may provide information of value in differentiating acute from chronic generalized renal disease.*

VIII. Renal biopsy

Microscopic evaluation of morphologic changes in renal biopsy samples may indicate the potential reversibility or irreversibility of primary renal disease since, in addition to establishment of a specific morphologic diagnosis, the stage (acute or chronic) and severity of the disease process may be established.

IX. Summary

Antemortem differentiation of potentially reversible from progressive irreversible urinary diseases is an essential prerequisite to establishment of a meaningful prognosis and intelligent choice of the proper regimen of therapy. With logical use and interpretation of the history, physical findings, pertinent laboratory data, radiographic findings, and biopsy findings, such an antemortem distinction can frequently be established.

DISEASES OF THE UPPER URINARY SYSTEM

Chapter 12
PATHOPHYSIOLOGY OF RENAL FAILURE

I. **There is a significant difference between renal disease and renal failure.**

　A. *Renal disease indicates the presence of renal lesions of any size, distribution (focal or generalized), or cause in one or both kidneys.*

　　Depending on the quantity of renal parenchyma involved and the severity of lesions, renal disease may or may not be associated with renal failure.

　B. *Renal failure indicates that three fourths or more of the functional capacity of the nephrons of both kidneys has been eliminated.*

　　Renal failure may be caused by functional or organic abnormalities (or both) which are acute or chronic, reversible or irreversible. The term renal failure is analogous to heart failure in that a level of organ function is described rather than a specific disease entity.

II. **Prerenal, postrenal, and primary renal failure**

　A. *Renal failure*

　　When the functional or structural integrity of both kidneys has been compromised to such a degree that signs of renal failure become manifest clinically, a relatively predictable symptom complex called uremia appears, regardless of underlying cause. Uremic crises may be precipitated in patients by acute or chronic, reversible or irreversible, prerenal, postrenal or primary renal disorders which alter the functional capacity of nephrons. In some instances, uremic crises may suddenly be precipitated by a combination of prerenal or postrenal factors which develop in patients with previously compensated primary renal failure.

　B. *From a clinical, diagnostic, prognostic, and therapeutic point of view, it is useful to divide renal failure into prerenal, primary (organic) renal, and postrenal categories.*

　　The validity of this classification is based on the fact that the pathophysiology of renal failure is dependent on the anatomic site of the predisposing cause.

　　1. Prerenal uremia is caused by abnormalities which reduce renal function by decreasing renal perfusion with blood (i.e., cardiac disease, shock, dehydration, hypoadrenalcorticism).

　　　a. Since blood pressure provides the force necessary for glomerular filtration, decrease in blood pressure below a critical level (approximately 60 mm. Hg) will result in cessation of glomerular filtration and anuria. Less severe reductions in renal perfusion pressure and glomerular filtration will result in oliguria.

　　　b. Prerenal uremia implies the presence of structurally normal kidneys

which are initially capable of quantitatively normal function, provided the prerenal cause is rapidly removed. If the prerenal cause is allowed to persist, primary ischemic renal disease may develop.
   c. A diagnosis of prerenal uremia may be established on the basis of abnormal elevation in the concentration of BUN or creatinine, and a high urine specific gravity (i.e., greater than 1.025).
      (1) It is theoretically possible to have an abnormal elevation of blood urea nitrogen or serum creatinine concentration associated with an elevated urine specific gravity in patients with primary renal failure. The renal lesion in such patients must be characterized by generalized glomerular damage which has not yet affected the renal tubules. Clinical experience has revealed that the probability of encountering a dog or cat with this type of primary renal disorder is not great.
2. Postrenal uremia is caused by diseases which prevent excretion of urine from the body.
   a. Causes include obstruction of the urethra, bladder, or both ureters, and rupture of the excretory pathway.
   b. Like prerenal uremia, a diagnosis of postrenal uremia implies the presence of structurally normal kidneys which are initially capable of quantitatively normal function provided the underlying cause is rapidly corrected. If the postrenal cause is allowed to persist, varying degrees of obstructive uropathy may develop, or the patient may die of fluid and electrolyte abnormalities (ruptured excretory pathway).
3. Primary uremia.
   a. Primary or organic uremia may be caused by a large number of disease processes (infection, ischemia, toxic agents, obstruction, congenital anomalies, neoplasia) which have in common destruction of at least three fourths of the parenchyma of both kidneys.
   b. Depending on the biological behavior of the disease in question, primary uremia may be reversible or irreversible.

III. Acute versus chronic renal failure

A. *Once the presence of primary renal failure has been established, it is often difficult to determine whether the underlying lesion is acute or chronic.*
   1. It is clinically useful to make such a distinction because, in general, a favorable prognosis is more often justified for patients with acute generalized renal failure than for those with chronic generalized renal failure.
   2. Usually, chronic generalized renal diseases of the dog are progressive and irreversible.

B. *The clinical findings associated with acute and chronic renal failure are more similar than dissimilar because functional and morphological abnormalities of the kidneys can be clinically manifested in only a limited number of ways.*
   1. Weakness, depression, anorexia, stomatitis, gastrointestinal disturbances, and central nervous system disturbances may occur in acute or chronic, reversible or irreversible renal failure.
   2. The presence of these signs does indicate the presence of generalized functional impairment, since approximately three fourths of the nephrons of both kidneys must be nonfunctional before signs become clinically manifest.

C. *Detection of progressive weight loss, anorexia, polyuria, nocturia, and polydipsia is reliable evidence of chronic generalized renal disease.*

Detection of abnormally small kidneys by digital palpation or radiography is also a finding which indicates the presence of irreversible generalized chronic renal disease.
  1. Chronicity may be inferred from the fact that all these clinical signs require time to develop.
  2. The generalized nature of the renal disease may be inferred from the fact that at least three fourths or more of the renal parenchyma must be functionally incapacitated before the signs become clinically apparent.
  3. Irreversibility of the renal disease may be inferred because most chronic generalized renal diseases of dogs and cats are progressive and irreversible.

D. *Certain exceptions to the above generalities exist, however, and should be considered when interpreting the significance of various signs of renal failure.*
  1. The absence of signs associated with chronic generalized renal disease does not consistently exclude its presence. Progressive renal diseases that destroy renal parenchyma at a relatively slow rate allow viable nephrons to undergo structural and functional compensation. Thus a numerically greater number of nephrons may be destroyed before renal function is reduced to such a degree that abnormalities become clinically detectable.
  2. Polyuria, nocturia, and polydipsia are cardinal signs of chronic generalized renal disease, but also may occur with acute generalized renal disease, and during the recovery phase of acute renal failure caused by ischemia or nephrotoxins. The history about the duration of polyuria and polydipsia may be of value in distinguishing between acute and chronic renal disease.
  3. Oliguria is the cardinal sign of the early phases of acute renal failure caused by generalized ischemic or nephrotoxic tubular disease; however, it also may occur as a terminal event in chronic generalized renal disease.

IV. Reversible versus irreversible renal failure

Ante-mortem differentiation of potentially reversible from progressive irreversible renal failure is an essential prerequisite to establishment of a meaningful prognosis and intelligent choice of therapy. The detection of renal diseases which are potentially reversible is justification for aggressive use of therapeutic regimens, whereas irreversible renal failure may not warrant such effort and expense. The distinction between potentially reversible from irreversible renal failure on the basis of clinical findings is usually difficult because of the nonspecificity of associated clinical signs. In order to differentiate potentially reversible renal failure from irreversible renal failure in the living patient, it is essential to consider basic morphologic and functional changes which occur in kidneys as a result of various types of injury, and the relationship of the latter to clinical manifestations of abnormal function. This knowledge and the intelligent use and interpretation of radiographic findings, laboratory data, and information obtained by biopsy are the most reliable means with which to consistently make such a distinction.

  A. *Renal reserve capacity*
  1. The kidneys have tremendous reserve capacity.
    a. Unilateral nephrectomy of patients with normal kidneys is not followed by clinical signs related to renal failure.

b. Impairment of urine concentrating capacity of canine kidneys is not detectable until approximately two thirds of the total renal parenchyma is surgically extirpated.
c. Although the serum concentration of nonprotein nitrogen (NPN) varies inversely with glomerular filtration rate, two thirds to three fourths of the nephrons of both kidneys must be nonfunctional before reduction in renal function is severe enough to be associated with significant elevations in NPN, BUN, or creatinine, as detected by routine laboratory methods.
  2. Because of the large functional reserve capacity of the kidneys, detection of renal disease before there is serious impairment of renal function is often difficult.

B. *Response of the kidneys to injury*
  1. Although the kidneys have a large functional reserve capacity in terms of numbers of nephrons necessary to maintain homeostasis, the ability of nephrons to regenerate following destruction by disease is limited.
  2. The kidneys cannot produce additional nephrons following maturation.
  3. Nephrons damaged as a result of ischemia or nephrotoxins may regain structural and functional competence provided the basement membranes of the tubules are not severely damaged, and provided a sufficient number of tubular epithelial cells have escaped injury so they can proliferate and reline denuded renal tubules.
    a. At first newly regenerated tubular epithelial cells develop cytoplasmic organelles necessary for protein synthesis and replication. At this stage the tubules are unable to concentrate or dilute urine.
    b. When necrotic epithelial cells have been replaced by newly regenerated epithelium, cytoplasmic organelles necessary for tubular reabsorption and secretion develop, and the ability to concentrate and dilute urine is eventually regained (see Chapter 17, Ischemic and Chemical Nephrosis).
    c. Intact tubular basement membranes are an essential prerequisite to tubular regeneration because they provide a framework which permits orderly reconstruction of the tubule by regenerated epithelial cells.
    d. Once fragmentation or dissolution of tubular basement membranes occurs, the lack of a continuous supporting scaffold may result in lack of orderly reepithelialization of the tubule, or obstruction of the tubular lumen as a result of ingrowth of granulation tissue from the interstitial tissue.
      (1) Extensive proliferation of tubular epithelium may still occur, but failure of restoration of a patent tubular lumen destroys the excretory capacity of the nephron.
      (2) The end result of such injury is usually replacement of affected nephrons by connective tissue.
  4. Severely damaged glomeruli have limited ability to regain normal structure and function.
    a. Minor inflammatory changes may be reversible.
    b. Severe atrophy and necrosis of glomeruli are irreversible lesions which ultimately lead to scarring of glomerular tufts.
    c. Renal amyloidosis typically causes progressive and irreversible destruction of glomeruli.

5. Lesions of the interstitial tissue may be reversible or irreversible, depending on the etiology and pathogenesis of the renal disease in question. For example, generalized interstitial edema may produce a profound alteration of renal function, but the changes are potentially reversible if the predisposing cause is rapidly eliminated.
6. Renal vasculature.
    a. Because the majority of the renal arteries are end arteries without significant collateral circulation, obstruction of blood flow by thrombi or emboli will result in infarction of the renal parenchyma supplied by the damaged vessels.
    b. Glomerular diseases which cause progressive reduction of blood flow will cause ischemic atrophy and necrosis of renal tubular cells since the latter are dependent on postglomerular peritubular capillaries for their blood supply.
7. The concept that the nephron is the structural and functional unit of the kidney is based upon the functional interdependence of glomeruli, tubules, peritubular capillaries, and surrounding interstitial tissue.
    a. If any portion of the nephron is irreversibly destroyed, the remaining portions become nonfunctional. Progressive irreversible lesions initially localized to the renal vascular system, glomeruli, tubules, or interstitial tissue are eventually responsible for the development of lesions in the remaining, but initially unaffected, portions of the nephron.
    b. Because of this structural and functional interdependency, differentiation of various renal diseases which have advanced to an end stage is difficult or impossible (see Chapter 20, End-Stage Kidneys).
    c. As a generality, the greater the degree of destruction of renal parenchyma by chronic progressive irreversible renal disease, the less evident are detectable differences in their gross and microscopic appearance.
    d. Since effective regeneration of renal parenchyma destroyed by progressive irreversible renal diseases does not occur, repair occurs by replacement fibrosis and scarring.

C. *Morphological and functional adaptation of the kidneys to injury*
    1. Although the kidneys cannot produce additional nephrons once maturation has occurred, or effectively repair nephrons severely damaged as a result of various disease processes, compensatory hypertrophy and hyperplasia are highly efficient adaptive mechanisms by which the functional capacity of surviving nephrons is increased.
        a. Unilateral nephrectomy is followed by a marked increase in size and function of the contralateral kidney.
        b. Microdissection of nephrons from dogs with chronic generalized renal disease revealed that proximal convoluted tubular (PCT) length had tripled, PCT volume had doubled, PCT thickness had increased by approximately one half, and glomerular surface area and volume had approximately doubled (Fig. 12–1).
        c. Effective renal blood flow, glomerular filtration rate, and tubular transport rate were observed to increase in remaining viable nephrons following experimental production of renal disease in dogs.
    2. The number of functional nephrons required to maintain homeostasis is dependent upon the rapidity with which the remainder are destroyed. Progressive renal diseases that destroy renal parenchyma at a relatively

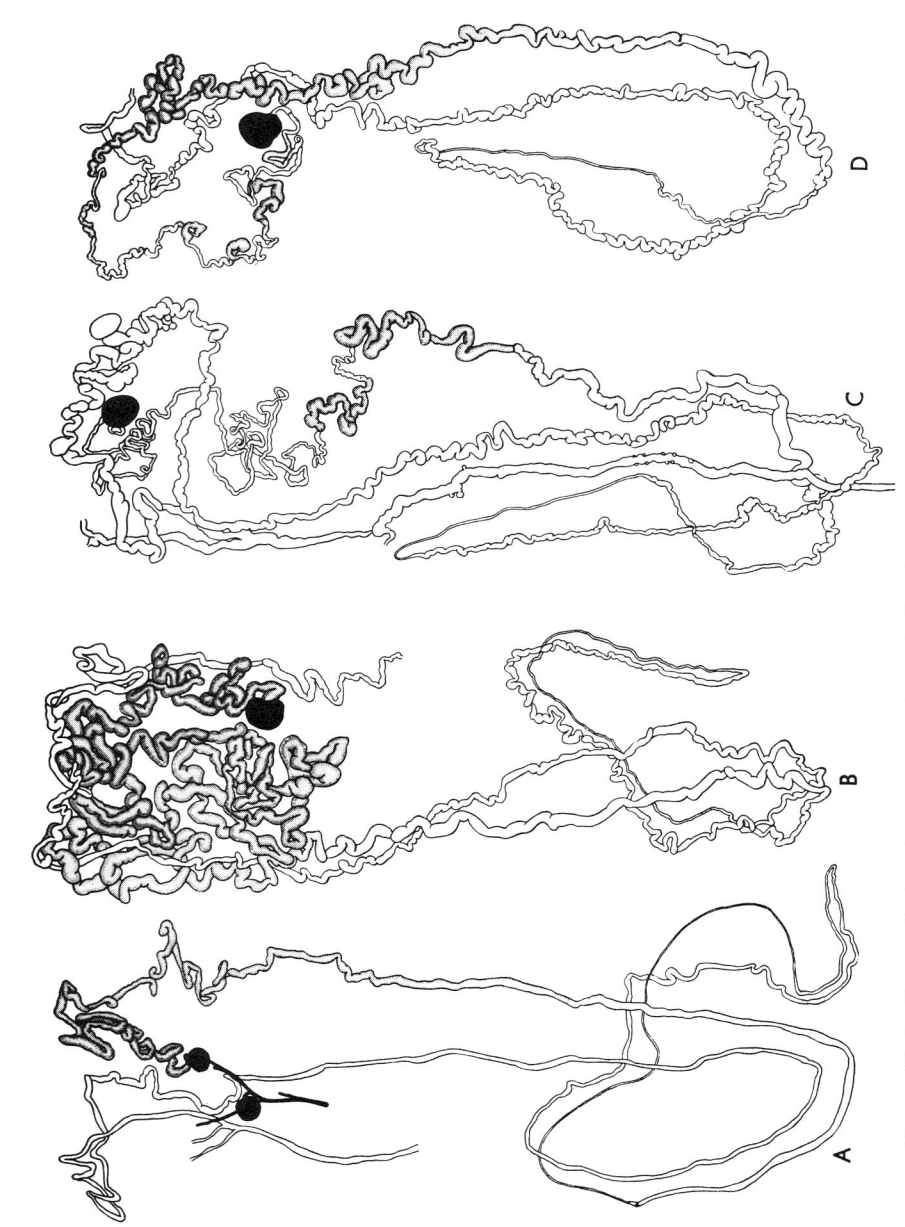

Figure 12–1. Camera lucida drawing of nephrons isolated by microdissection from dog kidneys and stained vitally with trypan blue. In all nephrons, the dye is localized only in the proximal convoluted tubules. *A* is from a normal dog kidney, and *B*, *C*, and *D* are from dog kidneys with compensated end-stage renal disease. In *B*, the proximal convolution shows marked hypertrophy and hyperplasia and is filled with dye granules in a normal manner throughout its course. In *C* and *D*, the proximal convolutions show atrophic dye-free stretches as well as hypertrophic dye-containing stretches. (Bloom, F.: Pathology of the Dog and Cat. The Genitourinary System, With Clinical Considerations. Evanston, Ill., American Veterinary Publications, Inc., 1954.)

slow rate allow viable nephrons time to undergo structural and functional transformation. Thus a larger number of nephrons may be destroyed before renal function is reduced to such a degree that functional abnormalities become detectable.

3. Viable nephrons undergo adaptive and compensatory changes as the nephron population progressively decreases, and retain a highly efficient and predictable degree of renal function.
   a. Because of the compensatory and adaptive changes which occur in residual viable nephrons of chronically diseased kidneys, the onset of progressive chronic renal diseases is typically insidious. Such diseases may remain asymptomatic for months or years.
   b. Once the limits of renal reserve and compensation have been exhausted, signs of renal failure typically appear in rapid succession and the condition of the patient often deteriorates rapidly even though there has been relatively little progression in the rate of pathologic destruction of the renal parenchyma.
   c. When renal failure occurs it is not characterized by disorganized function, but rather extremely efficient renal function by a population of nephrons which are too few in number to maintain homeostasis.
   d. Eventually the nephron number decreases below a critical level, and despite maximum compensation and adaptation by the remaining viable nephrons, life can no longer be sustained.
4. Diseases of the kidney which lead to progressive destruction and scarring of nephrons are characterized by a common pattern of metabolic and functional change called uremia.
5. The mechanisms responsible for inducing compensatory and adaptive changes of viable nephrons following destruction of renal parenchyma are poorly understood, but have been related to the following:
   a. Increased functional demands placed on viable nephrons.
   b. Hormonal stimulation by androgens.
   c. Stimulation by a tissue specific, species nonspecific, serum factor which is released following injury to the kidneys.

REFERENCES

Bloom, F.: A cytologic study of the tubular epithelium in acute and chronic Bright's disease with special reference to mitochondria. Amer. J. Path., *19*:957–975, 1943.

Bradford, J. R.: The results following partial nephrectomy and the influence of the kidney on metabolism. J. Physiol., *23*:415–496, 1898.

Bricker, N. S.: On the meaning of the intact nephron hypothesis. Amer. J. Med., *46*:1–11, 1969.

Bricker, N. S., Dewey, R. R., Lubowitz, H., Stokes, J., and Kirkensgaard, T.: Observations on the concentrating and diluting mechanisms of the diseased kidney. J. Clin. Invest., *38*:516–523, 1959.

Bricker, N. S., Kime, S. W., Morrin, P. A. F., and Orlowski, T.: The influence of glomerular filtration rate, solute excretion, and hydration on the concentrating mechanism of the experimentally diseased kidney in the dog. J. Clin. Invest., *39*:864–875, 1960.

Bricker, N. S., Morrin, P. A. F., and Kime, S. W.: The pathologic physiology of chronic Bright's disease. An exposition of the intact nephron hypothesis. Amer. J. Med., *28*:77–98, 1960.

Bucher, N. L. R., and Nalt, R. A.: Regeneration of Liver and Kidney. Boston, Mass., Little, Brown and Co., 1971.

Coburn, J. W., Gonich, H. C., Rubini, M. E., and Kleeman, C. R.: Studies of experimental renal failure in dogs. I. Effect of 5/6 nephrectomy on concentrating and diluting capacity of residual nephrons. J. Clin. Invest., *44*:603–614, 1965.

Cuppage, F. E.: Repair of the nephron in acute renal failure: Comparative regeneration following various forms of acute tubular injury. Path. Microbiol., *32*:327–344, 1968.

Dossetor, J. B., and Gault, M. H.: Nephron Failure. Conservation, Substitution, Replacement. Springfield, Illinois, Charles C Thomas, 1971.

Gonick, H. C., Coburn, J. W., Rubini, M. E., Maxwell, M., and Kleeman, C. R.: Studies of experimental renal failure in dogs. II. Effect of 5/6's nephrectomy on sodium conserving ability of residual nephrons. J. Lab. Clin. Med., 64:269–276, 1964.

Hayman, J. M., Shumway, N. P., Dumke, P., and Miller, M.: Experimental hyposthenuria. J. Clin. Invest., 18:195–212, 1939.

Kogan, J., and Kolberg, A.: Renal function as influenced by compensatory growth after subtotal nephrectomy in dogs. J. Medicine, 1:156–164, 1970.

Kolberg, A.: Relations of renal tubular and nephron function as influenced by 75% reduction of nephron number. Scandinav. J. Clin. Lab. Invest., 11(Suppl 41):1–152, 1959.

Liu, C. T., and Overman, R. R.: Effect of uninephrectomy on kidney weight and renal function in the dog. J. Urol., 100:215–219, 1968.

Morrin, P. A. F., Bricker, N. S., Kime, S. W., and Klein, C.: Observations on the acidifying capacity of the experimentally diseased kidney in the dog. J. Clin. Invest., 41:1297–1302, 1962.

Morrin, P. A. F., Joynt, M. S. K., and Frame, J.: The effect of a uremic environment on phosphate excretion by a small population of intact and severely diseased nephrons. Nephron, 7:248–257, 1970.

Nowinski, W. W., and Gross, R. J.: Compensatory Renal Hypertrophy. New York, N. Y., Academic Press, 1969.

Oliver, J., Bloom, F., and MacDowell, M.: Structural and functional transformations in tubular epithelium of dog's kidneys in chronic Bright's disease and their relation to mechanisms of renal compensation and failure. J. Exp. Med., 73:141–160, 1941.

Osborne, C. A., Low, D. G., and Finco, D. R.: Reversible versus irreversible renal disease in the dog. J.A.V.M.A., 155:2062–2078, 1969.

Rieselbach, R. E., Todd, L. E., Rosenthal, M., and Bricker, N. S.: Adaptive capacity of the chronically diseased kidney in the dog. J. Lab. Clin. Med., 62:1008, 1963.

Rous, S. N., and Wakim, K. G.: Kidney function before and after compensatory hypertrophy. J. Urol., 98:30–35, 1967.

Wagenknecht, L. V., Knuth, O. E., and Madsen, P. O.: Compensatory renal hyperfunction in the dog evaluated by continuous isotope clearance determinations. Invest. Urol., 8:502–506, 1971.

Chapter 13
EXTRARENAL MANIFESTATIONS OF UREMIA

I. Etiology of uremic syndrome

   A. *In the past, a variety of toxins were incriminated as the underlying causes of signs characteristic of uremia.*

      Most so-called "uremic toxins" (urea, guanidine, uric acid, sulphates, phosphates, phenols) are end products of protein and nucleoprotein metabolism which accumulate in the blood as a result of impaired renal clearance.

   B. *Clinical and experimental studies in man and animals which were designed to prove various "uremic toxin" hypotheses failed to reveal a single toxin which could produce signs typical of the uremic syndrome.*

   C. *More recently it has been hypothesized that uremia is caused by the interaction of multiple factors (multiple toxin concept) including:*
      1. Altered electrolyte balance.
      2. Altered fluid balance.
      3. Altered acid-base balance.
      4. Abnormal accumulation of nonelectrolyte, metabolic substances.
         a. Urea.
         b. Guanidines.
         c. Uric acid.
         d. Phenols.
      5. Altered activity of intracellular enzymes.
      6. Others.

   D. *When the structural and functional integrity of both kidneys has been compromised to such a degree that signs of renal failure become manifest clinically, a relatively predictable symptom complex called uremia appears regardless of underlying cause.*
      1. The clinical signs characteristic of uremia are manifestations of an interaction between autointoxication caused by reduction of renal function below that required to maintain homeostasis, and the body's compensatory attempts to maintain homeostasis.
      2. The clinical signs of uremia may vary from patient to patient depending on the nature, severity, duration, and rate of progression of the underlying disease. In most instances, however, uremia is the clinical state toward which all generalized progressive renal diseases ultimately converge, and associated signs are more similar than dissimilar.
      3. There is significant variability between the concentration of BUN or creatinine and the severity of clinical signs of uremia. The latter may be related, at least in part, to the duration of the renal disease. Progressive renal diseases that destroy renal parenchyma at a relatively slow rate allow the body to compensate for altered homeostatic states.

136 DISEASES OF THE UPPER URINARY SYSTEM

II. The following description of common signs of renal failure has been categorized according to various systems of the body.

Signs peculiar to a specific cause of renal failure are discussed with specific diseases of the kidney.

A. *Skin*
  1. Dehydration is often present in patients during a uremic crisis and is manifested clinically by varying degrees of loss of skin pliability (see Chapter 32, Fluid Therapy in Renal Failure) (Fig. 13–1).
  2. Uremic frost and pruritus have been mentioned in the veterinary literature. This appears to be an erroneous direct transfer from human literature.
     a. Perspiration in uremic people contains large amounts of urea, which contributes to the crystalline white deposit on the skin called uremic frost. Uremic frost may contribute to pruritus in man.
     b. Dogs and cats perspire only on very limited parts of their bodies. Urea does not accumulate on the surface of the skin.

B. *Respiratory system*

Because of anemia, acidosis, and, on occasion, terminal pulmonary edema, patients with advanced renal failure may have an increased respiratory rate. Changes in the rate and character of respiration associated with renal failure are usually difficult to detect. Unless there is coexisting heart failure, significant pulmonary edema does not occur, or develops as a terminal event. If present, moist rales may be ausculted.

C. *Cardiovascular system*
  1. Hypertension secondary to chronic renal failure in dogs and cats has not been adequately investigated. A reliable answer regarding its presence or absence has not been established. The limited amount of information

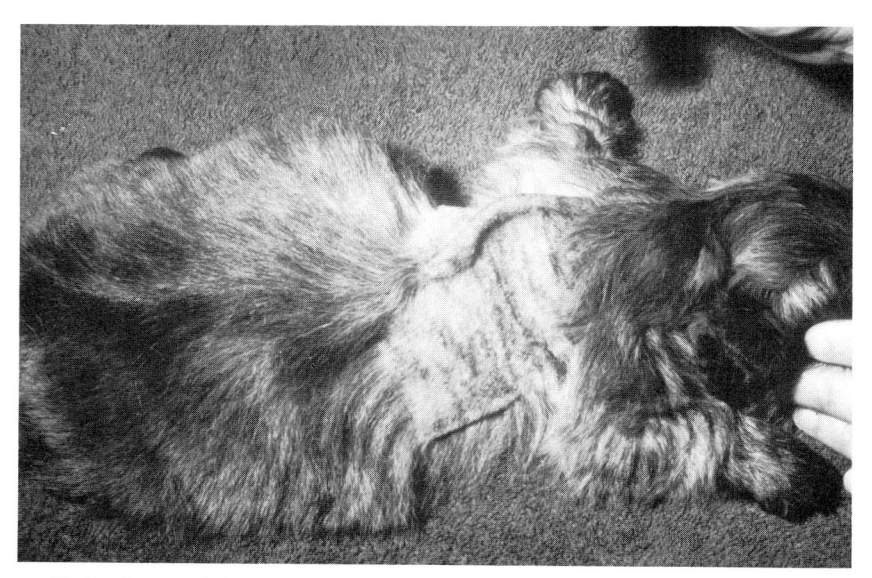

Figure 13–1. Severe dehydration in a 1-month-old male lhasa apso dog. The skin has retained the abnormal position to which it was displaced. The degree of dehydration was estimated to be in excess of 10 per cent of the dog's body weight.

EXTRARENAL MANIFESTATIONS OF UREMIA   137

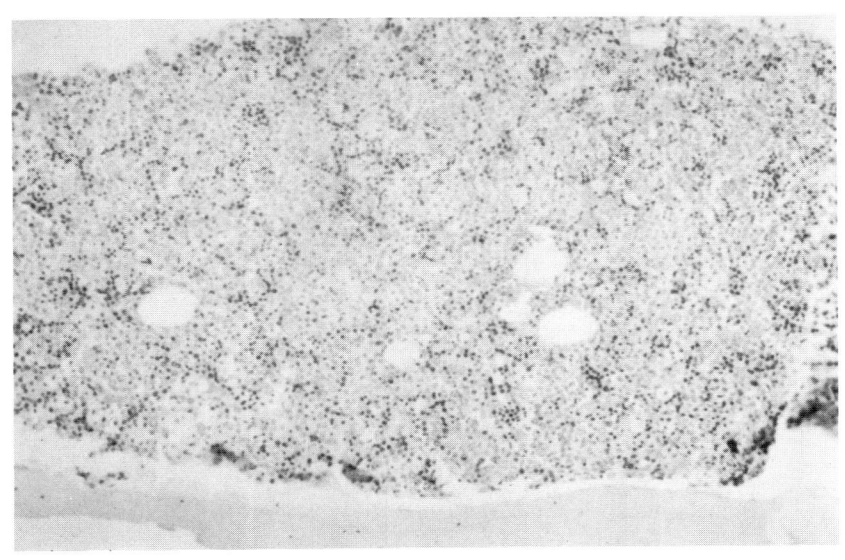

Figure 13-2. Photomicrograph of normal bone marrow obtained from an adult dog. Compare with Figure 13-3. H&E stain; × 25. (Courtesy of Dr. Victor Perman, College of Veterinary Medicine, University of Minnesota.)

available suggests that mild hypertension may occur in association with generalized chronic renal disease, but is not a consistent finding.
2. The heart rate may be accelerated in terminal renal failure as a result, at least in part, of the anemia which is frequently present.
3. Abnormalities in cardiac rate and conduction may occur as a result of potassium retention in oliguric or anuric uremic patients. Auscultation of these patients may reveal varying degrees of bradycardia, arrhythmias, and heart block. Cardiac conduction defects are reflected in the

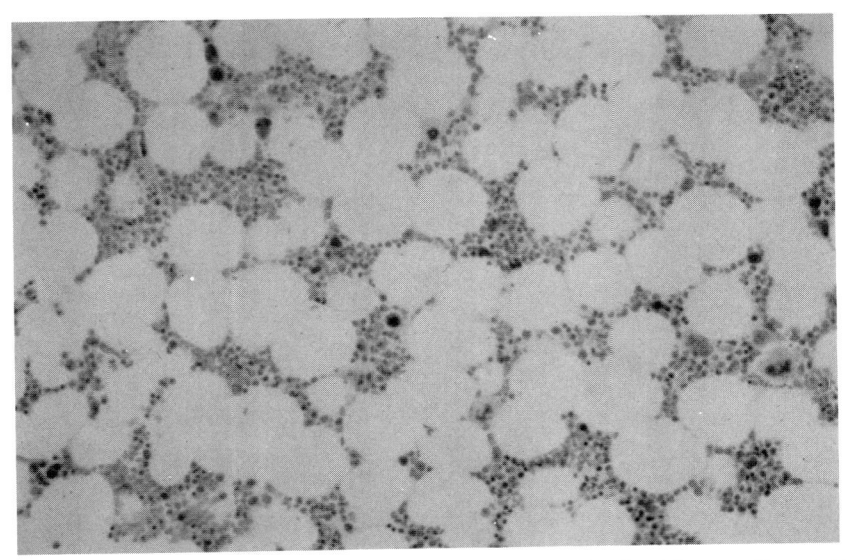

Figure 13-3. Photomicrograph of hypoplastic bone marrow obtained from an 8-year-old, female black Labrador retriever with chronic uremia. The marrow is hypocellular. H&E stain; ×25. (Courtesy of Dr. Victor Perman, College of Veterinary Medicine, University of Minnesota.)

electrocardiogram by increased amplitude and peaking of T waves, depression of the ST segment, prolongation of the P-R interval, widening of the QRS complex, and decreased amplitude and ultimate disappearance of the P wave.
   4. Left ventricular hypertrophy is a common necropsy finding in dogs with chronic generalized renal disease. Although its exact cause has not been established, it may be associated with anemia or hypertension.
D. *Hemic system*
   1. The kidneys are the source of renal erythropoietic factor (see Chapter 2, Applied Physiology of the Urinary System).
   2. In chronic generalized renal disease, a progressive nonregenerative anemia develops. This anemia is thought to be related, at least in part, to lack of a sufficient quantity of erythropoietin. It is associated with varying degrees of hypoplasia of erythroid cells in bone marrow (Figs. 13–2 and 13–3).
   3. A nonregenerative anemia is an unfavorable prognostic sign when associated with chronic uremia. Other causes of nonregenerative anemias, especially infection and neoplastic disease, should be considered when evaluating its diagnostic and prognostic significance.
E. *Digestive system*
   1. Mouth.
      a. Ulcers are sometimes observed in the gums, especially adjacent to canine and fourth premolar teeth coated with tartar. Ulcers which develop in these areas are probably caused by bacterial degradation of urea to ammonia (Fig. 13–4).
      b. Pale mucous membranes occur when marked anemia is present.
      c. Although it has been suggested that an ammoniacal odor to the breath may be detected in patients with uremia, this is an inconsistent and unreliable sign.

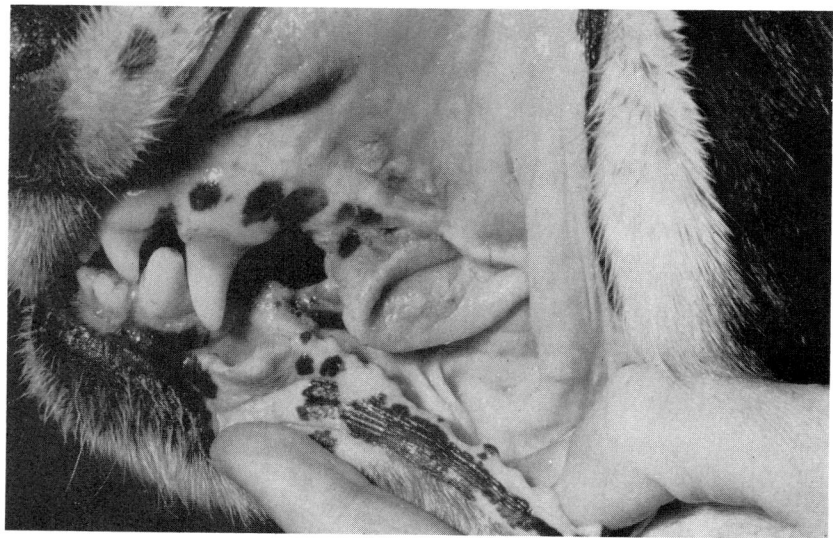

Figure 13–4. Ulceration of the tongue and buccal mucosa of an 11-year-old male springer spaniel with chronic uremia.

d. A red-brown discoloration of the anterior portion of the tongue may be observed. The pathogenesis of this alteration has not been established.
  2. Stomach.
     a. A hemorrhagic ulcerative gastritis (often called uremic gastritis) is often present. The microscopic appearance of this lesion is characterized by noninflammatory myoarteritis.
     b. Vomiting is a common sign in uremia. It is related to stimulation of the vomiting center in the medulla oblongata, and may also be related to ulcerative gastritis.
  3. Intestines and colon.
     a. Enterocolitis may be present, although it is less frequently encountered and is usually less severe than gastritis. When present, it may cause diarrhea.
     b. Constipation may also occur, and when present is probably related to compensatory conservation of water by the body in an effort to correct dehydration.

F. *Urinary system*
  1. In chronic renal failure, polydipsia and polyuria are commonly observed. As the underlying renal disease progresses, the volume of urine becomes inadequate to excrete waste products of metabolism even though urine volume may exceed that of normal animals.
     a. Polyuria is related, at least in part, to an obligatory osmotic diuresis in the surviving nephrons. Since the daily load of solute presented to the kidney for excretion must be handled by a reduced number of functioning nephrons, each viable nephron is undergoing continuous solute diuresis.

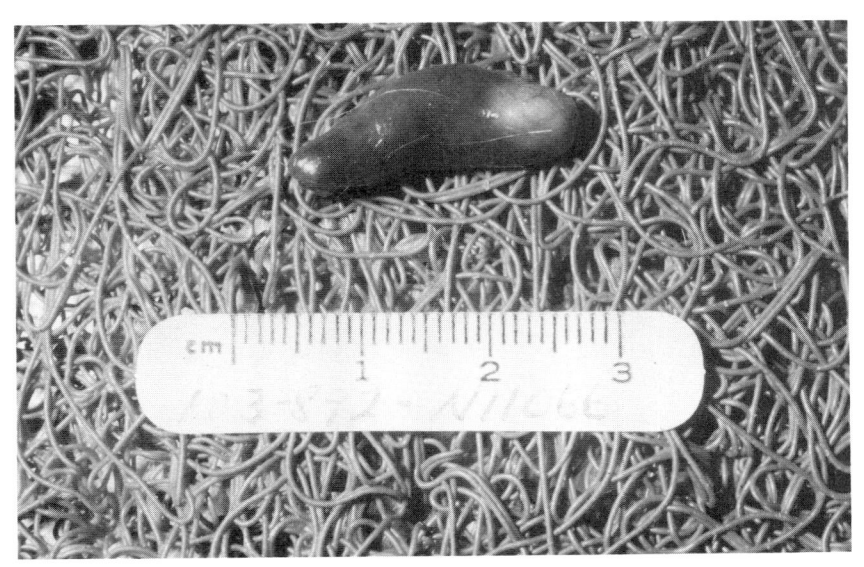

Figure 13-5. Hyperplastic parathyroid gland adjacent to thyroid gland obtained from an 11-year-old male springer spaniel dog with chronic generalized pyelonephritis. The serum concentration of phosphorus was 33.6 mg. per 100 ml. and the serum concentration of calcium was 7.5 mg. per 100 ml. The dog died of chronic renal failure.

b. The high osmolality present in medullary interstitial tissue, which is necessary for production of concentrated urine, may also be depressed. Continuous solute diuresis in nephrons results in washout of medullary solute (see Chapter 2, Applied Physiology of the Urinary System).
2. Patients with acute generalized nephrosis may have polyuria (see Chapter 17, Ischemic and Chemical Nephrosis).
3. Patients with acute generalized nephrosis, or terminal stages of chronic generalized renal disease may develop oliguria (see Chapter 17, Ischemic and Chemical Nephrosis).

G. *Endocrine system*
1. Secondary renal hyperparathyroidism.
   a. Secondary renal hyperparathyroidism is present in chronic renal failure.
      (1) A negative body balance of calcium may be caused by one or more of the following:
         (a) Impairment of renal metabolism of vitamin D.
         (b) Decreased intestinal absorption of calcium as a result of a decrease in vitamin D metabolites.
         (c) Increased urinary loss of calcium associated with renal diseases characterized by polyuria.
         (d) Excretion of abnormal quantities of phosphorus into the intestines with resultant formation of nonabsorbable calcium salts.
         (e) Imbalance of the normal calcium-phosphorus ratio in the body with resultant precipitation of calcium salts in various body tissues.
      (2) Hyperphosphatemia is a consistent finding in generalized renal

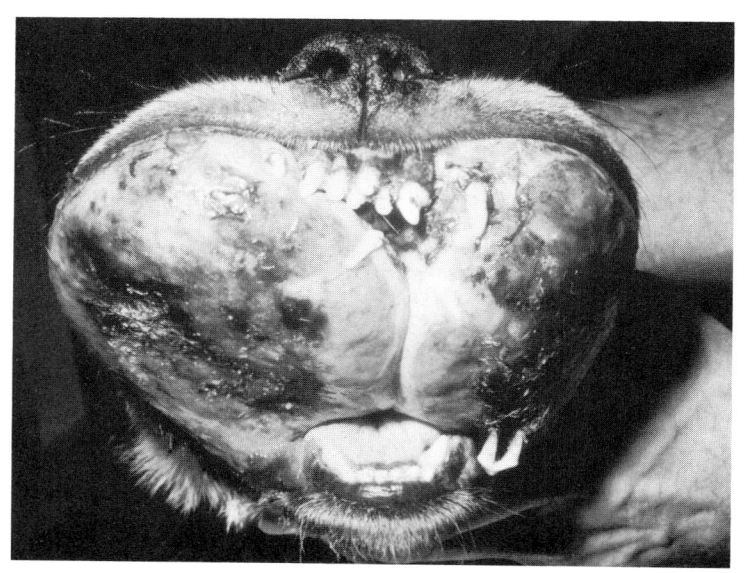

Figure 13-6. Advanced fibrous osteodystrophy of the head of a 9-month-old male mixed breed dog with chronic renal failure. The teeth are being extruded as a result of displacement by proliferation of fibrous connective tissue. Portions of the oral mucosa that were constantly exposed to air have ulcerated.

EXTRARENAL MANIFESTATIONS OF UREMIA 141

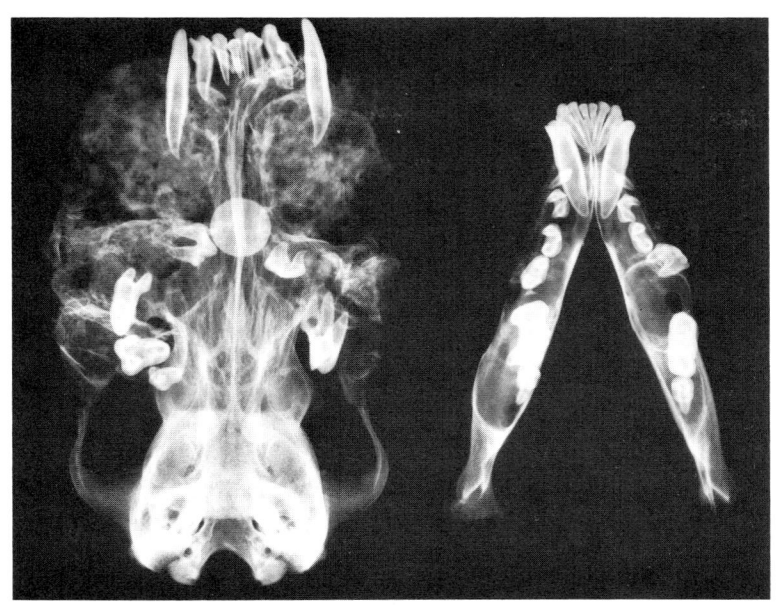

Figure 13-7. Radiograph of the demineralized skull of the dog described in Figure 13-6. The radiograph was taken following removal of soft tissue by a colony of beetles. The circular structure located on the midline of the maxillary bones is the outline of a piece of plastic used to support the skull. (Courtesy of Dr. Carl R. Jessen, College of Veterinary Medicine, University of Minnesota.)

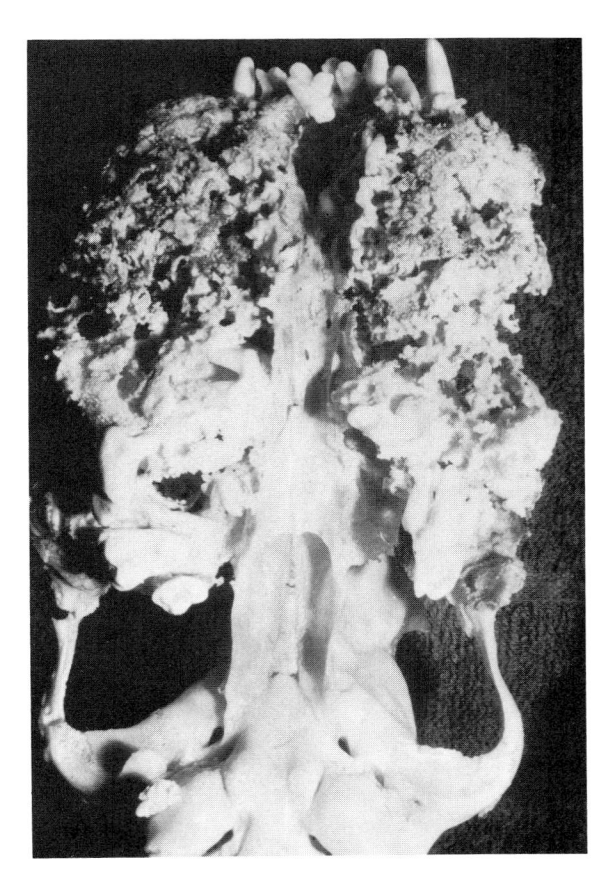

Figure 13-8. Skull of the dog described in Figure 13-6. Soft tissue has been removed by placing the head in a colony of beetles. (Courtesy of Dr. Walter Mackey, College of Veterinary Medicine, University of Minnesota.)

diseases of dogs and cats because phosphorus is normally eliminated by the kidneys.

b. The abnormally low serum calcium concentration stimulates the parathyroid glands to release parathormone, which mobilizes calcium from bones. After a sufficient period of time, demineralization of the skeleton and parathyroid hyperplasia develop (Fig. 13–5).

   (1) Skeletal changes associated with secondary renal hyperparathyroidism are most marked in immature dogs and cats because then bone is in an active state of growth.
   (2) Demineralization is especially prominent in the bones of the skull, and may be accompanied by marked proliferation of connective tissue (fibrous osteodystrophy) (Figs. 13–6, 13–7 and 13–8). The latter is not, however, a consistent finding (Fig. 13–9).
   (3) Demineralization of the skull may be associated with loosening of the teeth.
   (4) One of the earliest radiographic signs of demineralization of the skull is disappearance of the lamina dura.
   (5) Erosions of the tufts of the terminal phalanges and subperiosteal erosion of the middle and proximal phalanges may be detected radiographically.
   (6) In general, renal disease of sufficient severity to cause pathologic fractures, pain, or deformity of bones is uncommonly encountered

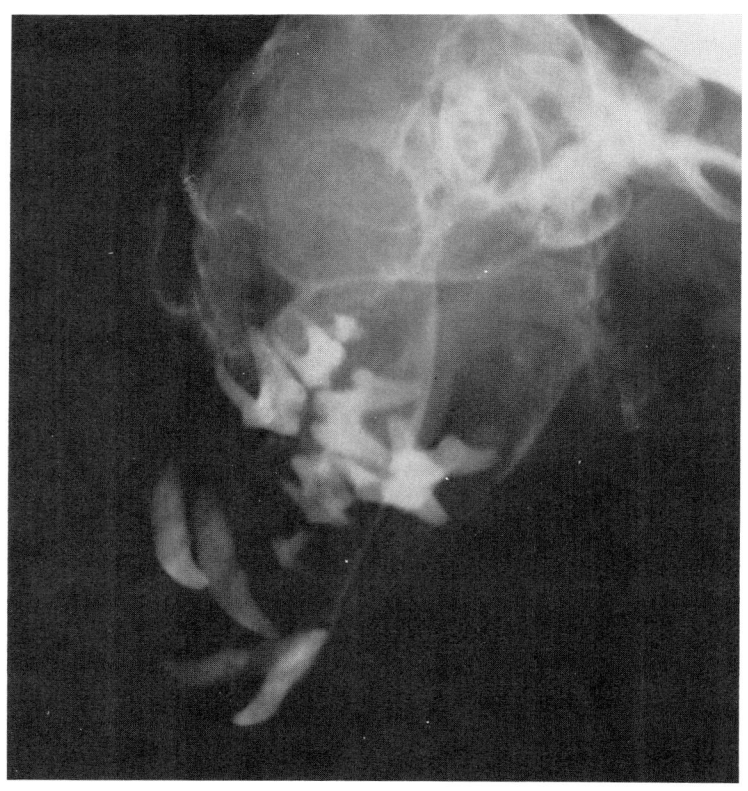

Figure 13-9. Radiograph of the skull of a 5.5-year-old male mixed breed dog with osteodystrophy secondary to chronic uremia. Marked proliferation of connective tissue was not observed.

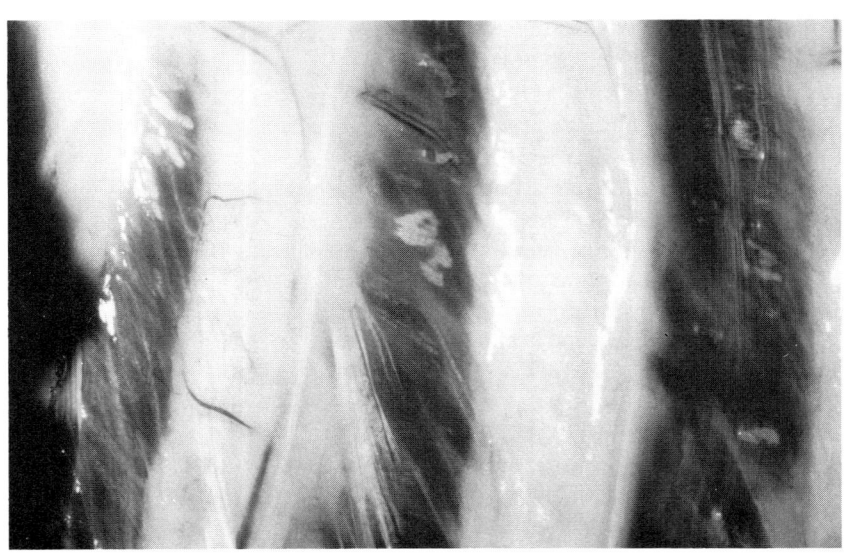

Figure 13-10. Uremic calcification in the parietal pleura of a 13-year-old male Irish setter with chronic uremia.

in association with spontaneously occurring renal disease of the dog and cat.
- (7) Metastatic and dystrophic calcification may occur.
  - (a) The kidneys of dogs and cats frequently contain calcium deposits.
  - (b) Extrarenal tissues of dogs, especially the gastrointestinal tract, pleura, lungs, myocardium and endocardium, frequently contain deposits of calcium (Fig. 13–10).
  - (c) Calcification of extrarenal tissues of cats has been reported to be an uncommon complication of uremia.
2. Atrophy of the germinal epithelium of the testicles results in sterility.

H. *Nervous system*
1. Patients with uremia are often depressed.
2. Tetanic convulsions caused by hypocalcemia may occur, but are uncommon. This is related to the fact that total serum calcium concentration usually does not decrease to dangerous levels. In addition, the concomitant presence of metabolic acidosis tends to prevent hypocalcemic tetany by conversion of nonionized calcium to the biologically active ionized form. As a result, nervous manifestations of hypocalcemia may not occur even though the serum concentration of calcium is abnormally low.
3. Non-hypocalcemic convulsions in uremic dogs and cats are extremely uncommon.

III. Potential causes of death in renal failure

A. *Urinary diseases caused by toxic agents, or which are associated with profound changes in fluid and electrolyte balance, have the potential of being lethal in a period of several hours to several days.*

B. *Dogs that have been nephrectomized and given no special therapy will survive for three to six days following surgery.*

144 DISEASES OF THE UPPER URINARY SYSTEM

 C. *Death associated with renal failure is probably caused by the interaction of multiple factors including altered fluid, acid-base, and electrolyte balance and accumulation of the waste products of protein metabolism.*
  1. Altered fluid balance.
   a. Deficit.
    (1) Dehydration may be a cause or an effect of renal failure.
     (a) Dehydration may cause prerenal uremia.
     (b) Dehydration may occur secondary to acute or chronic generalized renal disease as a result of impairment of the renal concentrating mechanism.
     (c) Polyuria unaccompanied by compensatory polydipsia, or complicated by vomiting and diarrhea, will also result in dehydration. Thus prerenal uremia due to dehydration may be superimposed on primary uremia.
    (2) Dehydration equivalent to a loss of 12 to 15 per cent of body weight will result in death from hypovolemic shock (see Chapter 32, Fluid Therapy in Renal Failure).
   b. Excess.
    (1) Primary uremia is uncommonly associated with overhydration in the dog and cat. When encountered, it is usually associated with either the nephrotic syndrome or parenteral administration of large quantities of fluid to uremic patients with oliguria or anuria.
    (2) Death due to spontaneous overhydration of uremic dogs and cats is unlikely to occur since the patients usually refuse to drink, and often vomit. Death due to iatrogenic overhydration of an oliguric patient is of greater likelihood.
  2. Altered acid-base balance.
   a. In renal failure, there is a tendency for development of metabolic acidosis because of impaired ability of the kidneys to excrete hydrogen ions and conserve buffer ions such as bicarbonate.
   b. The role of acidosis as a cause of death in uremic patients is dependent on its severity.
    (1) Blood pH values below 6.8 are incompatible with life, regardless of cause.
    (2) Uremic dogs in which acidosis has been corrected do not consistently recover.
    (3) Some dogs die of uremia without developing acidosis of sufficient magnitude to be incompatible with life.
    (4) There is no direct relationship between the concentration of BUN or creatinine and the degree of acidosis.
    (5) The preceding observations indicate that:
     (a) When the blood pH of a uremic patient approaches 6.8, death is probable.
     (b) A less severe state of acidosis may be contributory to the death of a uremic patient, but is not the sole cause.
  3. Altered electrolyte balance.
   a. Deficits.
    (1) Although uremic patients with polyuria tend to develop deficits of sodium, chloride, bicarbonate, and, in some instances, potassium, the loss of these ions usually is not of sufficient magnitude to cause death.

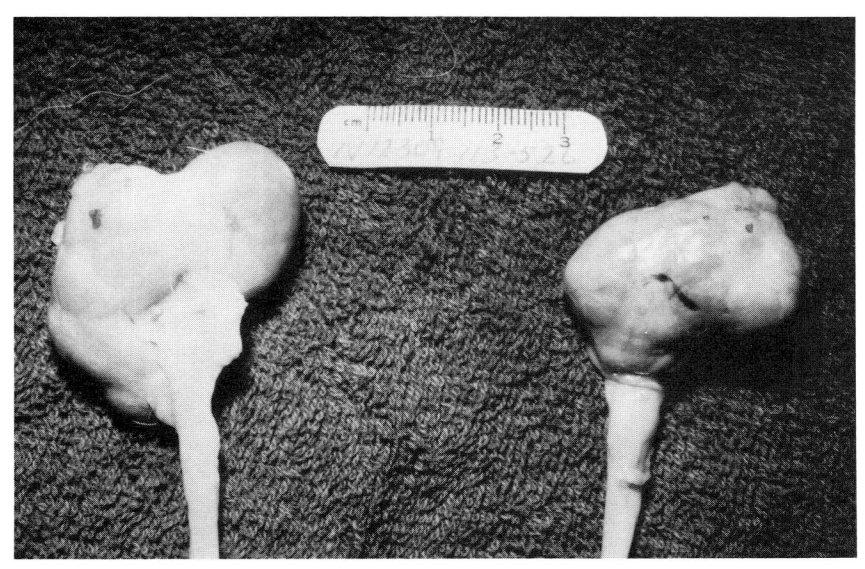

Figure 13-11. Kidneys with end-stage renal disease obtained from a 9-month-old male mixed breed dog (see Fig. 13-6). Following several months of conservative medical management of chronic renal failure, the dog died of hypocalcemic tetany. (Courtesy of Dr. Jerry B. Stevens, College of Veterinary Medicine, University of Minnesota.)

    (2) Mild to moderate hypocalcemia is a common finding in chronic uremia. Tetanic convulsions and death caused by hypocalcemia, however, are uncommon.
       (a) The latter is related to the fact that total serum calcium concentration usually does not drop to dangerous levels.
       (b) In addition, the concomitant presence of metabolic acidosis tends to prevent hypocalcemic tetany by conversion of nonionized calcium to the biologically active ionized form.
       (c) Death due to hypocalcemic tetany has been observed in two immature dogs with chronic renal failure. The total concentration of serum calcium was 5 to 6 mg. per 100 ml. Blood pH was normal in both dogs (Fig. 13-11).
  b. Excesses.
    (1) Uremia associated with oliguria or anuria will ultimately be associated with hyperkalemia. The severity of hyperkalemia may be aggravated by tissue catabolism.
    (2) Hyperkalemia can cause death from cardiac arrest if plasma concentration exceeds 10 mEq. per L.
    (3) Severe hyperkalemia is not a common complication of spontaneously occurring renal diseases in the dog and cat.

REFERENCES

Anderson, L. J., and Fisher, E. W.: The blood pressure in canine interstitial nephritis. Res. Vet. Sci., 9:304-313, 1968.
Black, D. A. K.: A perspective on uremic toxins. Arch. Int. Med., 126:906-909, 1970.
Bliss, S.: Cause of sore mouth in nephritis. J. Biol. Chem., 121:425-428, 1937.
Brodey, R. S., Medway, W., and Marshak, R. R.: Renal osteodystrophy in the dog. J.A.V.M.A., 139:329-341, 1961.

Cordy, C. R.: Apocrine cystic calcinosis in dogs and its relationship to chronic renal disease. Cornell Vet., 57:107–118, 1967.
Dammrich, K.: Pathological and histological studies on bones, kidneys, and parathyroids of dogs with renal disorders. Zbl. Vet. Med., 5:742–768, 1958.
Giovannetti, S.: Uremia like syndrome in dogs chronically intoxicated with methylguanidine and creatinine. Clin. Sci., 36:445–452, 1969.
Gray, R., Boyle, I., and DeLuca, H. F.: Vitamin D metabolism: The role of kidney tissue. Science, 172:1232–1234, June 18, 1971.
Grollman, E. F., and Grollman, A.: Toxicity of urea and its role in pathogenesis of uremia. J. Clin. Invest., 38:749–754, 1959.
Hoff, H. E., Smith, P. K., and Winkler, A. W.: The cause of death in experimental anuria. J. Clin. Invest., 20:607–624, 1941.
Hogg, A. H.: Osteodystrophic disease in the dog with special reference to rubber jaw (renal osteodystrophy) and its comparison with renal rickets in the human. Vet. Rec., 60:117–122, 1948.
Holmes, J. R.: A radiologic study of the digits in renal osteodystrophy in the dog. Vet. Rec., 69:642–643, 1957.
Humphreys, C. F.: Effects of diet and cation exchange upon survival of nephrectomized dogs. J. Urol., 82:208–211, 1959.
Krook, L.: Renal secondary hyperparathyroidism in the dog. Acta Path. Microbiol. Scand., Suppl. 122:40–58, 1957.
Lucke, V. M., and Hunt, A. C.: Renal calcification in the domestic cat. Path. Vet., 4:120–136, 1967.
Lumb, G. A., Mawer, E. B., and Stanbury, S. W.: The apparent vitamin D resistance of chronic renal failure. A study of the physiology of vitamin D in man. Amer. J. Med., 50:421–441, April, 1971.
McGill, H. C., Geer, J. C., Strong, J. P., and Holman, R. L.: Two forms of necrotizing arteritis in dogs related to diet and renal insufficiency. Arch. Path., 65:66–76, 1958.
Merrill, J. P., and Hampers, C. L.: Uremia. New England J. Med., 282:953–961, 1014–1021, 1970.
Murphy, G. P., Mirand, E. A., Kenny, G. M., Niemat, S., and Staubitz, W. J.: Extrarenal and renal erythropoietin levels in human beings and experimental animals in intact, anephric, and renal allotransplanted state. J. Urol., 103:686–691, 1970.
Persson, F., Persson, S., and Asheim, A.: Electrocardiographic changes in dogs with uremia. Acta Vet. Scand., 2:85–101, 1961.
Persson, F., Persson, S., and Asheim, A.: Blood-pressure in dogs with renal cortical hypoplasia. Acta Vet. Scand., 2:129–136, 1961.
Pirie, H. M., Mackey, L. J., and Fisher, E. W.: The relationship between renal disease and arterial lesions in the dog. Annals New York Acad. Sci., 127:861–873, 1965.
Platt, H.: Canine chronic nephritis II. A study of the parathyroid glands with particular reference to the rubber jaw syndrome. J. Comp. Path. Therap., 61:188–196, 1951.
Platt, H.: Canine chronic nephritis III. The skeletal system in rubber jaw. J. Comp. Path. Therap., 61:197–214, 1951.
Platt, H.: Morphological changes in the cardiovascular system associated with nephritis in dogs. J. Path. Bact., 64:539–549, 1952.
Schreiner, G. E., and Maher, J. F.: Uremia: Biochemistry, Pathogenesis, Treatment. Springfield, Ill., Charles C Thomas, 1962.
Slatopolsky, E., Cagler, S., Pennell, J. P., Taggart, D. D., Canterbury, J. M., Reiss, E., and Bricker, N. S.: On the pathogenesis of hyperparathyroidism in chronic experimental renal insufficiency in the dog. J. Clin. Invest., 50:492–499, 1971.
Sporri, H., and Leemann, W.: Blood pressure in dogs with chronic interstitial nephritis. Zbl. Vet. Med., 8:523–532, 1961.
Symposium on uremic toxins. Arch. Int. Med., 126:773–910, 1970.
Teschan, P. E.: On the pathogenesis of uremia. Amer. J. Med., 48:671–677, 1970.

Chapter 14
CAUSES OF POLYURIA—POLYDIPSIA COMPLEX

I. **Excessive water consumption**

   A. *Excessive water consumption may be reflected by a low specific gravity or osmolality in a randomly obtained urine sample.*

   B. *Proper evaluation may require the use of a urine concentration test (see Chapter 7, Tests of Renal Function).*

   C. *Some causes of excessive water consumption are physiologic, including:*
      1. Diets high in salt.
      2. Excessive body water loss as a result of high environmental temperature.

II. **End-stage renal disease (chronic interstitial nephritis)**

   A. *History*
      1. This disease complex occurs more commonly in older dogs.
      2. A higher incidence has been reported in males than in females.
      3. In the compensated state, polyuria, polydipsia, and nocturia are usually observed.
      4. In the decompensated state, anorexia, weight loss, depression, emesis, weakness, and diarrhea or constipation may be observed in addition to polyuria, polydipsia, and nocturia (see Chapter 13, Extrarenal Manifestations of Uremia).

   B. *Physical findings depend on the severity and the stage of disease. All findings do not invariably occur in all animals.*
      1. Significant physical findings may not be detected early in the course of events.
      2. Signs of the uremic syndrome may be observed, including:
         a. Signs related to the gastrointestinal system, such as anorexia, vomiting, stomatitis, mucosal ulceration, brick-red discoloration of tip of tongue, and diarrhea or constipation.
         b. Signs related to the nervous system, such as depression, apathy, coma, and sometimes fibrillary muscle twitching.
         c. Signs related to the hemic system, such as pallor of visible mucous membranes.
         d. Signs related to the musculoskeletal system, such as decalcification (renal osteodystrophy, renal secondary hyperparathyroidism).
         e. Signs related to the integumentary system, such as dehydration (loss of skin pliability).

148 DISEASES OF THE UPPER URINARY SYSTEM

    C. *Pertinent laboratory data*
- 1. Hemogram.
  - a. Progressive non-regenerative anemia.
  - b. Leucocytosis (mature).
  - c. Hemoconcentration (see Chapter 6, Laboratory Findings in Diseases of the Urinary System).
- 2. Urinalysis.
  - a. The specific gravity is usually low and may be fixed (1.008 to 1.012) even in the presence of:
    - (1) Water deprivation.
    - (2) Pitressin concentration.
    - (3) Clinical dehydration.
  - b. Protein may be absent, or present in minimal amounts (trace to 2 plus).
  - c. An occasional hyaline or granular cast may be present.
- 3. Blood chemistry.
  - a. BUN, creatinine, amylase, and phosphorus concentration are usually elevated.
  - b. Serum sodium, chloride, and bicarbonate concentrations may be decreased during advanced stages of the disease.
  - c. Renal excretion of phenolsulfonphthalein dye is usually decreased.
  - d. A significant leptospiral antibody titer is usually absent.

III. Renal amyloidosis

    A. *Clinical findings associated with renal amyloidosis are similar to those associated with end-stage kidneys, except for the marked and persistent proteinuria associated with amyloidosis.*

    B. *Amyloidosis may be associated with long-standing suppuration, necrosis, or neoplasia.*

    C. *Hypercholesterolemia is a consistent finding.*

    D. *See Chapter 26, Renal Amyloidosis.*

IV. Renal cortical hypoplasia

    A. *This disease occurs in young dogs (few months to several years of age).*

    B. *There is no sex prevalence.*

    C. *The clinical findings are similar to those associated with end-stage renal disease.*

    D. *See Renal cortical hypoplasia, in Chapter 15.*

V. Chronic pyelonephritis

    A. *The clinical findings are essentially the same as those associated with end-stage renal disease.*

    B. *In addition, mild pyuria, hematuria, proteinuria, casts, and bacteria may be found in the urine.*

    C. *See Chapter 19, Pyelonephritis.*

VI. Hyperadrenalcorticism

A. *There may be a higher incidence of this disease in toy and miniature poodles and dachshunds.*

B. *The history and physical findings are characterized by one or more of the following:*
   1. Polyuria, polydipsia, and nocturia. These abnormalities are often the first clinical signs observed by owners.
   2. Distention of the abdomen caused by muscular weakness.
   3. Skin changes, including:
      a. Dry skin, broken hair shafts, and hyperkeratosis.
      b. Symmetrical bilateral alopecia.
      c. Pigmentation of blisters and pustules.
      d. Secondary pyoderma.

C. *Pertinent laboratory data*
   1. An absolute and relative eosinopenia and lymphopenia are characteristic findings.
   2. A low urine specific gravity is often observed in randomly obtained samples of urine.
   3. Hyperglycemia and glucosuria sometimes occur but are not frequent findings.
   4. Water balance studies may reveal a:
      a. Two- to threefold increase in water intake.
      b. Two- to threefold increase in urine output.
   5. Increased urinary excretion of 17-ketogenic steroids is a constant finding.

D. *Similar findings may occur as a result of high or prolonged administration of adrenocorticoids (iatrogenic hyperadrenalcorticism).*

VII. Diabetes mellitus

A. *Clinical findings associated with diabetes mellitus depend on the stage of disease.*
   1. This disease occurs more commonly in older female dogs.
   2. The uncomplicated form of diabetes mellitus is characterized by:
      a. Polyuria, polydipsia, nocturia, polyphagia.
      b. Weight loss.
      c. Bilateral cataracts in approximately 10 to 15 per cent of the cases.
   3. The complicated (acidotic) form of diabetes mellitus is characterized by:
      a. Signs mentioned in uncomplicated form.
      b. Anorexia, depression, weakness.
      c. Vomition, dehydration.
   4. Signs referable to pancreatic disease may be present, including:
      a. Dehydration.
      b. Weight loss and steatorrhea associated with exocrine dysfunction.
      c. Anorexia and depression.

B. *Laboratory data*
   1. Uncomplicated form.
      a. Evaluation of urinalyses usually reveals a variable specific gravity (1.015 to 1.050+), marked glucosuria, marked ketonuria, and on occasion evidence of cystitis (see Urinalysis, in Chapter 6).
      b. Hyperglycemia and hypercholesterolemia are typical findings.

c. Evaluation of water balance studies usually reveals a significant increase in 24 hour urine output and 24 hour water intake.
    2. Complicated (acidotic) form.
        a. Evaluation of urinalysis will usually reveal an acid pH (5.5 or less) in addition to the findings seen in the uncomplicated form.
        b. The concentration of plasma bicarbonate and the blood pH are often decreased.
        c. The concentrations of cholesterol, BUN, creatinine, and amylase are often increased. The increase in amylase may be due to pancreatic disease, renal disease, or both (see Chapter 6, Laboratory Findings in Diseases of the Urinary System).
        d. Evaluation of hemograms may reveal an increase in PCV and WBC. The leucocytosis may be associated with pancreatitis, secondary infection, or the stress phenomenon.
        e. There may be a decrease in the quantity of exogenous pancreatic enzymes in the feces if diabetes mellitus is associated with generalized chronic pancreatitis.

C. See Diabetes mellitus, in Chapter 28.

VIII. Diabetes insipidus

A. The history is usually characterized by polydipsia, polyuria, and nocturia.

B. Physical examination usually reveals no significant findings. Signs associated with a CNS neoplasm may be detected.

C. Urinalysis
    1. The specific gravity is usually below the fixed range (1.001 to 1.006) since tubular reabsorption of solute is normal.
    2. There are no other abnormal findings.

D. Evaluation of hemograms and blood chemistry tests usually reveal no abnormalities.

E. Withholding water from the patient may result in slight elevation of urine specific gravity, but S.G. will not rise to values indicative of normal urine concentrating ability.

F. Water balance studies usually reveal a significant increase in 24 hour water intake and urine output.

G. Following parenteral administration of antidiuretic hormone, the ability to concencentrate urine returns (i.e. the specific gravity and osmolality become significantly elevated. See Chapter 7, Tests of Renal Function).

IX. Renal diabetes insipidus

A. Renal diabetes insipidus is often a "wastebasket" type of diagnosis.

B. The clinical findings associated with this disease are the same as those seen in diabetes insipidus, except the ability to concentrate urine does not return after parenteral administration of antidiuretic hormone.

C. PSP excretion is normal.

D. Many ill-defined syndromes associated with polyuria and polydipsia tend to be placed in this category.

E. Further evaluation of this disease syndrome is needed.

X. Pyometra

A. *History and physical findings*

1. This disease occurs more frequently in middle aged female dogs (six to seven years).
2. Patients usually have been in estrum three to six weeks previously.
3. A vaginal discharge composed of inflammatory elements may occur if pyometra is associated with an open cervix.
4. Abdominal enlargement may be observed.
5. Lethargy, depression, and weakness may occur.
6. Dehydration and vomition may occur.
7. Polydipsia, polyuria, and nocturia may occur.
8. Pallor of visible mucous membranes may occur.

B. *Pertinent laboratory data*

1. In the presence of renal involvement, urinalyses (when not contaminated with vaginal and uterine exudate) are characterized by:
   a. A low specific gravity (1.003 to 1.006) which is unresponsive to antidiuretic hormone.
   b. Proteinuria (mild).
2. There may be an elevation in BUN, creatinine, and serum amylase concentration, although the latter are nonconsistent findings.
3. Hemogram.
   a. Neutrophilic leucocytosis (20,000 to 100,000 WBC per cmm.) associated with immature neutrophils is a consistent finding.
   b. A nonregenerative anemia may be present.
4. The ability to concentrate urine may return to normal two to eight weeks following ovariohysterectomy.

C. *See Pyometra, in Chapter 28.*

XI. Severe liver disease

A. *Although the pathophysiology of polyuria associated with generalized liver disease has not been established, this syndrome has been observed in dogs with spontaneous liver disease.*

B. *Polyuria is not a consistent finding associated with liver disease.*

REFERENCES

Abbrecht, P. H.: Effects of potassium deficiency on renal function in the dog. J. Clin. Invest., *48*:432–442, 1969.
Adolph, D. F.: Measurements of water drinking in dogs. Amer. J. Physiol., *125*:75–86, 1939.
Dicker, S. E.: Polydipsia in relation to pyometra. J. Sm. Anim. Pract., *10*:479–489, 1969.
Earley, L. E., Kahn, M., and Orloff, J.: The effects of infusions of chlorothiazide on urinary dilution and concentration in the dog. J. Clin. Invest., *40*:857–866, 1961.
Giebisch, G., and Lozano, R.: The Effects of adrenal steroids and potassium depletion on the elaboration of osmotically concentrated urine. J. Clin. Invest., *38*:843–853, 1959.
Gillenwater, J. V.: Antidiuretic properties of chlorothiazide in diabetes insipidus. Metabolism, *14*:539–558, 1965.
Henry, W. B., and Sieber, S. E.: Traumatic diabetes insipidus in a dog. J.A.V.M.A., *146*:1317–1322, 1965.
Kunau, R. T.: Function of the ascending loop of Henle in the potassium deficient dog. Amer. J.Physiol., *219*:1071–1079, 1970.
Manitius, A., Levitin, H., Beck, D., and Epstein, F. H.: On the mechanism of impairment of renal concentrating ability in potassium deficiency. J. Clin. Invest., *39*:684–692, 1960.

Mulinos, M. G., Springarn, C. L., and Lojkin, M. E.: A diabetes insipidus-like condition produced by small doses of desoxycorticosterone acetate in dogs. Amer. J. Physiol., 135:102–112, 1941.

O'Conner, W. J., and Potts, D. J.: Water exchange in normal dogs. Quart. J. Exp. Physiol., 54:244–265, 1969.

Osbaldiston, G. W.: Renal effects of long term administration of triamcinolone acetonide in normal dogs. Canad. J. Comp. Med., 35:28–35, 1971.

Osborne, J. C., and Harns, J. E.: Chromophobe adenoma in a dog. V. M./S.A.C., 11:1079–1081, 1970.

Richards, M. A.: Differential diagnosis of polyuric syndromes. J. Sm. Anim. Pract., 10:651–667, 1969.

Saunders, L. Z., Stephenson, H. C., and McEntee, K.: Diabetes insipidus and adiposo-genital syndrome in a dog due to infundibuloma. Cornell Vet., 41:445–458, 1951.

Siegel, E. T., Kelly, D. F., and Berg, P.: Cushing's syndrome in the dog. J.A.V.M.A., 157:2081–2090, 1970.

Vaamonde, C. A., Vaamonde, L. S., Morosi, H. J., Klinger, E. L., and Papper, S.: Renal concentrating ability in cirrhosis. I. Changes associated with the clinical status and course of the disease. J. Lab. Clin. Med., 70:179–194, 1967.

Chapter 15
CONGENITAL AND INHERITED RENAL DISEASE

A. *Renal aplasia*
 1. Renal aplasia refers to the complete lack of development of one or both kidneys.
 2. When bilateral, it is incompatible with life, and therefore it is a necropsy finding in the newborn.
 3. When unilateral, clinical abnormalities are usually absent unless renal disease develops in the contralateral kidney.
    a. The right kidney is absent more often than the left.
    b. Males are affected more often than females.
    c. The opposite kidney undergoes compensatory hypertrophy and hyperplasia.
    d. A diagnosis is usually established by:
       (1) Exploratory laparotomy.
       (2) Necropsy.
       (3) Excretory urography performed for other purposes.
 4. Renal aplasia has been uncommonly reported in the dog and cat.
 5. It is considered to be a congenital defect, but it may be inherited in beagles.
 6. Treatment.
    a. None is available for bilateral renal aplasia.
    b. In instances of unilateral aplasia and concomitant disease of the remaining kidney, treatment must be directed toward the etiology of the concomitant disease.
 7. Prognosis.
    a. Death is invariable in patients with bilateral renal aplasia.
    b. The prognosis is good for patients with unilateral renal aplasia, provided the opposite kidney is normal.

B. *Renal hypoplasia*
 1. Renal hypoplasia refers to defective formation of one or both kidneys with the end result of a decreased number of nephrons.
 2. Clinical signs depend on the degree of renal involvement.
    a. When unilateral or mild, it is usually an incidental finding.
    b. When bilateral and severe, uremia usually develops at a young age.

3. The frequency with which hypoplastic renal diseases have been reported in cats, and especially in dogs, has been increasing in recent years.
    a. The condition is often alleged to be a congenital defect, but proof of this is often lacking.
    b. Familial predisposition has also been incriminated, but again this is usually not based on reliable fact.
    c. Experimental investigations in a variety of animals have revealed that renal aplasia and renal hypoplasia may develop in association with a variety of nonheritable abnormalities.
        (1) Renal agenesis and hypoplasia have been produced in fetal pigs and rats from mothers fed diets deficient in vitamin A.
        (2) Arrested nephrogenesis associated with moderately hypoplastic kidneys can be induced in cats by intrauterine injection of fetuses with panleucopenia virus.
4. Diagnosis.
    a. When present, associated clinical signs usually occur at a young age.
    b. A tentative diagnosis may be based on kidney size established by radiography or necropsy. Renal hypoplasia, however, must be differentiated from end-stage kidneys due to acquired renal disease (see Chapter 20, End-Stage Kidneys).
5. Only palliative treatment is available (see Chapter 31, Treatment of Renal Failure).
6. For patients with unilateral renal hypoplasia, the prognosis is good, provided the opposite kidney is normal. For patients with bilateral renal hypoplasia, a guarded to poor prognosis is justified since even though the clinical course may be relatively long, the renal changes are progressive and irreversible.
7. At necropsy, the prominent feature is very small kidneys (Fig. 15–1). Alterations secondary to uremia may also be noted (see Chapter 13, Extrarenal Manifestations of Uremia).

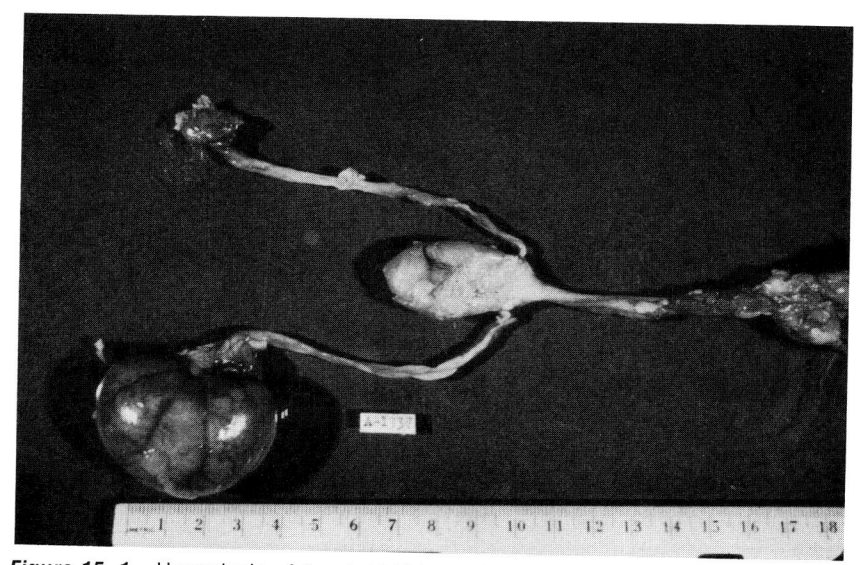

Figure 15–1. Hypoplasia of the right kidney of an adult domestic short-haired cat.

CONGENITAL AND INHERITED RENAL DISEASE   155

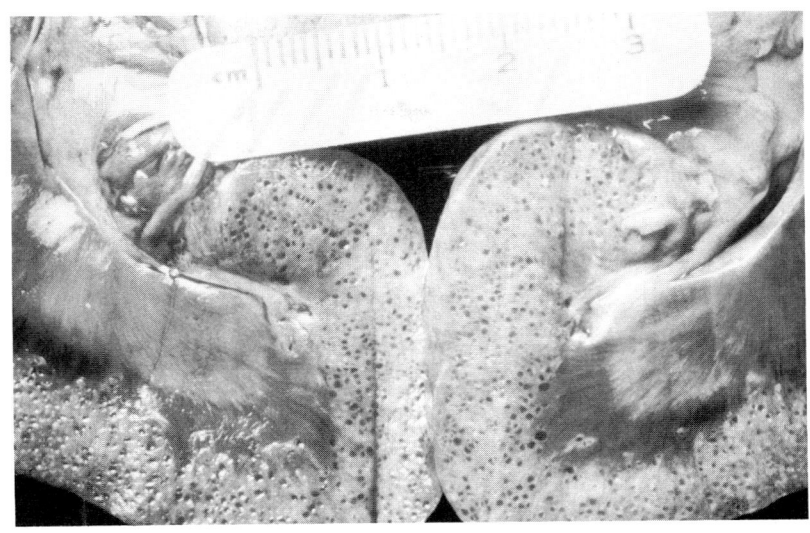

Figure 15–2. Polycystic left kidney obtained from a 2.5-year-old female Norwegian elkhound dog. The right kidney did not contain cysts, but was markedly reduced in size. The dog died of chronic renal failure. (Courtesy of Dr. Harold J. Kurtz, College of Veterinary Medicine, University of Minnesota.)

C. *Polycystic disease*
1. Polycystic disease is characterized by replacement of a variable quantity of renal parenchyma with multiple cysts of varying sizes (microscopic to several cm. in diameter) (Figs. 15–2 and 15–3).
2. The disease may involve one or both kidneys.
3. It is considered to be a congenital defect in the dog and cat, although clinical investigation of this disease has been meager. In man, both adult and infantile types of polycystic disease are inherited. Previous theories concerning the pathogenesis of polycystic kidney disease in man have been

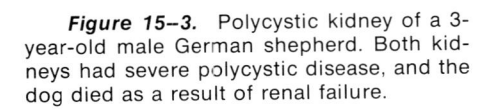

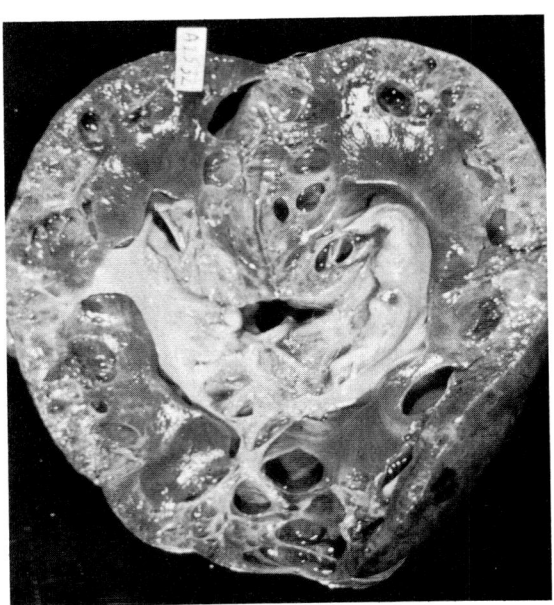

Figure 15–3. Polycystic kidney of a 3-year-old male German shepherd. Both kidneys had severe polycystic disease, and the dog died as a result of renal failure.

supplanted by microdissection studies. These investigations have established that polycystic kidneys may occur as a result of any one of the following:
   a. Dilatation and hyperplasia of collecting ducts.
   b. Inhibition of ureteral ampullary activity associated with failure of the ampullary regions to branch into collecting ducts.
   c. Multiple abnormalities anywhere along the nephrons.
4. Clinical findings are variable, being dependent on the number of cysts and the degree to which the adjacent renal parenchyma is involved.
   a. Generalized bilateral renal involvement leads to progressive and irreversible destruction of the renal parenchyma and is manifested clinically by signs of uremia in the young.
   b. Unilateral kidney involvement is usually not associated with clinical manifestations if the contralateral kidney is functionally normal.
   c. Kidneys which have become abnormally enlarged, multilobulated masses as a result of severe involvement may be detected by abdominal palpation.
   d. If cysts become infected, fever, leukocytosis, pyuria, hematuria, and proteinuria may be observed.
5. Gross pathology.
   a. Multiple cysts of varying size and number are scattered throughout the renal parenchyma (Figs. 15-2 and 15-3).
   b. Cysts contain clear, cloudy, or viscid fluid. On occasion cystic fluid may be red or brown as a result of hemorrhage or infection.
6. Histopathology.
   a. Renal cysts are separated by renal parenchyma which may be normal or abnormal.
   b. The cysts may be lined with flattened or cuboidal epithelium or the lining may be comprised of inflammatory tissue.
   c. Superimposed renal disease may be detected.
7. A diagnosis of polycystic renal disease may be established by:
   a. Renal biopsy.
   b. Supportive evidence gained by radiology.
   c. Exploratory laparotomy.
   d. Necropsy.
8. Treatment.
   a. The progressive renal insufficiency due to generalized bilateral involvement of the kidneys is irreversible.
   b. Symptomatic and supportive therapy may be provided for renal failure (see Chapter 31, Treatment of Renal Failure).
   c. If unilateral pyelonephritis refractive to medical treatment complicates the underlying disease, unilateral nephrectomy may be indicated, provided the opposite kidney is capable of sustaining life.
9. Prognosis.
   a. A guarded to poor prognosis is justified in the presence of generalized severe bilateral involvement of both kidneys.
   b. A guarded to good prognosis is justified in the presence of unilateral or mild bilateral involvement of the kidneys.

D. *Renal cortical hypoplasia (RCH)*
   1. RCH has been reported in certain genetic lines of cocker spaniels as an inherited trait.

2. It has been reported in several breeds of dogs from several months of age to about three years of age.
3. This disease affects both males and females.
4. The underlying mechanisms responsible for development of the abnormality are unknown.
5. The clinical history is usually characterized by progressive polydipsia, polyuria, weight loss, anorexia, and depression. Vomiting may occur but is not a consistent finding. If uremia occurs during the growth phase of the dog's life, stunted growth may also be present.
6. Laboratory features.
    a. Urinalysis.
        (1) A specific gravity between 1.002 and 1.012 is often observed.
        (2) Glucosuria may be present.
        (3) Protein is present in trace to moderate amounts.
    b. Hematology.
        (1) Profound nonregenerative anemia may occur in later stages.
        (2) WBC are often affected by the uremic stress response (see Chapter 6, Laboratory Findings in Diseases of the Urinary System).
    c. Blood chemistry.
        (1) BUN and creatinine are elevated.
        (2) Serum electrolytes are altered as in other causes of chronic uremia (see Chapter 6, Laboratory Findings in Diseases of the Urinary System).
7. Diagnosis.
    a. Occurrence of chronic progressive renal disease at a young age provides supportive evidence.
    b. Acquired causes of renal disease such as leptospirosis must be eliminated.
    c. Renal biopsy. The histopathology is characterized by:
        (1) Marked interstitial fibrosis and nephron destruction.
        (2) A paucity of interstitial lymphocytic or neutrophilic infiltrate.
        (3) These findings are similar to those seen in acquired generalized renal disease (see Chapter 20, End-Stage Kidneys).
    d. Necropsy. The most significant gross necropsy finding is marked decrease in the width of the renal cortex. Other causes of shrunken kidneys must be considered in the diagnosis of this disease (see Chapter 20, End-Stage Kidneys).
8. Treatment (see Chapter 31, Treatment of Renal Failure).
9. Prognosis.
    a. In general, the progress of the disease is relatively slow. Even after the onset of clinical signs of renal disease, patients may live for several months (see Chapter 12, Pathophysiology of Renal Failure).
    b. Reversal of the process does not occur, and thus the long term prognosis is poor.

E. *Horseshoe kidneys*
    1. Etiology. Although the cause of spontaneously occurring fusion of the kidneys in man and animals has not been established, horseshoe kidneys have been observed in a significant percentage of the offspring of maternal rats fed a vitamin A deficient diet.

2. Pathophysiology.
   a. Congenital fusion of the kidneys is thought to occur as a result of abnormal fusion of embryonic kidneys at an early stage of development.
   b. Since fusion occurs prior to rotation and ascent of the kidneys in the abdominal cavity, fused kidneys seldom ascend to their normal position (T–13 to L–2), and are not tilted cranioventrally.
   c. In most of the reported cases of fused kidneys in man and animals, the ureters remained separate and each kidney received its own blood supply.
   d. Human patients with fused kidneys are predisposed to ureteral obstruction because of a high incidence of associated aberrant vasculature, and because of the necessity of one or both ureters to arch over fused renal tissue.
   e. Malformations resulting from embryonic fusion of nephrogenic blastemas may be symmetrical or asymmetrical.
      (1) Symmetrical fusion is exemplified by the horseshoe kidney. In man, 90 per cent of the horseshoe kidneys are fused at their caudal poles.
      (2) The kidneys may be united by a thin fibrous band of connective tissue, or they may be connected by renal parenchyma.
      (3) The fused kidneys may be divided equally between the two flanks, or the entire structure may be located on one side.
      (4) When fusion between kidneys is extensive, the anomalous structure is usually located adjacent to the bony pelvis and is commonly called a cake, disc, shield, or dumbbell kidney.
3. Clinical findings.
   a. Generalities concerning the spectrum of clinical findings associated with congenital fusion of the kidneys in dogs and cats cannot be made because of the lack of a sufficient number of reported cases in which clinical manifestations have been discussed.
   b. In man, the majority of patients with fused kidneys have no clinical signs referable to the urinary system. When signs attributable to renal disease are encountered, they usually occur secondary to varying degrees of ureteral obstruction.

F. *Primary renal glucosuria*
   1. This disease is characterized by glucosuria which occurs secondary to a renal tubular enzymatic defect in active glucose reabsorption.
   2. History.
      a. Affected patients are usually asymptomatic.
      b. The disease may be detected because:
         (1) Urinalysis reveals glucosuria.
         (2) Bacterial cystitis occurs secondary to the glucosuria.
   3. The physical examination usually reveals no abnormal findings, except in some patients with secondary cystitis.
   4. Laboratory results.
      a. The fasting blood sugar concentration is normal (90 to 110 mg. per 100 ml.).
      b. Evaluation of a glucose tolerance test usually reveals glucose levels which are normal or below normal.

c. Urinalysis.
   (1) Persistent glucosuria is invariably present. A method which specifically detects glucose should be used.
   (2) Evidence of urinary tract infection may be present (see Urinalysis, in Chapter 6).
d. Renal function tests.
   (1) BUN and serum creatinine concentrations are normal.
   (2) Urinary PSP excretion is normal.
5. Diagnosis.
   a. Persistent glucosuria in the presence of normal blood glucose levels provide strong supportive evidence. Other causes of glucosuria must be eliminated, including:
      (1) Transient glucosuria secondary to physiologic hyperglycemia.
      (2) Diabetes mellitus.
      (3) Administration of dextrose by parenteral or oral routes.
      (4) Renal diseases such as renal cortical hypoplasia and familial renal disease in elkhounds which may be associated with glucosuria.
   b. Normal values for BUN and PSP excretion provide supportive evidence by eliminating generalized renal dysfunction as a cause of the glucosuria.
6. Treatment.
   a. No treatment is available that will reverse the glucosuria, since it is secondary to a specific enzymatic defect for glucose reabsorption.
   b. Bacterial cystitis should be treated if present (see Chapter 38, Bacterial Cystitis).
7. The prognosis is good since the disease does not adversely affect the dog, except for an increased susceptibility to cystitis.
8. Necropsy.
   a. No necropsy findings have been reported for dogs.
   b. Gross or microscopic renal lesions have not been observed in human patients with renal glycosuria.
9. A familial tendency may exist for canine renal glucosuria.

G. *Cystinuria*
   1. Cystinuria refers to a specific defect in the renal tubules that results in defective reabsorption of certain amino acids including cystine.
   2. History and clinical features.
      a. Affected dogs may be asymptomatic.
      b. Cystine uroliths occur in some dogs (see Chapter 34, Urolithiasis).
      c. Male dogs are predominantly, if not exclusively, affected. A sex-linked inheritance probably exists.
      d. The abnormality occurs in numerous breeds and mongrels.
   3. Diagnosis. A diagnosis of cystinuria may be established by:
      a. Detection of uroliths composed of cystine.
      b. Detection of increased urinary excretion of cystine.
         (1) Common screening tests for urine cystine used in man may give false negative readings in the dog.
         (2) Urine amino acid analysis, paper chromatography, and high voltage electrophoresis can be used, but are relatively expensive.
   4. Treatment.
      a. The renal defect cannot be altered.

  b. See Chapter 34, Urolithiasis, for prophylaxis and treatment of cystine calculi.
5. The prognosis is good unless uroliths develop.
6. At necropsy no renal abnormalities will be observed unless uroliths are present.

H. *Familial renal disease in Norwegian elkhound dogs*
1. This disease is a generalized renal disease characterized by development of uremia and death at an early age.
2. History and clinical features.
 a. Polydipsia and polyuria are consistent findings.
 b. Stunted growth may occur in severe cases with early onset.
 c. Depression, weight loss, and vomiting occur as the disease progresses.
 d. Affected dogs may live from a few months to three to five years.
3. This disease appears to differ from renal cortical hypoplasia in that kidneys appear to be normal in size early in the course of the disease, but decrease in size later in the course of the disease due to destruction of renal parenchyma.
4. Laboratory findings.
 a. Urinalysis.
  (1) A specific gravity of 1.003 to 1.012 is typical.
  (2) Glucosuria may be present.
  (3) Evidence of urinary tract infection is usually absent.
 b. Blood chemistry.
  (1) BUN and creatinine concentrations are elevated in advanced cases.
  (2) PSP excretion is depressed early in the course of the disease.
 c. Hematology.
  (1) A nonregenerative anemia occurs prior to the onset of uremia.
  (2) A profound anemia occurs late in the course of the disease.
5. Renal biopsy. The histopathology of biopsy samples is characterized by:
 a. Periglomerular fibrosis, and thickening of the basement membranes of Bowman's capsule and tubules.
 b. Interstitial fibrosis.
 c. A paucity of interstitial lymphocytic or neutrophilic infiltrate.
6. Diagnosis. A diagnosis of familial renal disease in Norwegian elkhounds can usually be based on the following:
 a. Breed.
 b. Young age at onset of renal failure.
 c. Clinical signs of renal failure.
 d. Laboratory findings consistent with chronic renal failure.
 e. Renal biopsy findings.
 f. Necropsy findings.
7. Treatment.
 a. No specific treatment will reverse the disease process.
 b. Palliative (see Chapter 31, Treatment of Renal Failure).
8. Prognosis.
 a. The clinical course may vary from a few weeks to two to three years, depending on the stage at which the disease was diagnosed and the rate of its progression (see Chapter 12, Pathophysiology of Renal Failure).
 b. The long-term prognosis is poor.

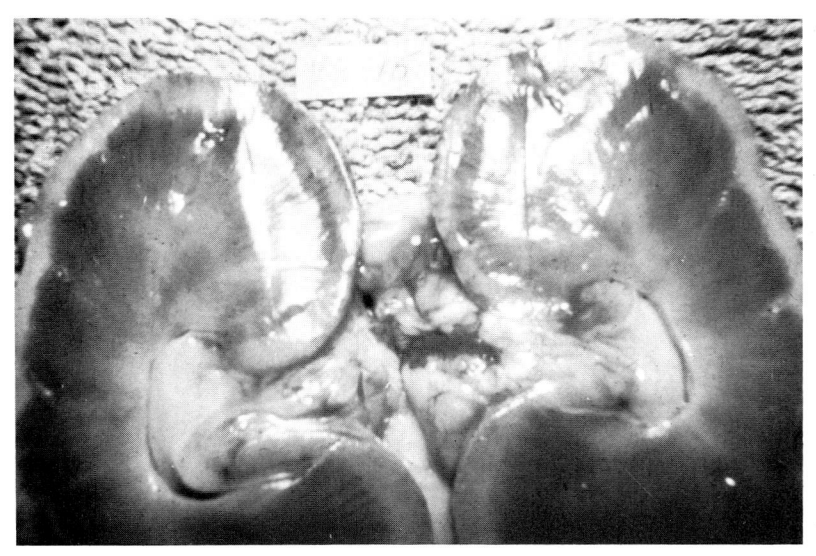

Figure 15–4. Kidney obtained from a 4-month-old male Norwegian elkhound with end-stage renal disease.

9. Necropsy.
    a. The kidneys are small and fibrotic with adherent renal capsules. (see Chapter 20, End-Stage Kidneys).
    b. The renal cortices are thin (Fig. 15–4).
    c. Findings secondary to uremia may be observed (see Chapter 13, Extrarenal Manifestations of Uremia).
10. This disease is probably inherited as a recessive trait. It is apparently not prevalent in the elkhound breed.

I. *Familial disease in Lhasa Apso dogs*
    1. History and clinical features.
        a. Depression, crying, and retarded growth have been noted by owners during the nursing period.
        b. Marked dehydration has been noted on examination of the pups.
        c. Untreated pups may die at this stage of the disease.
        d. Treated pups may survive the nursing period, but develop uremia when they are several months of age.
    2. Laboratory features.
        a. Urinalysis.
            (1) A low specific gravity (1.003 to 1.012) occurs.
            (2) Evidence of urinary tract infection is absent.
        b. Blood chemistry.
            (1) BUN and creatinine concentrations are elevated.
        c. Hematology.
            (1) A nonregenerative anemia is present in uremic pups.
    3. Treatment is palliative.
        a. Dehydration of pups has been treated with polyionic, balanced, isotonic electrolyte solutions parenterally and with water orally.
        b. Treatment of uremia may be instituted (see Chapter 31, Treatment of Renal Failure).

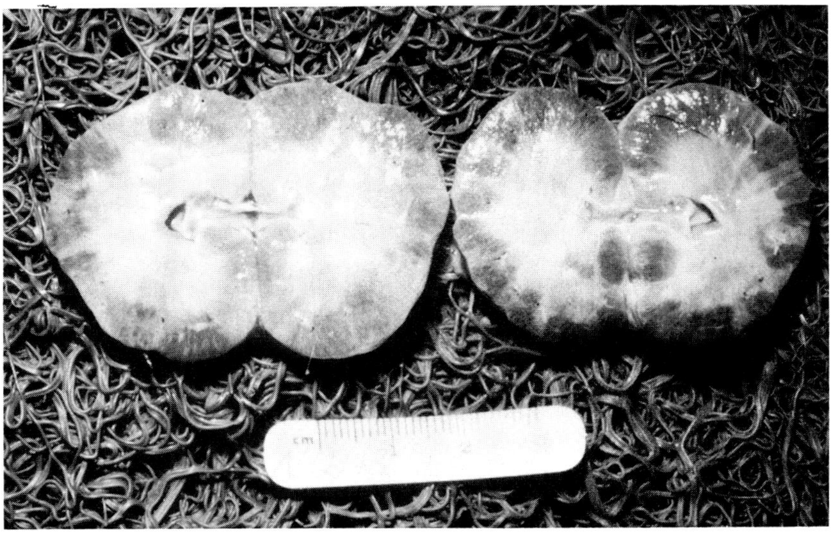

Figure 15-5. Kidneys obtained from a 6-month-old male lhasa apso dog with end-stage renal disease. The dog died of chronic renal failure (BUN = 300 mg. per 100 ml.). (Courtesy of Dr. Harold J. Kurtz, College of Veterinary Medicine, University of Minnesota.)

4. Diagnosis. A diagnosis of familial disease in lhasa apsos can usually be based on the following:
   a. Breed involved.
   b. Young age at time of onset.
   c. Signs and laboratory findings typical of generalized renal disease.
5. Prognosis.
   a. The prognosis is guarded to good for temporary improvement of dehydrated pups.
   b. The long-term prognosis is poor.
6. Necropsy.
   a. Contracted kidneys are evident macroscopically (Fig. 15-5).
   b. Microscopic alterations of renal tissue are characterized by nephron destruction and generalized fibrosis.

J. *At the present, knowledge concerning congenital and hereditary renal diseases of the dog and cat is in its infancy.*
   1. Numerous renal diseases of a hereditary or congenital nature probably occur in the dog and cat, but have not been adequately studied. Some have erroneously been diagnosed as chronic interstitial nephritis.
   2. The presence of disease in specific genetic lines of any breed, and an increase in incidence of the disease associated with inbreeding provides strong evidence that the defect is inherited. Acquired factors such as subclinical viral infection, exposure to drugs or chemicals, and altered calcium and vitamin D metabolism, warrant consideration and further investigation for the possibility of breed idiosyncrasy or vulnerability to these agents.
   3. Renal diseases described in cocker spaniels, Norwegian elkhounds, and lhasa apsos have not been studied in sufficient detail to establish if all breeds have the same disease. In addition, similarities or differences in

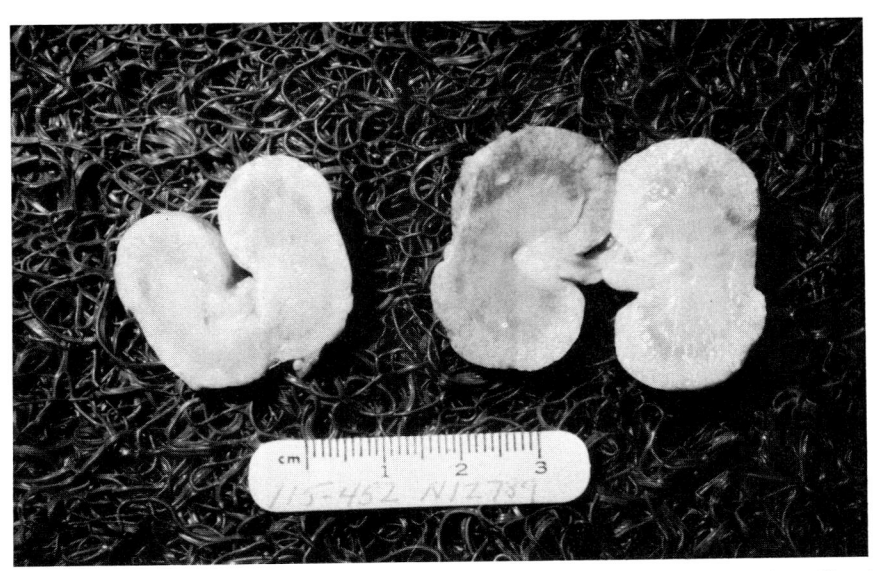

Figure 15–6. End-stage kidneys obtained from an immature, female shih tzu dog. The dog died of chronic renal failure. (Courtesy of Dr. J. E. Mosier, College of Veterinary Medicine, Kansas State University.)

etiology and pathogenesis of the disease in each affected breed have not been critically evaluated.

4. Inherited renal disease has also been suspected in German shepherd dogs, dachshunds, miniature schnauzers, and shih tzus, on the basis of occurrence of generalized renal disease in these breeds early in life (Fig. 15–6). The fact that more than one member of the litter (and in some instances the entire litter) is often affected has added to this suspicion.
5. The possibility of inherited or congenital renal disease should be considered when:
   a. Renal disease occurs at a young age.
   b. Environmental agents (infectious disease, chemical agents, drugs) cannot be incriminated as a causative factor.
   c. Related dogs are affected.

REFERENCES

Brand, E., Cahill, G. F., and Kussell, B.: Canine cystinuria. 5. Family history of two cystinuric Irish terriers and cystine determination of dog urine. J. Biol. Chem., *133*:431–436, 1940.

Brouwers, J., and Dewaele, A.: Congenital absence of a kidney in dogs and cats. Ann. Med. Vet., *104*:229–231, 1960.

Cordes, D. O., and Dodd, D. C.: Bilateral renal hypoplasia of the dog. Pathologica Vet., *2*:37–48, 1965.

Cornelius, C. E., Bishop, J. A., and Schaffer, M. H.: Aminoaciduria in dachshunds. Cornell Vet., *57*:177–183, 1967.

Crane, C. W., and Turner, A. W.: Amino-acid patterns of urine and blood plasma in a cystinuric Labrador dog. Nature, *177*:237–238, 1956.

Crocker, J. F. S., Brown, D. M., and Vernier, R. L.: Developmental defects of the kidney. A review of renal development and experimental studies of maldevelopment. Pediatric Clin. N. Amer., *18*:355–376, May, 1971.

Finco, D. R., Kurtz, H. J., Low, D. G., and Perman, V.: Familial renal disease in Norwegian elkhound dogs. J.A.V.M.A., *156*:747–760, 1970.

Fox, M. W.: Inherited polycystic mononephrosis in the dog. J. Hered., *55*:29, 1964.

Frimpter, G. W., Thouin, P., and Ewalds, B.: Penicillamine in canine cystinuria. J.A.V.M.A., *151*:1084–1086, 1967.

Johnson, C. E.: Pelvic and horseshoe kidneys in the domestic cat. Anat. Anz., *46*:69–78, 1914.

Kaufman, C. F., Soirez, R. F., and Tasker, J. P.: Renal cortical hypoplasia with secondary hyperparathyroidism in the dog. J.A.V.M.A., *155*:1679–1685, 1969.

Kilham, L., Margolis, G., and Colby, E. D.: Congenital infections of cats and ferrets by feline panleucopenia virus manifested by cerebellar hypoplasia. Lab. Invest., *17*:465–480, 1967.

Krook, L.: The pathology of renal cortical hypoplasia in the dog. Nord. Vet-Med., *9*:161–176, 1957.

Murti, G. S.: Renal agenesis and dysgenesis. J.A.V.M.A., *146*:1120–1124, 1965.

Osathanondh, V., and Potter, E. L.: Pathogenesis of polycystic kidneys. Arch. Path., *77*:459–512, 1964.

Persson, F., Persson, S., and Asheim, A.: Renal cortical hypoplasia in dogs. I. A clinical study of uremia and secondary hyperparathyroidism. Acta Vet. Scand., *2*:68–84, 1961.

Persson, F., Persson, S., and Asheim, A.: Blood-pressure in dogs with renal cortical hypoplasia. Acta Vet. Scand., *2*:129–136, 1961.

Pollock, S.: Cystinuria in the dog. J.A.V.M.A., *126*:188–191, 1955.

Robbins, G. R.: Unilateral renal agenesis in the beagle. Vet. Rec., *77*:1345–1347, 1965.

Storey, H. E.: A case of horseshoe kidney and associated vascular anomalies in the domestic cat. Anat. Rec., *86*:307–319, 1943.

Treacher, R. J.: The etiology of canine cystinuria. Biochem. J., *90*:494, 1964.

Vymetal, F.: Renal aplasia in beagles. Vet. Rec., *77*:1344–1345, 1965.

Chapter 16
ACUTE RENAL DISEASE

I. Definition

Acute renal disease is a nonspecific term used to designate a class of diseases with many common clinical characteristics. It includes causes of acute nephritis (inflammatory lesions of the nephron) and acute nephrosis (degenerative lesions of the kidney characterized primarily by damage to tubules).

II. Etiology

A. Infectious agents
1. Bacterial infection.
   a. Leptospira serotypes.
   b. *Escherichia coli.*
   c. Streptococci.
   d. Staphylococci.
   e. *Proteus* spp.
   f. Others.
2. Viral diseases (viral effects on the kidneys are often subclinical).
   a. Infectious canine hepatitis.
   b. Canine distemper.
   c. Herpes virus.

B. Chemical agents
1. Ethylene glycol and diethylene glycol.
2. Arsenic.
3. Mercury.
4. Lead.
5. Bismuth.
6. Thallium.
7. Nephrotoxic antibacterial drugs including sulfonamides, neomycin, kanamycin, gentamicin, vancomycin, polymyxin B, and amphotericin B.
8. Uranium salts.
9. Carbon tetrachloride.

C. Renal ischemia
1. Shock.
2. Any cause of severe impairment of renal perfusion with blood.

166 DISEASES OF THE UPPER URINARY SYSTEM

III. History

   A. *The history is dependent, at least in part, on the specific etiology.*

   B. *Observations frequently made by owners regardless of etiology include:*
      1. Signs of uremia including depression, anorexia, vomiting, and sometimes diarrhea.
      2. Scanty or voluminous urine production.

   C. *The abruptness in onset of signs and their duration may be of aid in differentiating acute from chronic renal diseases.*

   However, it is probably only in the instance of astute observations by owners that the insidious onset of chronic renal disease will be detected prior to the onset of a uremic crisis.

IV. Physical examination findings

   A. *Some findings may be related directly to the specific etiology (see Chapter 17, Ischemic and Chemical Nephrosis; Chapter 36, Physical Injuries; and Leptospirosis, in Chapter 28).*

   B. *Physical findings associated with uremia include:*
      1. Scleral injection.
      2. Dehydration.
      3. Oliguria or polyuria.
         a. Urine volume may be scanty (oliguria) during the early phases of acute renal disease, but may be voluminous during the convalescent phase.
         b. During the early phases oliguria may be present in association with a urine of either high or low specific gravity.
            (1) Oliguria with a low specific gravity suggests that a very small number of nephrons are functional at that time, and that massive renal injury has occurred.
            (2) Oliguria with a high specific gravity indicates a marked decrease in glomerular filtration rate, but retention of some tubular function.
         c. Voluminous urine volume following oliguria suggests that repair to damaged nephrons is occurring. This is usually a good prognostic sign; however, death from uremia may occur during this phase.

   C. *Pain in the area of the kidneys is not diagnostic of acute renal disease.*

   The absence of pain in the area of the kidneys does not eliminate the possibility of acute renal disease.

V. Laboratory findings

   A. *Hemogram*
      1. No significant changes are usually present except those:
         a. Unique to the specific etiology of the acute renal disease.
         b. Due to stress (see Chapter 6, Laboratory Findings in Diseases of the Urinary System).

ACUTE RENAL DISEASE

    2. The absence of anemia in a uremic dog may occur in acute renal disease or relatively early in the course of chronic renal disease.

B. *Urinalysis*
1. The specific gravity may be high or low. In subclinical cases associated with prerenal uremia, the specific gravity is high because the kidney has retained its ability to concentrate urine, and is required to do so to maintain water balance. In cases associated with generalized damage to nephrons, it is low because of loss of concentrating ability by the nephrons.
2. Proteinuria is much more common and is frequently more profuse on qualitative tests in acute renal disease than chronic renal diseases. (see Urinalysis, in Chapter 6).
3. Microscopic examination of urine sediment.
   a. Increased numbers of RBC, WBC, and casts may occur, but may be present only transiently.
   b. Their presence may depend on the etiology; their absence does not eliminate the possibility of acute renal disease.

C. *Blood chemistry (see Chapter 6, Laboratory Findings in Diseases of the Urinary System).*

VI. Diagnosis

A. *The history and physical examination may be helpful in isolating a specific cause of acute renal disease.*

B. *Laboratory findings and urinalysis may provide supportive evidence.*

C. *Renal biopsy may reveal morphologic alterations of diagnostic significance.*

D. *Response to therapy may provide supportive or specific evidence, depending on the disease being considered and the treatment given.*

VII. Treatment

A. *Therapy should be directed at the specific etiologic agent when known.*

B. *Palliative (see Chapter 31, Treatment of Renal Failure).*

VIII. Prognosis

A. *The prognosis is dependent on the etiology, severity, and duration of the disease.*

B. *In general, the potential for reversal of acute renal disease is much greater than for the reversal of chronic renal disease.*

IX. Pathology

A. *Gross lesions*
1. Macroscopic changes are somewhat variable depending on the etiology of the renal disease.
2. Morphologic alterations of kidneys affected with acute renal disease which help differentiate acute from chronic generalized disease include:

DISEASES OF THE UPPER URINARY SYSTEM

      a. Size. The kidneys are usually enlarged and swollen in acute generalized renal disease.
      b. Consistency. The tissue bulges when cut or when the capsule is stripped, and the tissue imparts little resistance when cut in acute generalized renal disease.
      c. The cortical tissue is often swollen and appears wider than normal in acute generalized renal disease.

B. *The appearance of a microscopic lesion is dependent on the specific cause.*
Consult veterinary pathology texts for specific details.

Chapter 17
ISCHEMIC AND CHEMICAL NEPHROSIS

I. **Nephrosis is a disease of the kidneys characterized by degenerative lesions of the renal tubules.**

It may be caused by a variety of agents, the most common of which are ischemia and nephrotoxins. Clinical signs of acute nephrosis are similar regardless of etiology, and are of little or no value in indicating the underlying cause.

II. **Renal ischemia versus nephrotoxins**
   A. *Although renal failure caused by ischemia is clinically indistinguishable from renal failure caused by nephrotoxins, each in pure form produces a different type of tubular lesion.*
   1. Microscopic and microdissection studies in kidneys of dogs have revealed that structural damage induced by severe renal ischemia is characterized by irregular or patchy distribution of lesions throughout the tubules.
      a. The lesions consist of varying degrees of disruption, fragmentation, or dissolution of tubular basement membranes and necrosis of tubular epithelial cells.
      b. Variable numbers of nephrons are damaged, but rarely is an entire nephron damaged.
      c. With the possible exception of a paucity of RBC in glomerular capillaries and the presence of platelet thrombi, the glomeruli of affected kidneys are morphologically normal.
      d. The severity of morphologic changes produced by ischemia induced by hypotension is variable, but the sequence of alterations is the same. Variables affecting the severity of morphologic lesions include:
         (1) The degree of hydration of the patient prior to hypotension.
         (2) The period of time which has elapsed from the onset of ischemia to examination of the tissue.
         (3) The duration and degree of inadequate renal perfusion.
         (4) The presence or absence of concomitant renal diseases.
      e. The tubules are the major site of pathologic alterations because the high metabolic activity of tubular epithelial cells makes them more susceptible to the effects of ischemia than glomeruli, blood vessels, and interstitial tissue.
   2. Structural damage induced by nephrotoxic nephrosis in pure form is characterized by cellular degeneration and necrosis which is primarily confined to the epithelium of the proximal portions of the tubules. Un-

like renal ischemia, all of the nephrons may be affected and the basement membranes of the damaged portions of the renal tubules are not significantly altered.
- a. Explanation of the distribution of lesions caused by nephrotoxins may be related to the fact that nephrotoxins can be filtered by all glomeruli, and thus can be concentrated by renal tubular cells in sufficient quantity to cause cell death.
- b. Since most nephrotoxins cause damage to cells of other organs, they may also cause renal ischemia and associated tubular basement membrane lesions as a result of generalized fluid loss and hypotension.

B. *These morphologic differences in lesions induced by renal ischemia and nephrotoxins are clinically significant since tubular basement membranes must be relatively intact to allow structural and functional restoration of damaged nephrons.*

Because of the nature of the renal lesions they produce, the potential for nephron repair may be greater following injury by nephrotoxins than by ischemia.

III. Etiopathogenesis of ischemic nephrosis

A. *Etiology*
1. In the past, ischemic nephrosis has been called acute tubular necrosis, acute renal failure, lower nephron nephrosis, hypoxic nephrosis, and anoxic nephrosis. Most of these names were chosen because they emphasized a common clinical or pathological finding, or reflected a proposed etiopathogenic cause.
2. Any factor or combination of factors which causes prolonged and severe renal hypoperfusion has the potential to cause ischemic nephrosis.
   - a. Some of the more commonly incriminated causes include hemorrhage, trauma, anesthesia, profound fluid and electrolyte disturbances, and major surgery.
   - b. The significance of spontaneously occurring hypovolemic shock as a cause of ischemic nephrosis in dogs and cats has not been established.
     (1) Attempts to produce acute oliguric renal insufficiency in experimental dogs similar to that associated with hypovolemic shock in human beings were not successful.
     (2) Hemorrhagic or traumatic shock in dogs which was of sufficient severity and duration to cause acute renal failure consistently resulted in death of the dog due to circulatory failure before renal failure had time to develop.
     (3) The prevalence of acute oliguric renal failure due to spontaneous hypovolemic shock in dogs and cats has not been documented.

B. *Pathophysiology*
1. The exact mechanisms by which renal failure occurs in any species following hemorrhage, trauma, surgery, etc., have not been established.
   - a. Prolonged renal ischemia due to vasospasm, obstruction of tubules with casts and cellular debris, intravascular coagulation and direct toxic effects of abnormal substances in blood and urine on tubular cells have been hypothesized.
   - b. With the exception of prolonged renal ischemia due to vasospasm, there is little data to support the aforementioned hypotheses.

2. A common denominator of all causes of ischemic renal failure appears to be renal ischemia caused by poor perfusion of the renal microcirculation.
    a. Reduction in effective circulatory volume and secondary renal vasoconstriction can be induced by:
        (1) External or internal hemorrhage.
        (2) Sequestration of large volumes of fluid into damaged areas of the body (traumatic wounds, surgical sites, gastrointestinal tract).
    b. In surgical patients, the risk of renal failure is related to the adequacy of renal function that exists prior to surgery.
        (1) The usual hazards associated with surgery and the postoperative period are often exaggerated in the presence of compromised renal function.
        (2) Patients with generalized renal disease are especially susceptible to the renal effects of volume depletion, a condition which frequently occurs during or immediately following surgery.
        (3) In addition to alterations in peripheral blood flow and cardiac output associated with preexisting disease or anesthesia, major surgical procedures performed on dehydrated patients may be associated with additional reduction in volume as a result of internal sequestration of fluid in the operative area.
        (4) In addition, manipulation of abdominal organs in dogs is known to be associated with a reflex depression of renal blood flow.
    c. Despite the potential for occurrence, most patients do not develop significant azotemia following surgery, trauma, or shock.
        (1) Hypotension must be severe and prolonged in order to cause irreversible damage to previously normal kidneys.
        (2) The sensitivity of the kidneys to ischemia appears to be intermediate between the skin and skeletal muscles (which can withstand long periods of ischemia without detrimental effects), and the central nervous system (which cannot withstand ischemia for more than a few minutes).
        (3) In normothermic experimental dogs, renal ischemia produced by complete occlusion of the renal pedicle for a period of 30 minutes was not associated with the development of significant renal lesions.
        (4) Complete normothermic occlusion of the renal pedicle for a period of two hours usually, but not invariably, produced a significant degree of reversible functional and morphologic renal damage. Gradual recovery of renal function usually occurred over a period of two to three weeks.
        (5) Complete normothermic renal ischemia of more than four hours duration consistently caused irreversible renal injury leading to death from renal failure in a period of four to eight days.
        (6) Experimental dogs in which renal perfusion at a pressure of less than 30 mm. Hg (which is less than that required to produce irreversible shock) was allowed to persist for as long as three hours following partial occlusion of the renal pedicle did not develop significant functional impairment.
        (7) The aforementioned experimental data is of clinical value in that it provides some perspective to the amount of time which

can elapse before the kidneys are irreversibly damaged by renal ischemia. If adequate blood volume is restored and maintained in patients known or suspected to have renal hypoperfusion, renal failure may be corrected or prevented.

IV. Etiopathogenesis of nephrotoxic nephrosis

  A. *Etiology*

   Nephrotoxins which have the potential to produce nephrosis in dogs and cats include:
   1. Heavy metals and their compounds.
       a. Mercury.
       b. Lead.
       c. Bismuth.
       d. Arsenic.
       e. Thallium.
       f. Uranium.
   2. Organic solvents.
       a. Carbon tetrachloride.
       b. Tetrachlorethylene.
   3. Glycols.
       a. Ethylene glycol.
       b. Diethylene glycol.
   4. Drugs.
       a. Sulfonamides.
       b. Neomycin.
       c. Kanamycin.
       d. Vancomycin.
       e. Gentamicin.
       f. Polymyxin B.
       g. Amphotericin B.
       h. Bacitracin.

  B. *Pathophysiology*
   1. Some chemical injuries to the kidneys, especially those associated with drugs, are often mild and self-limiting upon withdrawal of the therapeutic agent.
   2. Most nephrotoxins are generalized cell poisons, and therefore may be associated with polysystemic disorders. For example, renal failure usually does not become a clinical problem in patients poisoned with ethylene glycol unless they survive toxic damage to the gastrointestinal and nervous systems, and disorders in fluid, electrolyte, and acid-base balance.
   3. Following filtration by glomeruli, it has been hypothesized that nephrotoxins are concentrated by the reabsorptive action of tubular cells. In this fashion, they accumulate in sufficient concentration to cause tubular cell necrosis.

V. Clinical findings

  A. *Clinical findings associated with renal failure caused by acute nephrosis are partially dependent on the underlying cause.*

B. *Patients with acute nephrosis may have a history of recent shock, major surgery, or exposure to nephrotoxins.*

In some instances, however, a predisposing cause may not be detected.

C. *Several hours or even days may elapse from the onset of the predisposing condition to recognition of the onset of renal failure.*

D. *Early signs of acute renal insufficiency may be obscured by clinical signs related to the precipitating cause.*

E. *Depending on the stage of the disease process, oliguria or polyuria may be present.*
   1. During the early phases of the disease urine volume may be scanty.
      a. The presence of oliguria may not be recognized for some time, however, since daily urine output is not routinely evaluated except by subjective estimation.
      b. Although oliguria associated with acute nephrosis has been attributed to passive reabsorption of filtrate through damaged tubules and tubular obstruction by casts, these hypotheses have not been substantiated by clinical or experimental evidence.
      c. Although the exact pathophysiology involved in the production of oliguria has not been established, marked reduction in glomerular filtration rate is apparently an important factor.
      d. Oliguria usually persists for hours or days, but in some instances it is so transient that it is not detected.
      e. Oliguria per se is not pathognomonic of acute nephrosis since it may occur in association with prerenal uremia. In order to be meaningful, urine volume must be correlated with other parameters of renal function (e.g., urine specific gravity, BUN). A concentrated urine sample (S.G. = 1.025 or greater) indicates the presence of functional nephrons which are far greater in number than is compatible with uremia due to primary uremia.
      f. Anuria is uncommonly associated with acute nephrosis. Its presence should lead one to suspect the presence of obstructive uropathy.
   2. If the patient survives, diuresis will develop during the convalescent stage of the disease process.
      a. Diuresis associated with acute nephrosis may be attributed, at least in part, to the fact that newly regenerating tubular epithelial cells are unable to concentrate or dilute urine (see Chapter 12, Pathophysiology of Renal Failure).
      b. Diuresis may also be attributed to obligatory osmotic diuresis caused by retention of solute due to renal failure.
      c. The onset of the diuretic phase does not abruptly terminate all the problems associated with renal failure. In fact, renal function may continue to decline for the first several days following its onset.
      d. Although diuresis following oliguria indicates that repair is occurring, death from uremia may still occur.

F. *Information extrapolated from experimental studies of acute ischemic and nephrotoxic nephrosis in dogs suggests that if the patient survives the initial stages of the uremic crisis and is properly treated, functional recovery adequate to sustain life can usually be expected in two to four weeks.*

In some instances, however, permanent but inactive renal lesions may remain.

174   DISEASES OF THE UPPER URINARY SYSTEM

VI. Laboratory findings

A. *Evaluation of various renal function tests will reveal findings consistent with renal dysfunction.*

B. *Abnormal quantities of casts, tubular epithelial cells, RBC, WBC, and protein may be observed in the urine sediment.*

C. *Oxalate crystals may be observed in the urine sediment obtained from patients with ethylene glycol toxicity, but are not a consistent finding.*

D. *The specific gravity of the urine (regardless of volume) obtained from patients with renal failure secondary to nephrosis will be similar to that of glomerular filtrate (1.008 to 1.012) if a sufficient quantity of nephrons have been incapacitated to prevent concentration or dilution of urine.*

    1. If the S.G. is above 1.025 in a patient with renal failure, at least one third of the nephrons must be capable of function. In this instance, a prerenal cause of uremia should be suspected until proved otherwise.

    2. One must avoid being misled by evaluation of residual urine formed prior to the onset of an episode of acute nephrosis. When the results do not correlate with clinical findings, urinalyses should be repeated.

E. *The hemogram will not reveal a nonregenerative anemia if the disease is acute.*

F. *Oliguric uremic patients in states of accelerated tissue catabolism may have markedly abnormal concentrations of serum potassium.*

VII. Radiographic findings

A. *In dogs in which there is no history of a predisposing cause of a uremic crisis, radiographic evaluation of kidney size may be of value (see Chapter 8, Radiographic Evaluation of the Urinary System).*

    1. If the kidneys are bilaterally contracted, an acute episode of nephrosis superimposed on chronic renal disease should be suspected.

    2. If the kidneys are normal or enlarged in size and are bilaterally symmetrical, acute nephrosis caused by ischemia or nephrotoxins should be considered.

B. *Radiographic evaluation of kidney size in cats is usually unnecessary since both kidneys can routinely be evaluated by digital palpation.*

Radiography may be of value in obtaining more accurate information about kidney size if the latter is compared to the size of other normal anatomic structures on the radiograph (see Chapter 8, Radiographic Evaluation of the Urinary System).

VIII. Renal biopsy findings

A. *In cases in which a diagnosis of acute nephrosis cannot be established on the basis of clinical and laboratory findings, renal biopsy should be considered.*

B. *In addition to establishing a specific diagnosis, renal biopsies may be of value in establishing the presence or absence of concomitant renal diseases which may be causing or potentiating renal failure, and they may indicate the potential reversibility of the underlying lesions.*

    1. The morphology of biopsy samples obtained from kidneys of patients with renal failure caused by ischemia or nephrotoxins may be remark-

ably normal, even though renal function tests reveal the presence of primary renal failure. Even though establishment of a specific diagnosis may not be possible, such findings suggest that recovery is feasible, and thus provide justification for aggressive therapy.
2. If the renal morphology of a uremic patient is such that repair appears to be improbable, the decision to support the patient with therapy in the hope that spontaneous recovery will occur may be altered.

IX. Diagnosis

A. *A history of recent trauma or shock, or exposure to potentially nephrotoxic agents is especially helpful in establishing a diagnosis of acute nephrosis since the clinical findings associated with this disorder may be only suggestive of renal failure.*

B. *Positive identification of a toxic agent in blood or urine provides proof of exposure and absorption.*

C. *Renal biopsy samples may reveal significant morphological alterations, and often may allow assessment of the potential reversibility of nephron damage.*

D. *Response to specific therapy may also provide support for the tentative diagnosis, and in some instances may indicate a specific cause.*

E. *A variable period of time must elapse from the onset of the precipitating cause of acute nephrosis to the development of clinical and laboratory abnormalities associated with renal failure.*

  1. Early recognition of impending acute renal failure in the absence of overt clinical signs is dependent on knowledge of when and how it develops.
  2. Asymptomatic patients with the potential to develop acute nephrosis should be re-evaluated at appropriate intervals.

X. Treatment

A. *Prophylactic therapy*

  1. Prophylactic therapy must be timely to be effective and therefore must be considered before, during, and immediately following the onset of an abnormality with the potential to cause acute nephrosis.
  2. In order to avoid precipitating a uremic crisis, elective surgical procedures should be preceded by evaluation of renal function. The latter may be accomplished by means of information obtained from the:
     a. History.
     b. Physical examination.
     c. Complete urinalysis.
     d. BUN or serum creatinine concentration.
     e. If the aforementioned procedures reveal abnormalities, a more detailed evaluation of the urinary system should be performed in order to evaluate the significance of the renal disease in the light of impending surgery.
     f. Additional justification for preoperative evaluation of the urinary system lies in the fact that evaluation of the significance of complications in the postoperative patient by means of various diagnostic tests is enhanced if preoperative data is available for comparison.

3. Prerenal uremia.
   a. In an experimental study in dogs, it was observed that moderate dehydration was associated with an increased susceptibility of the kidneys to ischemic injury. Rehydration associated with diuresis provided significant protection against ischemic renal damage.
   b. In patients with prerenal uremia, abnormalities causing poor renal perfusion should be corrected prior to, during, and following surgery in order to prevent or minimize the development of tubular cell necrosis (see Chapter 32, Fluid Therapy in Renal Failure).
4. Primary renal uremia.
   a. Major surgery may be successfully performed in patients with renal insufficiency provided careful attention is paid to fluid and electrolyte balance and the potential complications which may develop during the postoperative period.
   b. If surgery becomes necessary in patients with impaired renal function, such as azotemic patients with pyometra, or in patients in which the surgical procedure is associated with a high risk of complicating renal failure (major trauma, cardiac surgery), prophylactic renoprotective therapy should be employed.
      (1) As was the situation with prerenal uremia, deficits in fluid and electrolyte balance should be corrected by parenteral fluid therapy prior to, during, and following surgery. Adequate hydration must be maintained in order to insure adequate renal perfusion during surgery.
      (2) Clinical experience and experimental investigations have revealed that timely induction and maintenance of diuresis at the time of surgery has often been effective in minimizing or preventing renal failure in high risk patients.
         (a) The use of diuretics such as hypertonic dextrose (10 or 20%), hypertonic mannitol (20 to 25%), furosemide, and ethacrynic acid, either singly or in various combinations, has provided the most consistent results (see Chapter 31, Treatment of Renal Failure). The effectiveness of these diuretics is related to their ability to promptly induce and sustain diuresis.
         (b) It is stressed that diuretics are not effective substitutes for adequate hydration and electrolyte replacement.
         (c) Diuretics can be detrimental to renal homeostatic defense mechanisms unless adequate fluid and electrolyte balance are maintained.
         (d) Although the exact mechanisms by which the aforementioned diuretics protect renal function are controversial, increased renal blood flow associated with expansion of extracellular fluid volume and increased cardiac output, and augmentation of intratubular volume and flow have been suggested as the most probable mechanisms. Greatest emphasis has been placed on increased tubular flow, this occurring in response to a marked decrease in tubular reabsorption of solute. These diuretics may prevent the formation of tubular casts and interstitial edema by increasing urine volume.
         (e) If properly hydrated patients do not promptly develop a diuresis in response to test trials with the diuretics mentioned

above, it can be concluded that primary generalized renal dysfunction has occurred. Continued use of diuretics in attempts to re-establish urine flow in such instances are contraindicated since such therapy will be ineffective and may be associated with severe overhydration. Other modes of therapy such as peritoneal dialysis or hemodialysis should be considered.

B. *Specific therapy of ischemic nephrosis*
 1. As a working hypothesis, the development of oliguria in traumatic, postoperative or severely dehydrated patients should be considered to be of prerenal origin until proved otherwise.
    a. There is no sharp clinical dividing line which indicates the period of transition from a state of prerenal uremia to a state of primary uremia.
    b. Even after organic renal failure develops, it is not an all or none phenomenon.
        (1) The severity of renal damage caused by ischemia increases in proportion to the duration of the state of renal hypoperfusion.
        (2) For this reason timely administration of renoprotective therapy may reduce or prevent the development of a functional state of acute ischemic nephrosis.
        (3) Early treatment is imperative, as the likelihood of successful response decreases with time.
 2. Even though renal function tests indicate dysfunction, and primary renal failure is considered as a possibility, correction of deficits in fluid and electrolytes and the intelligent use of test trials with certain diuretics (dextrose, mannitol, furosemide, ethacrynic acid) may be followed by significant patient response.
 3. If fluid and diuretic therapy are not associated with significant diuresis, a regimen of therapy characterized by restriction of fluid should be adopted (see Chapter 32, Fluid Therapy in Renal Failure).

C. *Specific therapy of nephrotoxic nephrosis*
 1. Treatment of nephrotoxic nephrosis should consist of the use of specific chemical or pharmacologic antidotes if available.
    a. Recent investigations have revealed that administration of ethyl alcohol soon after exposure may be of therapeutic value in patients poisoned with ethylene glycol. Ethyl alcohol is thought to be a competitive inhibitor of the oxidation of ethylene glycol by hepatic alcohol dehydrogenase.
    b. British antilewisite (BAL) may be of value in the treatment of arsenic toxicity.
 2. In addition to antidotes, the source of the toxic agent must be eliminated.
    a. If exposure has been via the oral route, emetics, adsorbants, gastric lavage, or laxatives should be considered in effort to remove residual quantities of the toxic agent from the gastrointestinal tract.
    b. Removal of toxic agents from the body by peritoneal dialysis may be of value in some cases. The following toxic agents are known to be dialyzable in man:
        (1) Ethylene glycol.

(2) Arsenic.

(3) Neomycin, streptomycin, kanamycin, sulfonamides.

3. If the toxic agent cannot be identified, or if a specific antidote is not available, the only alternative is to employ symptomatic and supportive therapy with the hope that the patient can be kept alive until spontaneous repair of the kidneys occurs.

D. *Symptomatic and supportive therapy of acute nephrosis*

1. Once organic renal failure has developed, no regimen of therapy will eliminate the renal lesions. Although the precipitating causes must be eliminated if life is to be maintained, the renal damage which has occurred must heal spontaneously over a period of days to weeks, and remaining viable nephrons must undergo compensatory adaptation.

2. If patients with organic renal failure are in need of extensive supportive and symptomatic therapy, every effort should be made to determine the potential reversibility of the underlying lesion.

    a. The detection of renal diseases which are potentially reversible is justification for vigorous employment of available therapeutic techniques.

    b. Irreversible renal failure may not warrant such effort and expense.

3. The objective of therapy for patients with reversible renal failure must be to keep the patient alive until the processes of regeneration, repair, and compensatory adaptation allow the kidneys to regain sufficient function to re-establish homeostasis. This may be accomplished by minimizing changes in fluid, electrolyte and acid-base balance with various combinations of conservative medical management, diuresis, and peritoneal dialysis (see Chapter 31, Treatment of Renal Failure).

4. The objective of therapy for patients with irreversible renal failure must be to re-establish and maintain biochemical homeostasis (see Chapter 31, Treatment of Renal Failure).

    a. The therapeutic principles are the same as those required to treat reversible renal failure, but therapy must be continued for the life of the patient.

    b. Although there is no cure, symptomatic and supportive treatment of renal failure may allow the patient to survive comfortably for a period of months and sometimes years.

5. Because there are significant differences in the type and magnitude of excesses and deficits of fluids and electrolytes that develop in oliguric and nonoliguric uremic patients, it is imperative to divide candidates for therapy of renal failure into those with oliguria and those with polyuria (see Chapter 32, Fluid Therapy in Renal Failure).

    a. Oliguria.

        (1) Once potentially reversible extrarenal causes of oliguria (e.g., prerenal uremia) have been eliminated, and test trials with diuretics have proved to be unsuccessful, a regimen of therapy characterized by fluid, electrolyte, and protein restriction should be adopted. Severe persistent oliguria is typically associated with fluid retention, hyperkalemia, and marked metabolic acidosis (see Chapter 32, Fluid Therapy in Renal Failure).

        (2) One must avoid overloading an oliguric patient with excessive quantities of fluids and electrolytes or drugs; this may be just as detrimental as the condition being treated.

(a) Fluid balance should be monitored by periodic evaluation of the patient's physical status, body weight, and urine volume.

(b) Drugs which are dependent on the kidneys for excretion in active or metabolized form should be given with caution in order to prevent accumulation of the drug and possible development of toxic side reactions (see Chapter 33, Drug Therapy in Renal Failure).

(3) Since the goal of therapy is to ameliorate signs of renal failure until the kidneys heal, the precise change in the concentration of BUN or creatinine should not be overemphasized. The direction and rate of change of the concentration of these substances is probably of greater significance than actual values. In addition, patient response is more significant than absolute laboratory values indicating abnormal renal function.

b. Polyuria.

(1) Provided the patient survives, oliguria will cease after a variable period of time and polyuria will develop. As the degree of polyuria increases, potential complications change from those of overhydration and hyperkalemia to those of excessive loss of fluids and electrolytes, especially sodium. While hyperkalemia is a common finding in oliguric renal failure, it is usually not a feature of polyuric renal failure, since viable nephrons undergo compensatory adaptation and are capable of maintaining potassium balance.

(2) Patients with polyuric renal failure should receive a regimen of medical therapy characterized by:

(a) Unlimited access to water, unless they are vomiting. Maintenance of fluid and electrolyte balance may also require parenteral administration of isotonic, polyionic fluids such as lactated Ringer's solution.

(b) Use of diets containing reduced quantities of protein of high biological value, and liberal quantities of fat and carbohydrate.

(c) Oral administration of sodium chloride and sodium bicarbonate tablets.

(d) Oral administration of vitamins.

(e) Oral or parenteral administration of anabolic steroids.

(f) Avoidance of stress.

(3) For specific details regarding conservative medical management of uremic patients with polyuria, see Chapter 31, Treatment of Renal Failure.

XI. Prognosis

A. The prognosis for uremic patients with acute nephrosis is dependent on:

1. The specific nature of the underlying cause(s).
2. The duration of the disease process.
3. The severity and character of nephron injury.
4. The presence or absence of concomitant renal diseases.

B. The prognosis for patients with prerenal uremia is favorable provided the underlying cause is amenable to therapy.

C. The prognosis for patients with primary uremia which responds to diuretic therapy is guarded to good.

D. The prognosis for patients with primary uremia which is unresponsive to fluid and diuretic therapy is unpredictable (i.e., guarded).

1. Although lesions induced by nephrotoxins or ischemia may be potentially reversible, the likelihood of keeping the patient alive until adequate renal function returns to maintain homeostasis is usually determined in retrospect.
2. Recovery of adequate renal function to maintain life may require days or several weeks.
3. Uremic patients with extensive trauma or infection have a less favorable prognosis for survival than previously healthy patients exposed to nephrotoxins.

E. In general, transition from a state of oliguria to a state of polyuria is a favorable prognostic sign.

REFERENCES

Balint, P.: Pathogenesis of mercuric chloride induced renal failure in the dog. Acta Med. Acad. Sci. Hung., 25:287–297, 1968.
Beckett, S. D., and Shields, R. P.: Treatment of acute ethylene glycol (antifreeze) toxicosis in the dog. J.A.V.M.A., 158:472–476, 1971.
Belt, A. E., and Joelson, J. J.: The effect of ligation of branches of the renal artery. Arch. Surg., 10:117–149, 1925.
Ben-Ishay, Z., Wiener, J., Sweeting, J., Bradley, S. E., and Spiro, D.: Fine structural alterations in the canine kidney during hemorrhagic hypotension. Effects of osmotic diuresis. Lab. Invest., 17:190–210, 1967.
Berg, P., Nunamaker, D., Amand, W., Harvey, C., and Klide, A.: Renal allograft in a dog poisoned with ethylene glycol. J.A.V.M.A., 158:468–471, 1971.
Bowles, W. T., and Koehler, P. R.: Acute renal vein ligation in dogs. Invest. Urol., 4:341–345, 1967.
Carriere, S., Thornburn, G. O., O'Morchure, C. E. C., and Barger, A. C.: Intrarenal distribution of blood flow in dogs during hemorrhagic hypotension. Circ. Res., 19:167–179, 1966.
Cuppage, F. E., and Tate, A.: Repair of the nephron following injury with mercuric chloride. Amer. J. Path., 51:405–429, 1967.
Friedman, S. M., Johnson, R. L., and Friedman, C. L.: The pattern of recovery of renal function following renal artery occlusion in the dog. Circ. Res., 2:231–235, 1954.
Gourley, I. M. G.: Prevention and treatment of acute renal failure in the canine surgical patient. J.A.V.M.A., 157:1722–1728, 1970.
Hamilton, P. B., Phillips, R. A., and Hiller, A.: Duration of renal ischemia required to produce uremia. Amer. J. Physiol., 152:517–522, 1948.
Jonsson, L., and Rubarth, S.: Ethylene glycol poisoning in dogs and cats. Nord. Vet Med., 19:265–276, 1967.
Kersting, E. J., and Nielsen, S. W.: Ethylene glycol poisoning. J.A.V.M.A., 146:113–118, 1965.
Kersting, E. J., and Nielsen, S. W.: Ethylene glycol poisoning. Amer. J. Vet. Res., 27:574–582, 1966.
Kramer, K.: Renal failure in hemorrhagic shock. In Shock: Biochemical, Pharmacological and Clinical Aspects. Edited by A. Bertelli, and N. Back. New York, N. Y., Plenum Press, 1970.
Ladd, M.: A comparison of acute renal insufficiency following toxic and traumatic injuries in the dog. Surg. Forum, 4:446–453, 1953.
Litwin, M. S., Walter, C. W., and Jackson, N.: Experimental production of acute tubular necrosis. Ann. Surg., 152:1010–1025, 1960.
MacNider, W.: The pathological changes which develop in the kidney as the result of occlusion by ligature of one branch of the renal artery. Part II. J. Med. Res., 24:425–454, 1911.
Moyer, J. H., Heider, C., Morris, G. C., and Handley, C.: Renal failure. I. The effect of complete renal artery occlusion for variable periods of time as compared to exposure to sub-filtration arterial pressures below 30 mm. Hg for similar periods. Ann. Surg., 145:41, 1957.
Nordstoga, K.: Spontaneous bilateral renal cortical necrosis in animals. Path. Vet., 4:233–244, 1967.
Nunamaker, D. M., Medway, W., and Berg, P.: Treatment of ethylene glycol poisoning in the dog. J.A.V.M.A., 159:310–314, 1971.

Oliver, J., MacDowell, M., and Tracy, A.: The pathogenesis of acute renal failure associated with traumatic and toxic injury. Renal ischemia, nephrotoxic damage, and the ischemuric episode. J. Clin. Invest., 30:1307–1439, 1951.

Phillips, R. A., Dole, V. P., Hamilton, P. N., Emerson, K., Archibald, R. M., and Van Slyke, D. D.: Effects of acute hemorrhagic and traumatic shock on renal function of dogs. Amer. J. Physiol., 145:314–336, 1946.

Roof, B. S., Lauson, H. D., Bella, S. T., and Edler, H.: Recovery of glomerular and tubular function, including p-aminohippurate extraction, following two hours of renal artery occlusion in the dog. Amer. J. Physiol., 166:666, 1951.

Sheehan, H. L., and Davis, J. C.: Complete permanent renal ischemia. J. Path. Bact., 76:569–587, 1958.

Sheehan, H. L., and Davis, J. C.: Renal ischemia with failed reflow. J. Path. Bact., 78:105–120, 1959.

Sheehan, H. L., and Davis, J. C.: Renal ischemia with good reflow. J. Path. Bact., 78:351–377, 1959.

Sheehan, H. L., and Davis, J. C.: Patchy permanent renal ischemia. J. Path. Bact., 77:33–46, 1959.

Sheehan, H. L., and Davis, J. C.: Intermittent complete renal ischemia. J. Path. Bact., 79:77–87, 1960.

Sheehan, H. L., and Davis, J. C.: Minor renal lesions due to experimental ischemia. J. Path. Bact., 80:259–270, 1960.

Sherwood, T., Lavender, J. P., and Greenspan, R. H.: Renal magnification angiograms in the dog. Observations on responses to vasodilators and surgical trauma. Brit. J. Radiol., 42:241–246, 1969.

Van Slyke, D. D.: The effects of shock on the kidney. Ann. Int. Med., 28:701–722, 1948.

Vinnicombe, J., and Stamey, T. A.: The relative nephrotoxicities of polymyxin-B sulfate, sodium sulfomethyl-polymyxin B, sodium sulfomethyl-colistin (Colymycin) and neomycin sulfate. Invest. Urol., 6:505–519, 1969.

Wertlake, P. T., Hill, G. J., and Butler, W. T.: Renal histopathology associated with different degrees of amphotericin B toxicity in the dog. Proc. Soc. Exp. Biol. Med., 118:472–476, 1965.

Wilson, D. H., Barton, B. B., Parry, W. L., and Hinshaw, L. B.: Effects of intermittent versus continuous renal arterial occlusion on hemodynamics and function of the kidney. Invest. Urol., 8:507–515, 1971.

Chapter 18

CHRONIC INTERSTITIAL NEPHRITIS (CIN)

I. **Definition**

Chronic interstitial nephritis is a term initially used by pathologists to describe the morphological appearance of the kidneys of dogs and cats affected with chronic, progressive, and irreversible renal disease of unknown cause. Chronic interstitial nephritis is a condition in which tubular and interstitial lesions are disproportionately more severe than lesions of glomeruli. The term is related to the morphologic lesions present, and is not restricted to a single disease with a single cause. Chronic interstitial nephritis is the final stage of a variety of renal diseases of different etiologies which have in common a chronic, progressive, irreversible course and a similar morphological appearance at the time of renal failure (see Chapter 20, End-Stage Kidneys).

II. **Etiology**

  A. *Unknown*
  1. The causative relationship which has been suggested to exist between leptospirosis and chronic interstitial nephritis has not been well established.
      a. At the University Veterinary Hospital, University of Minnesota, detectable antibodies against common strains of *Leptospira* have been consistently absent in dogs with CIN.
      b. Cats, which rarely develop leptospirosis, do develop CIN.
      c. Dogs recovered from experimentally induced acute leptospirosis and evaluated with respect to kidney function for up to four and one half years did not develop chronic progressive renal disease (see Leptospirosis, in Chapter 28). At necropsy the kidneys of these dogs were morphologically normal.
      d. Leptospiral organisms have not been demonstrated in the kidneys of dogs which have died of CIN.
      e. Progression of lesions associated with acute and subacute interstitial nephritis caused by leptospirosis to the lesions characteristic of CIN has not been demonstrated.

  B. *It has been hypothesized that CIN may be caused, at least in part, by autoimmune mechanisms, but little evidence has been presented to support this hypothesis.*

  C. *As stated previously, CIN is the final stage of the pathologic progression of a variety of different renal diseases.*

III. Prevalence

A. Age

CIN may occur at any age, but is more commonly encountered in older dogs and cats.

B. Sex

Male dogs have been reported to be affected about four times more frequently than female dogs. The significance, if any, of these observations has not been established.

C. Prevalence of CIN has not been well established.

Generalized, progressive, irreversible CIN associated with clinical signs of renal failure occurs less commonly than the literature implies.
1. Some studies of the incidence of CIN have been based on surveys of necropsy material in which mild, subclinical cases without generalized involvement of both kidneys were included. This data has been misinterpreted by some to suggest that all cases of CIN evaluated in such surveys were characterized by overt signs of chronic renal failure (see Chapter 12, Pathophysiology of Renal Failure).
2. Other generalized renal diseases are commonly included in a CIN category.
3. When chronic progressive renal diseases have reached an "end stage" which is associated with chronic renal failure, even experienced pathologists cannot distinguish between many of the diseases which can result in chronic renal failure (see Chapter 20, End-Stage Kidneys).

IV. Clinical and laboratory findings, diagnosis, treatment, and prognosis (see Chapter 20, End-Stage Kidneys)

REFERENCES

Anderson, L. J.: Experimental reproduction of canine interstitial nephritis. J. Comp. Path., 77:413–418, 1967.

Bloom, F.: Pathology of the Dog and Cat. The Genitourinary System with Clinical Considerations. Evanston, Ill., American Veterinary Publishers, Inc., 1954.

Krohn, K., Mero, M., Oksanen, A., and Sandholm, A.: Immunologic observations on canine interstitial nephritis. Amer. J. Path., 65:157–177, Oct., 1971.

Lucke, V. M., and Hunt, A. C.: Interstitial nephropathy and papillary necrosis in the domestic cat. J. Path. Bact., 89:723–728, 1965.

Oliver, J., Bloom, F., and MacDowell, M.: Structural and functional transformations in the tubular epithelium of the dog's kidney in chronic Bright's disease and their relation to mechanisms of renal compensation and failure. J. Exp. Med., 73:141–160, 1941.

Platt, H.: Canine Chronic Nephritis. I. Observations on the pathology of the kidney. J. Comp. Path. and Therap., 61:140–149, 1951.

Waisbren, B. A., Hensley, G., Lutsky, I., and Farmer, S.: Experimental interstitial nephritis in the dog. J. Lab. Clin. Med., 70:989, 1967.

Chapter 19
PYELONEPHRITIS

I. **Definition**

Pyelonephritis is an inflammatory disease of the renal parenchyma and renal pelvis.

II. **Pyelonephritis in dogs and cats**

  A. *Published information concerning spontaneously occurring pyelonephritis in the dog and cat is meager.*

  B. *Most of the available information is difficult to interpret because pyelonephritis has been confused with, or used synonymously with, so-called chronic interstitial nephritis.*

III. **Incidence**

  A. *The incidence of pyelonephritis in dogs and cats is not known.*

  B. *Its frequency is reported to increase with age.*

IV. **Pathogenesis**

  A. *Pyelonephritis is caused by bacterial infection.*
   1. *Escherichia coli* and *Proteus* spp. are commonly incriminated.
   2. Staphylococci and Streptococci spp. are less commonly encountered.

  B. *Organisms may reach the kidney by:*
   1. Ascending via the ureters or periureteral lymphatics.
   2. Hematogenous route.
   3. Direct extension from infection of adjacent structures (uncommon).

  C. *Predisposing causes*
   1. Urinary stasis or obstruction are considered to be important predisposing causes, regardless of route of infection (see Obstructive ureteropathy in Chapter 35). The latter enhance growth of bacteria and allow ascending migration of organisms to the kidneys via stagnated urine.
   2. Experimental studies in rodents have revealed that the renal medulla is more susceptible to bacterial infection than the renal cortex. This predisposition may be related to one or more of the following:
      a. The anatomic location of the medulla predisposes it to ascending bacterial infections.
      b. The hyperosmotic environment characteristic of normal medullary tissue inhibits the migration of granulocytes to the infection site and thus deprives the medulla of a major body defense mechanism against bacteria.
         (1) In rats, mobilization of granulocytes in the renal medulla is increased when dilute urine is being excreted.

(2) In one study, water restriction increased the incidence of coliform nephritis in the rat.

(3) In another study, diuresis diminished the severity of induced pyelonephritis in rats.

c. Sluggish blood flow inherent to medullary tissue may impair transport of endogenous and exogenous antimicrobial substances to this area.

d. Acidosis predisposes the rat medulla to bacterial infection. It has been hypothesized that the action of complement is inhibited in an acid environment.

3. Vesico-ureteral reflux is a significant predisposing cause of pyelonephritis in man. Although spontaneously occurring vesico-ureteral reflux does occur in dogs, its significance with respect to pyelonephritis has not been established.

4. Calculi may be associated with pyelonephritis, but it has not been determined whether they are a cause or a sequela to this disease.

5. Predisposing causes may not be detected in every patient suspected of having pyelonephritis.

D. *Pathogenic organisms invade the renal parenchyma and cause suppuration and necrosis.*

E. *Infection may remain focal or become disseminated; tubular lumens often serve as a pathway for dissemination of organisms.*

F. *Destroyed nephrons are replaced by fibrous connective tissue (see Chapter 12, Pathophysiology of Renal Failure, and Chapter 20, End-Stage Kidneys).*

V. Pathology

A. *Pyelonephritis may be present in one or both kidneys. When it is bilateral, one kidney may be more severely affected than the other (Fig. 19–1).*

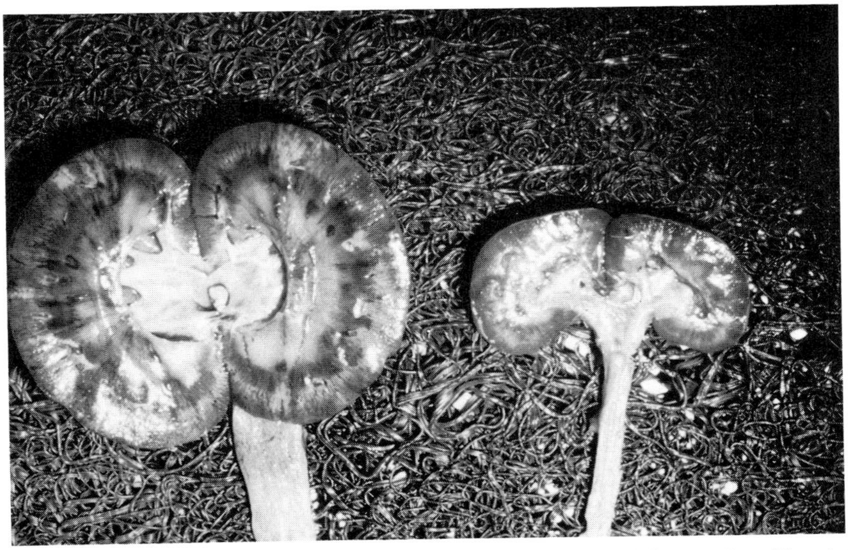

Figure 19–1. Kidneys obtained from a 6½-year-old female English pug dog. The right kidney contains a renolith and has mild hydronephrosis. The left kidney is contracted as a result of chronic generalized pyelonephritis. (J.A.V.M.A., *157*:837–840, 1970.)

B. *Pyelonephritis may be characterized by focal lesions, or it may become widespread and destroy sufficiently large quantities of renal parenchyma to cause renal failure.*

C. *Haphazard distribution of the renal lesions is characteristic.*

D. *Pyelonephritis is often classified as acute, chronic, or healed on the basis of morphologic lesions.*

Such classifications are arbitrary, however, since sharp divisions between various stages of renal diseases often do not exist.
1. Acute stage.
    a. The acute stage is characterized grossly by foci of suppuration in the renal parenchyma. A radial distribution of grayish-yellow streaks may be observed in the medulla. The renal capsules are not adherent to the underlying parenchyma.
    b. The acute stage is characterized microscopically by suppurative necrosis of the renal parenchyma. Abscesses may be discrete and focal in one or both kidneys, or form areas of coalescing suppuration which destroy large segments of the entire kidney.
2. Healed stage.
    a. Areas of fibrosis may be minute and focal, or generalized.
    b. The renal capsule may be adherent to subcapsular lesions. The asymmetry of the renal surface contour induced by scarring of the renal parenchyma tends to be coarse in character.
    c. The healed stage is characterized microscopically by replacement of destroyed renal parenchyma with connective tissue, and the presence of chronic inflammatory cells.
3. Chronic stage.
    a. Chronic pyelonephritis is a composite of the acute and healed stages. Acute suppurative necrosis and scarring are present.
    b. When chronic and generalized, the kidneys appear as small granular contracted kidneys which are similar in gross appearance to kidneys with so-called chronic interstitial nephritis, chronic amyloidosis, or chronic generalized glomerulonephritis (see Chapter 20, End-Stage Kidneys).

E. *Both acute and chronic forms may be associated with renal calculi.*

VI. Clinical findings are dependent on the stage of the disease.

A. *Acute, healed, and chronic stages may not be recognized ante mortem, especially if the renal parenchyma is not affected in a generalized fashion.*

B. *Any one or more (or none) of the following laboratory findings may be detected in patients with pyelonephritis.*
1. Urinalysis may reveal pyuria, bacteriuria, proteinuria, hematuria, and granular or WBC casts. Significant numbers of casts are especially meaningful because they indicate damage to the kidneys. In the absence of casts or laboratory findings indicating renal failure, it is difficult to distinguish pyelonephritis from other inflammatory lesions of the urinary tract.
2. Leucocytosis. Neutrophilia will occur if a large quantity of renal tissue is actively infected but will not occur if only a small portion of the renal parenchyma is involved.
3. Fever.

C. Signs of renal failure may develop when both kidneys are severely affected (see Chapter 13, Extrarenal Manifestations of Uremia).

D. Signs referrable to kidney disease may be combined with or obscured by a predisposing cause.

VII. **Diagnosis**

A. Renal biopsy. The biopsy sample will appear normal if the lesions have a focal distribution (see Limitations of renal biopsy, in Chapter 9).

B. History, physical examination, and pertinent laboratory data provide supportive evidence.

VIII. **Treatment**

A. Antibiotic therapy
  1. The choice of antibiotic(s) should be made on the basis of bacterial culture and antibiotic sensitivity of the organism. Organisms may be isolated from urine or renal biopsy samples (see Chapter 9, Percutaneous Renal Biopsy).
  2. Antibiotic treatment should be continued until urinalyses are normal.
     a. Remission of clinical signs is not a reliable index of cure.
     b. Post-treatment urinalyses should be performed at periodic intervals for the purpose of detecting recurrence.
  3. Therapy may be required for several months, and in some instances indefinitely.
     a. In instances where infection cannot be eliminated, continuous suppression of bacterial growth with antibacterial drugs may minimize progressive damage to the renal parenchyma.
     b. Antibacterial drugs should be administered to uremic patients with caution (see Chapter 33, Drug Therapy in Renal Failure).
  4. For choice of antibiotic, see Treatment of bacterial cystitis in Chapter 38.

B. If present, predisposing causes (urinary obstruction, calculi, or others) should be eliminated.

C. Information extrapolated from experimental studies in rats suggests that inducing a diuresis with the objective of reducing the hypertonicity of the renal medulla may be of therapeutic benefit.
     a. Do not restrict water consumption.
     b. Administer sodium chloride (enteric coated tablets) orally with the objective of increasing urine volume and decreasing urine specific gravity.

D. If the patient is uremic, provide conservative medical therapy for renal failure (see Chapter 31, Treatment of Renal Failure).

IX. **Prognosis**

A. Patients with minimal involvement of the renal parenchyma, and patients with acute generalized pyelonephritis which responds to treatment, should receive a guarded to favorable prognosis.

B. *Patients with acute generalized pyelonephritis that is unresponsive to therapy, and patients with chronic generalized pyelonephritis, should receive a guarded to poor prognosis since the damage to the renal parenchyma is usually progressive and irreversible.*

REFERENCES

Andriole, V. T.: Acceleration of the inflammatory response of the renal medulla by water diuresis. J. Clin. Invest., *45*:847–854, 1966.

Andriole, V. T.: Water, acidosis and experimental pyelonephritis. J. Clin. Invest., *49*:21–30, 1970.

Gold, A. C., Jeffs, R. D., and Wilson, R. B.: Experimental pyelonephritis. Canad. J. Comp. Med., *32*:450–453, 1968.

Kaye, D.: The effect of water diuresis on spread of bacteria through the urinary tract. J. Infect. Dis., *124*:297–305, 1971.

Kleine, L. J.: An unusual case of pyelonephritis. J. Amer. Vet. Rad. Soc., *5*:54–57, 1964.

Pachaly, L., Vivaldi, E., and Belmar, M.: Lesions of spontaneous pyelonephritis. Zbl. Vet. Med., *14*:371–382, 1967.

Rocha, H.: Experimental pyelonephritis. Characteristics of the infection in dogs. Yale J. Biol. Med., *36*:183–190, 1963.

Ross, G., and Thompson, J. M.: The relationship of nonobstructive reflux and chronic pyelonephritis. An experimental study. J. Urol., *90*:391–394, 1963.

Samellas, W., and Szymber, J.: Experimental pyelonephritis: The influence of reduced pulse pressure on susceptibility of the dog kidney to infection. J. Urol., *86*:507–509, 1961.

Schechter, R. D.: Acute and chronic pyelonephritis in the dog. *In* Current Veterinary Therapy. Vol. 4. Edited by R. W. Kirk. Philadelphia, Pa., W. B. Saunders Co., 1971.

Shapiro, A. P. Scheib, E. T., and Croker, B. P.: The effect of water diuresis on blood pressure and renal damage in male and female rats with chronic pyelonephritis due to Proteus. J. Lab. Clin. Med., *75*:970–979, 1969.

Waisbren, B. A., Hensley, G., Lutsky, I., and Farmer, S.: Experimental interstitial nephritis in the dog. J. Lab. Clin. Med., *70*:989, 1967.

Wettimuny, S. G.: Pyelonephritis in the dog. J. Comp. Path., *77*:193–197, 1967.

Chapter 20
END-STAGE KIDNEYS

I. Definition

The term "end-stage kidney" is commonly used to refer to all inflammatory and ischemic renal diseases which are generalized, progressive, irreversible, and at an advanced stage in development. Because the functional and morphological response of the kidneys to injury by a variety of causes is similar, the clinical manifestations and lesions associated with end-stage kidneys are not diagnostic. This term has been adopted because of the inability to differentiate antecedent causes of end-stage kidneys.

II. Pathophysiology

A. *The concept that the nephron is the functional unit of the kidney is based upon the functional interdependence of the glomeruli, their tubules, peritubular capillaries, and surrounding interstitial tissue.*

If any portion of the nephron is irreversibly destroyed, the remaining portions become nonfunctional. Progressive irreversible lesions initially localized to the renal vascular system, glomeruli, tubules or interstitial tissue are eventually responsible for the development of lesions in the remaining but initially unaffected portions of the nephron. Since effective regeneration of renal parenchyma destroyed by progressive irreversible renal diseases does not occur, repair occurs by replacement fibrosis and scarring.

B. *The common denominator of all causes of end-stage kidneys is progressive reduction in the number of functioning nephrons.*

C. *Because of the structural and functional interdependency of components of the nephron, differentiation of various renal diseases which have advanced to an end stage is difficult or impossible.*

Although varying degrees and types of structural alteration may be prominent features during some phases of chronic generalized renal diseases, varying degrees of atrophy, inflammation, fibrosis, and calcification of diseased nephrons which are superimposed on compensatory and adaptive structural changes of viable nephrons provide a gross and microscopic similarity of end-stage kidneys. As a generality, the greater the degree of destruction of renal parenchyma by chronic, progressive, and irreversible renal diseases, the less obvious are detectable differences in their gross and microscopic appearance.

D. *Causes of end-stage kidneys*

1. So-called chronic interstitial nephritis is the most common cause of end-stage kidneys in dogs and cats. Many veterinary authors apparently use the terms chronic interstitial nephritis and end-stage kidneys synonymously.

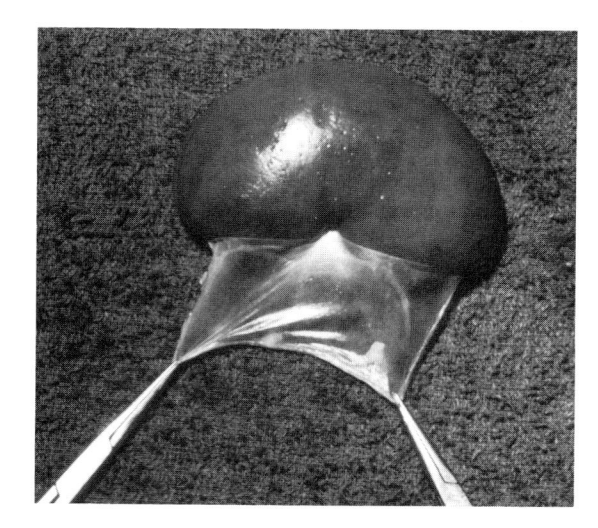

Figure 20–1. Normal kidney from an adult dog. The surface contour of the kidney is smooth. When the renal capsule was removed, it did not adhere to the underlying renal parenchyma. Compare this kidney to those in Figures 20–2 through 20–7.

2. Renal cortical hypoplasia.
3. Familial renal disease in Norwegian elkhound and lhasa apso dogs.
4. Chronic generalized pyelonephritis.
5. Chronic generalized renal amyloidosis.
6. Chronic generalized glomerulonephritis.
7. Progressive renal ischemia due to vascular disease may cause end-stage kidneys provided the patient survives for a sufficient period of time for morphologic changes to develop. Although vascular disease (benign nephrosclerosis) is a common cause of end-stage kidneys in man, it is uncommon in the dog and cat.
8. Other causes of end-stage kidneys undoubtedly exist, but have not yet been defined.

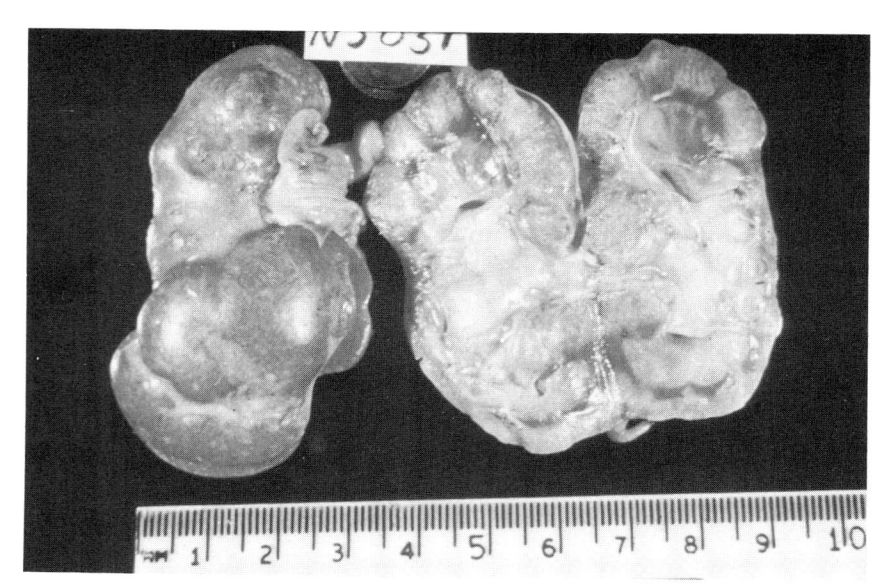

Figure 20–2. Kidneys obtained from a 7-year-old female golden retriever with end-stage renal disease.

END-STAGE KIDNEYS 191

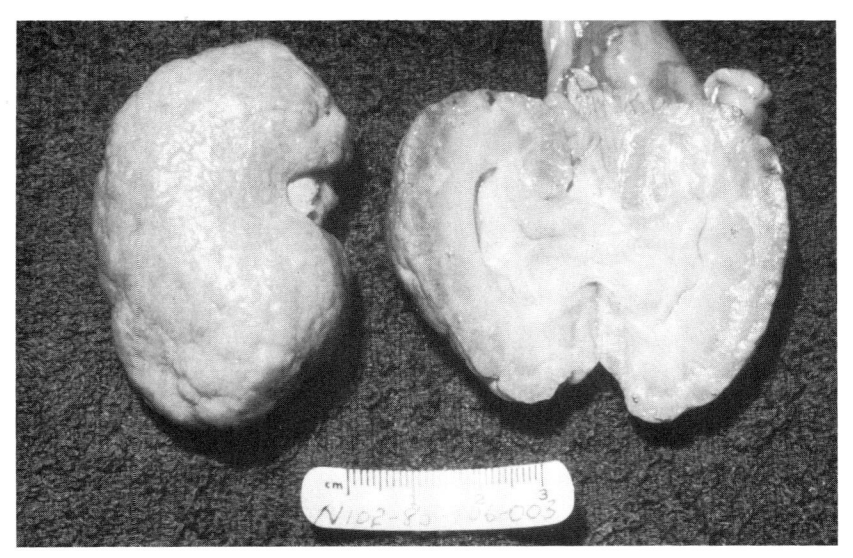

Figure 20–3. Abnormally small, pitted asymmetrical kidneys obtained from an 8-year-old female black Labrador retriever with end-stage renal disease.

E. *Gross appearance of end-stage kidneys*

It is usually not possible to differentiate the underlying cause(s) of end-stage kidneys on the basis of gross morphology (Figs. 20–1 to 20–7).
1. The gross appearance of kidneys affected with an end stage of the aforementioned diseases is characterized by abnormal reduction in size, pitted capsular surfaces, adherent renal capsules, and retention cysts.
2. Decreased size, capsular adhesions, and generalized pitting of the capsular surface of the cortex occur in response to replacement of damaged renal parenchyma with mature collagenous connective tissue. Retention cysts develop when replacement fibrosis of damaged parenchyma causes partial or complete obstruction of some of the remaining tubules.

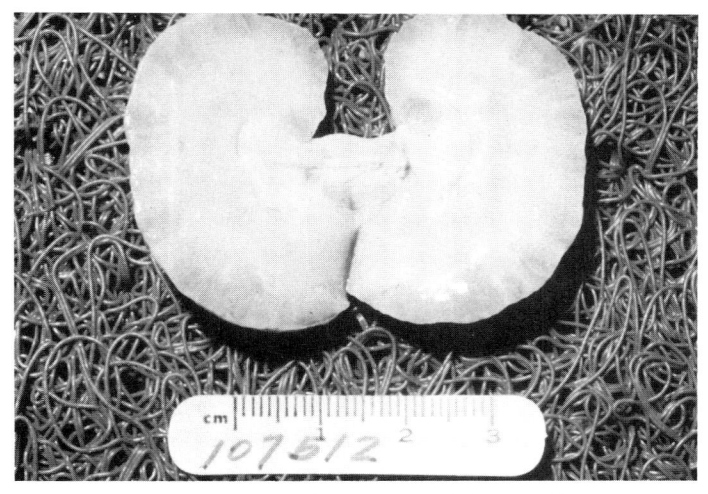

Figure 20–4. Kidney obtained from a 6½-month-old female Norwegian elkhound dog with end-stage renal disease.

192   DISEASES OF THE UPPER URINARY SYSTEM

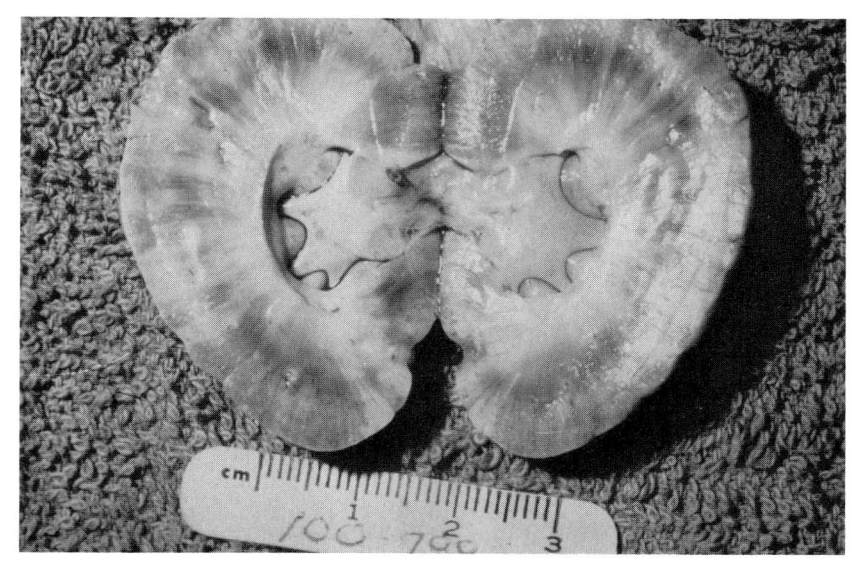

Figure 20–5. End-stage right kidney obtained from a 7-year-old male miniature schnauzer with chronic uremia. The left kidney was removed 2 years previously because it contained a calculus. Microscopic examination of sections of the left kidney revealed lesions consistent with chronic pyelonephritis. Despite antibacterial therapy, recurrent pyuria was observed on numerous occasions prior to death. Microscopic examination of sections of bladder obtained at necropsy revealed no abnormal findings. Microscopic examination of sections of the right kidney revealed the presence of end-stage renal disease.

F. *Microscopic appearance of end-stage kidneys*

Renal diseases which have progressed to an end stage in development have architectural similarity since they are characterized morphologically by hyperplasia and hypertrophy of viable nephrons which is superimposed on severe and generalized inflammatory, ischemic, regressive, and fibrous changes.

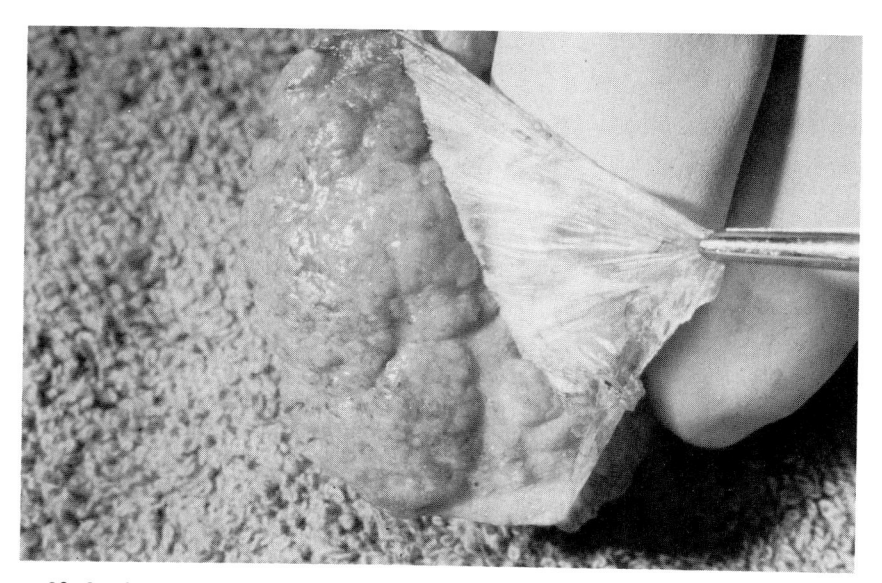

Figure 20–6. Abnormally small, pitted, asymmetrical kidney obtained from an 11-year-old springer spaniel with chronic generalized pyelonephritis. The renal capsule is adherent to the cortex.

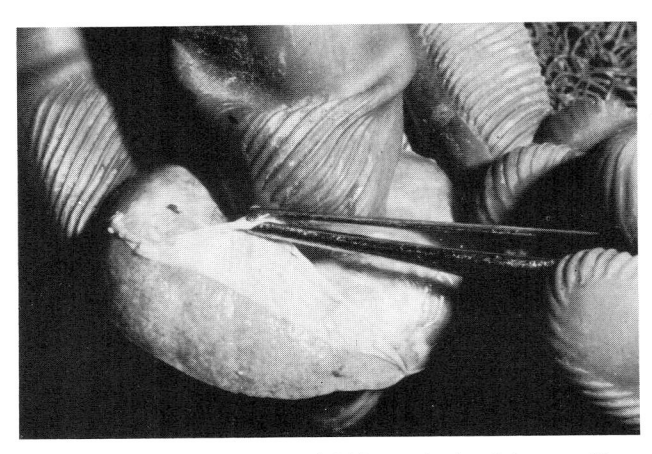

Figure 20-7. End-stage amyloid contracted kidney obtained from a 12-year-old male cocker spaniel dog. The renal capsule is adherent to the cortex and the external surface of the cortex is pitted and irregular in contour. (J.A.V.M.A., *157*:203-219, 1970.)

1. End-stage canine kidneys with amyloid usually can be differentiated from other types of end-stage kidneys by the characteristic accumulation of amyloid in the glomerular tufts.
2. Morphological changes in glomeruli which have not been replaced with scar tissue often allow chronic generalized glomerulonephritis to be differentiated from other causes of end-stage kidney disease.

III. History

The first signs that owners notice may be polyuria, polydipsia, and nocturia. When circumstances prevent the owner from making these observations, signs associated with the development of uremia, such as vomiting, anorexia, depression, weakness, and weight loss, are likely to be the first abnormalities detected.

IV. Physical findings

A. *Because of the reserve capacity and functional adaptation of the kidneys, the early lesions are not associated with clinical signs of renal disease.*

B. *Late in the course of the disease various combinations of signs characteristic of chronic renal failure may be present, including:*
   1. Polydipsia.
   2. Anorexia.
   3. Weight loss.
   4. Vomiting.
   5. Diarrhea, or constipation.
   6. Dehydration.
   7. Ulcerations of the buccal mucosa, especially adjacent to the canine teeth and upper fourth premolar teeth.
   8. Brownish deposits on the teeth.
   9. Brownish-red discoloration of the tongue.
   10. Asthenia.
   11. Scleral injection.

DISEASES OF THE UPPER URINARY SYSTEM

12. Polyuria. Oliguria may develop as a terminal event. If the concentration of BUN or creatinine is progressively increasing, it may be concluded that urine production, regardless of volume, is inadequate to excrete waste products of metabolism.
13. Anemia.
14. Secondary renal hyperparathyroidism. The latter may be characterized by:
    a. Pathologic fractures.
    b. Loose teeth.
    c. Increased radiotranslucency of bones.
15. Depression. A coma-like state commonly occurs when the patient is near death.

V. Laboratory findings

See Chapter 6, Laboratory Findings in Diseases of the Urinary System.

VI. Diagnosis

A. *The history, physical findings, and pertinent laboratory data provide supportive evidence.*

B. *A diagnosis of end-stage kidney disease may be confirmed by histologic evaluation of a renal biopsy sample.*

VII. Treatment

A. *There is no specific treatment available.*

B. *See Chapter 31, Treatment of Renal Failure, for supportive measures that may prolong life.*

VIII. Prognosis

A. *A meaningful prognosis can usually be established if it is based on pertinent physical findings and laboratory data.*

The following findings are justification for establishment of a guarded to poor prognosis:
1. Severe non-regenerative anemia.
2. Advanced secondary renal hyperparathyroidism.
3. Progressive increase in serially determined BUN or creatinine concentrations.
4. Progressive decrease in serially determined urinary excretion of PSP dye.
5. Progressive weight loss.
6. Detection of morphologic changes characteristic of end-stage kidneys by renal biopsy.

B. *The prognosis for patients with end-stage kidneys is unfavorable because of the progressive and irreversible nature of the disease.*

Comfortable survival for periods of months or years may be achieved, however, by careful medical management of the patient.

IX. Significance of end-stage kidneys

A. Once various renal diseases have progressed to an end stage of development, the lesion invariably represents a progressive and irreversible disease, and determination of the cause or evolution of the disease process contributes little to the prognosis.

B. Because destruction of the kidneys is often irreversible by the time most generalized renal diseases have progressed to a chronic stage, future progress is dependent upon clinical detection and treatment of progressive renal diseases at an early stage.

1. Before diagnostic criteria can be established which will facilitate consistent clinical detection of renal diseases at a potentially reversible stage, definition of their cause and pathogenesis is essential.
2. The correlation of clinical findings and laboratory data with progressive histopathologic, immunochemical, and electron microscopic changes of diseased kidneys, and a more complete understanding of the pathophysiology of the nephron are necessary for improvement of diagnosis, prognosis, and treatment of renal disorders.

REFERENCES

Gold, A. C., Jeffs, R. D., and Wilson, R. B.: Experimental pyelonephritis. Canad. J. Comp. Med., *32*:450–453, 1968.

Hepinstall, R. H.: Pathology of end-stage kidney disease. Amer. J. Med., *44*:656–663, May, 1968.

Osborne, C. A., and Johnson, K. H.: End-stage kidneys in dogs and cats. J. Amer. Anim. Hosp. Assoc., *6*:174–181, 1970.

Ross, G., and Thompson, J. M.: The relationship of nonobstructive reflux and chronic pyelonephritis: An experimental study. J. Urol., *90*:391–394, 1963.

Chapter 21
RENAL CYSTS

I. Solitary cysts (simple cysts)

  A. *The pathogenesis of solitary cysts is obscure.*

  B. *Morphologically, solitary cysts are characterized by the presence of one or more large cysts, usually not less than 1 cm. or more than 5 cm. in diameter, which are usually found in the renal cortex.*

  The cysts usually contain fluid with physical characteristics similar to those of urine.

  C. *Significance*
   1. Solitary cysts are usually of no clinical significance.
   2. Uncommonly, extremely large cysts may be palpated per abdomen or detected radiographically. One must differentiate large solitary cysts from more significant renal diseases such as renal neoplasms or hydronephrosis.
   3. Rarely, simple cysts may become infected and cause hematuria, pyuria, proteinuria, or other disease conditions.

  D. *Diagnosis*
   1. Radiology.
      a. Solitary cysts may be detected as abnormalities of the surface contour of kidneys on survey radiographs.
      b. A nephrogram, nephrotomogram, or intravenous urogram may aid in radiographic evaluation of solitary cysts.
      c. Injection of a radiopaque dye into a cyst following aspiration of its contents may enhance radiographic visualization.
   2. Percutaneous renal cyst puncture. Cyst contents obtained by percutaneous or modified percutaneous aspiration with a 22 to 26 gauge needle and syringe should be examined with the aid of a microscope (see Chapter 9, Percutaneous Renal Biopsy).
   3. Exploratory laparotomy. Solitary renal cysts may be an incidental finding during abdominal surgery.

  E. *Treatment*
   1. Treatment of solitary cysts is usually unnecessary.
   2. Partial nephrectomy or nephrectomy may be performed if cysts are causing serious renal dysfunction.
   3. Aspiration of fluid and injection of 3 to 5 ml. of Pantopaque* has been reported to be of therapeutic value in human patients with solitary cysts.

  F. *Prognosis*

  Because simple cysts are not usually associated with clinical signs, the prognosis is favorable.

---

*Iophendylate Injection U.S.P., Keleket X-Ray Corporation, Waltham, Massachusetts.

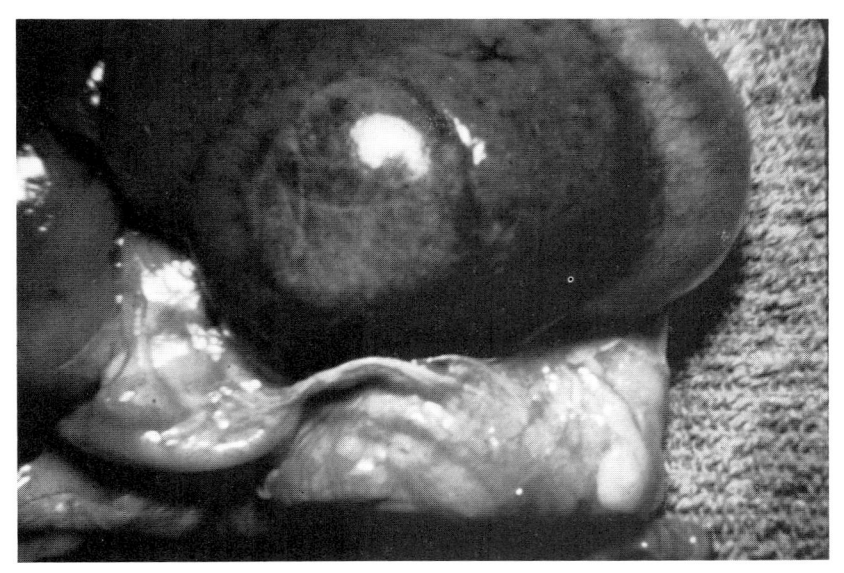

Figure 21-1. Retention cysts in an end-stage amyloid contracted kidney obtained from a 10.5-year-old, male German shepherd dog.

II. Retention cysts (acquired cysts)

 A. *Retention cysts arise secondary to inflammation and replacement fibrosis of the renal parenchyma which causes partial or complete obstruction of the renal tubules.*

 The portion of the tubular lumen proximal to the site of obstruction becomes distended with urine, and eventually dilates.

 B. *Pathology*

 The cysts are usually multiple and small (less than 1 cm. in diameter) and are associated with changes characteristic of severe chronic renal disease such as small, contracted, granular, end-stage kidneys (Fig. 21-1).

 C. *Significance*

 Retention cysts indicate the presence of advanced chronic irreversible renal disease.

 D. *Diagnosis*

 Retention cysts are usually observed at necropsy. They may be palpated during renal biopsy performed in association with the keyhole technique.

 E. *Treatment is dependent upon the nature and biological behavior of the underlying renal disease.*

 F. *The prognosis associated with retention cysts is usually poor since they indicate the the presence of chronic, generalized, progressive, irreversible renal disease.*

Chapter 22
HYDRONEPHROSIS

I. **Definition**

Hydronephrosis is an abnormality of the kidney that is characterized by progressive dilatation of the renal pelvis and progressive atrophy of the renal parenchyma. It occurs as a result of obstruction to urine outflow due to any cause.

II. **Etiology**

   A. *Congenital*

   Hydronephrosis may occur as a result of:
   1. Torsion or kinking of the ureters due to abnormal displacement of the kidneys.
   2. Stenosis or atresia of the ureters or urethra.
   3. Aberrant renal vessels that constrict ureters.

   B. *Acquired*

   Hydronephrosis may occur as a result of any disease that impairs urine outflow, including:
   1. Abdominal masses (neoplastic or inflammatory) which impinge upon the ureters or urethra and which partially or completely obstruct urine outflow (Figs. 22–1, 22–2 and 22–3).
   2. Urinary calculi in any location.
   3. Inflammation and stricture of the ureter or urethra due to any cause.
   4. Accidental ligation of a ureter during surgery.
   5. *Dioctophyma renale*.

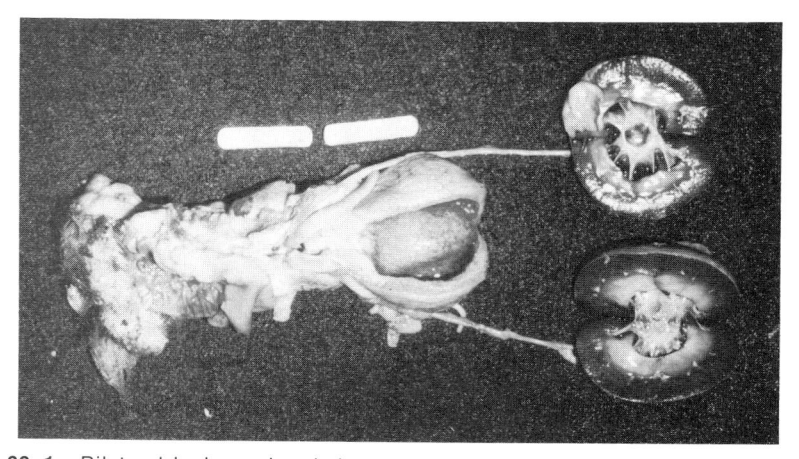

Figure 22–1. Bilateral hydronephrosis in a 12-year-old male collie dog caused by urethral obstruction. The lumen of the urethra was compressed by an invasive scirrhous adenocarcinoma that originated in the rectum.

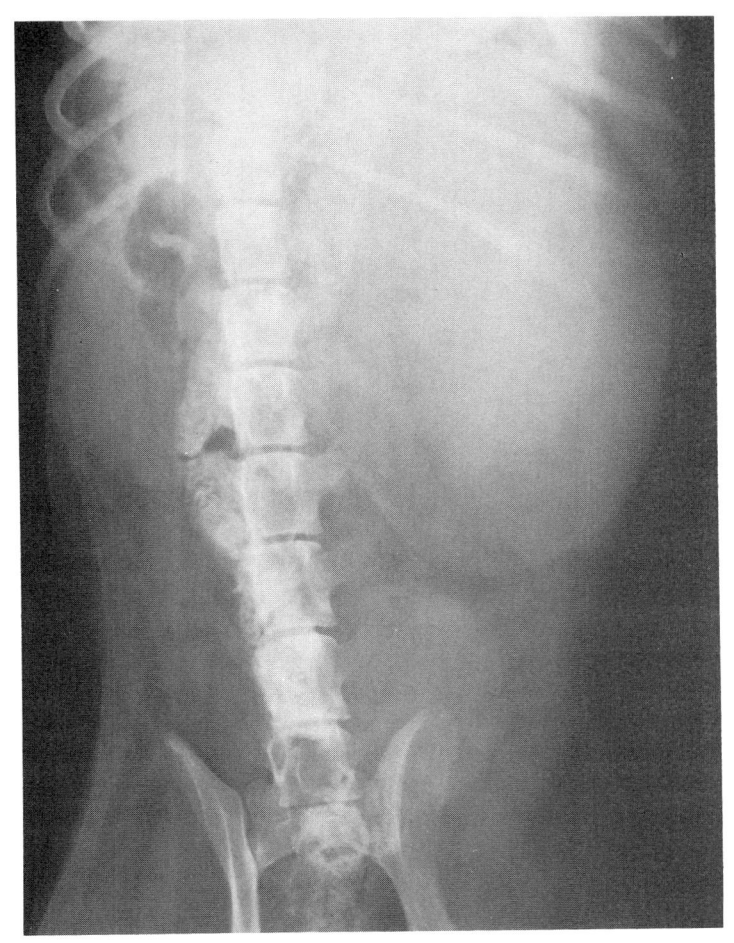

Figure 22-2. Survey radiograph of the abdomen of a 3.5-year-old female mixed breed dog with bilateral hydronephrosis. Obstruction to urine flow occurred as the result of occlusion of the ureters by a spay granuloma which developed at the region of the trigone.

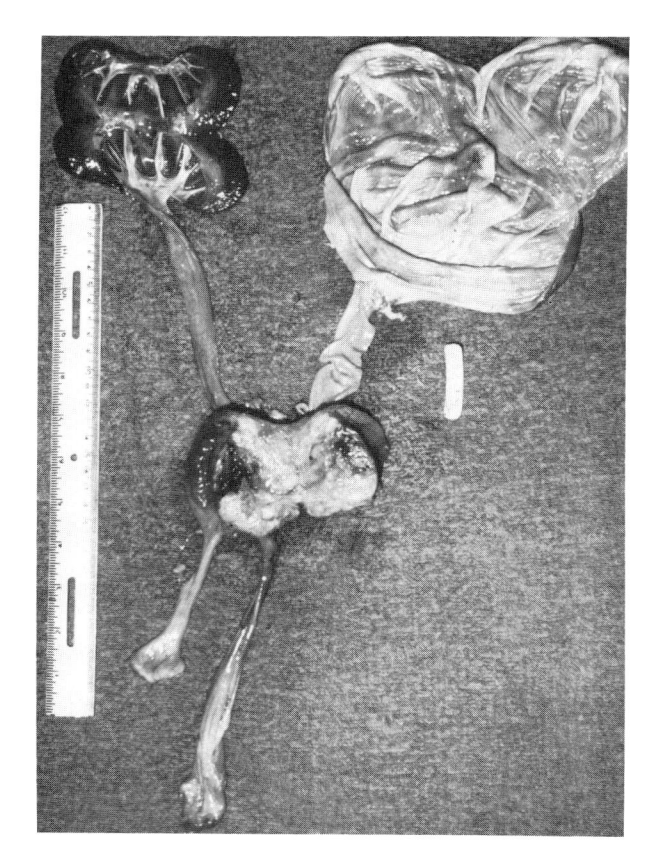

Figure 22-3. Bilateral hydronephrosis of the kidneys of the dog described in Figure 22-2. Both ureters were obstructed by a granuloma that occurred at the site of ligation of the body of the uterus. Ovariohysterectomy was performed 15 months previously.

C. *Predisposing causes may not be detected in every patient with hydronephrosis.*

In cats, several cases of hydronephrosis have been reported in which a large quantity of fluid collected between the external surface of the renal cortex and the capsule. Affected kidneys were abnormally enlarged and could be palpated per abdomen. The etiology of this form of "capsular hydronephrosis" has not been defined, although a relationship to lymphatic obstruction has been hypothesized.

III. Pathogenesis

A. *Hydronephrosis occurs as a result of partial or complete obstruction to urine flow anywhere from the renal pelvis to the urethral orifice.*

If the obstructive lesion persists, and if the patient survives, obstruction to urine outflow will initiate a sequence of changes that have the potential to destroy the kidney.

B. *The pathologic changes of hydronephrotic atrophy are caused by pressure and ischemia, and are peculiar to the kidney.*

Complete obstruction of the excretory ducts of other glands in the body produces almost immediate cessation of secretion and disuse atrophy.
1. Maintenance of abnormal back pressure in the kidneys is dependent on continuing renal secretion and backflow.
   a. Even when urine excretion is completely blocked, stagnation of fluid in the obstructed portion of the urinary system does not occur.

b. Fluid formed by renal secretion is reabsorbed via communication with:
   (1) Veins.
   (2) Lymphatics.
   (3) Interstitial tissue.
c. Provided backflow is established, secretory pressure is maintained until the renal parenchyma is destroyed. The latter may take several months.

2. If backflow fails to occur following complete obstruction to urine flow, the resultant changes will be characterized by primary atrophy. The kidneys will become smaller in size rather than enlarged.

C. *Because of the anatomical relationship of components of the urinary system, and the presence of a relatively inexpansible renal capsule, urine retention results in increased back pressure in that portion of the urinary system proximal to the site of obstruction.*

1. Increased pressure causes dilation of the renal pelvis and distention of tubular lumens. In some instances Bowman's space may also be distended.
2. Compression and collapse of portions of the renal vasculature occur as a result of increased renal back pressure. The resultant ischemia causes ischemic atrophy and necrosis of the renal parenchyma.
3. The renal tubules are the major site of pathologic change during the

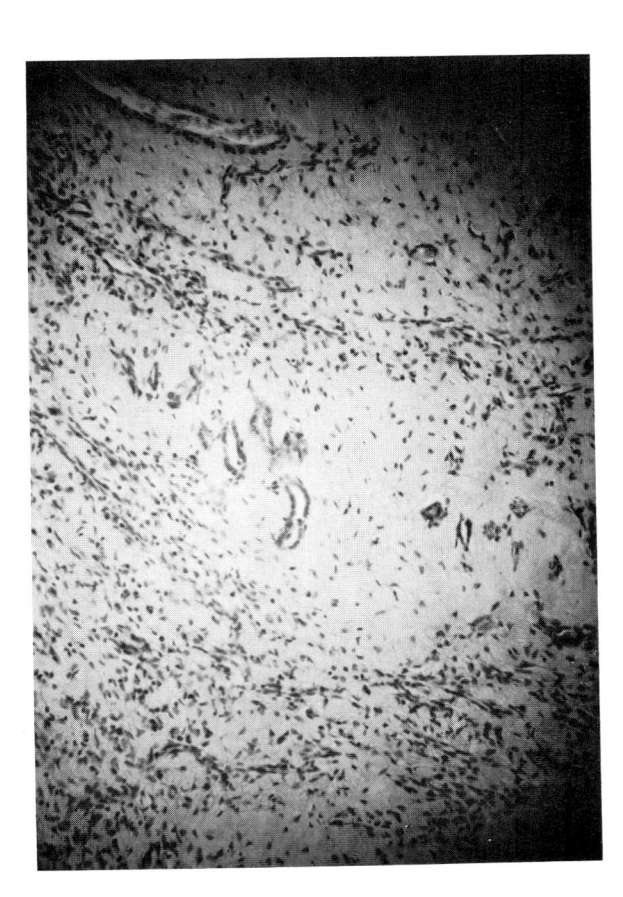

Figure 22-4. Photomicrograph of a section of right hydronephrotic kidney obtained from a 15-month-old female golden retriever dog. Only a few renal tubules can be identified. The remainder have been replaced by fibrous connective tissue. H&E stain; ×400. (J.A.V.M.A., *155*:605–620, 1969.)

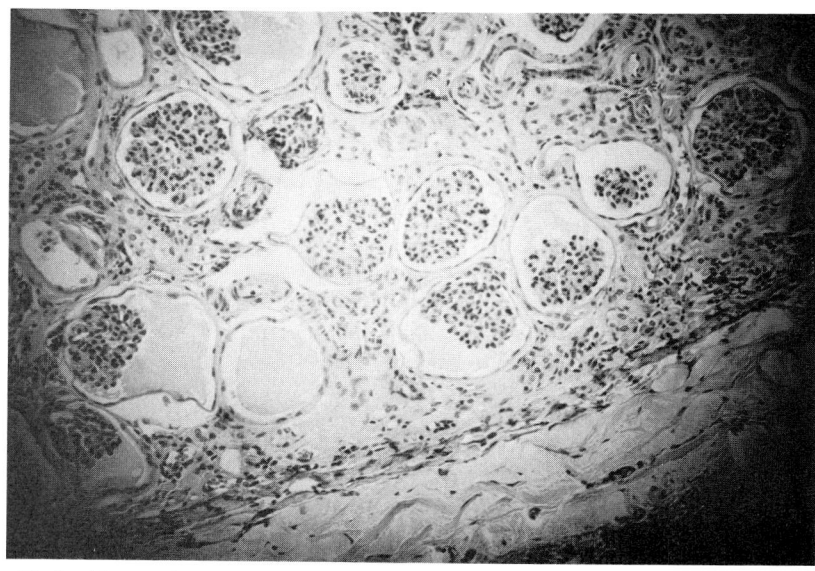

Figure 22–5. Photomicrograph of a section of a hydronephrotic right kidney obtained from a 15-month-old female golden retriever dog. Glomeruli appear numerous as a result of destruction of renal tubules. H&E stain; × 400. (J.A.V.M.A., *155*:605–620, 1969.)

early course of the disease because the high metabolic activity of tubular epithelial cells makes them more susceptible to the effects of ischemia and pressure than glomeruli, blood vessels, or interstitial tissue (Fig. 22–4).
4. Glomeruli persist the longest, but eventually they are destroyed (Fig. 22–5).
5. The severity of renal lesions is not uniform throughout the kidneys.
   a. Because of differences in blood flow, certain groups of nephrons are affected more severely than others.
   b. Since renal arterioles are end arteries, ischemic atrophy and necrosis are more severe in parenchyma which is farthest from interlobular arteries.

D. *The degree of change in the renal parenchyma is related to the location, degree, and duration of obstruction.*
   1. A direct relationship exists between the degree of obstruction to urine outflow (i.e., partial or complete) and the severity of hydronephrosis. Depending on the latter variables, obstruction may be associated with:
      a. No significant change.
      b. Asymptomatic hydronephrosis.
      c. Functional (symptomatic) hydronephrosis.
   2. Experimental studies in dogs in which the ureters were ligated yielded the following observations.
      a. A small degree of partial obstruction over a sufficient length of ureter (25 per cent obstruction over 1.5 cm. of ureter) will produce functional hydronephrosis.
      b. Focal areas of ureteral obstruction must occlude 75 to 80 per cent of the lumen to produce functional hydronephrosis.

c. Partial constriction of a ureter which affects a significant length of the lumen can produce the same degree of hydronephrosis as complete obstruction.

E. *The most severe morphologic changes occur when hydronephrosis is unilateral.*

Dilatation and atrophy are less severe in bilateral hydronephrosis because patients die of uremia before extensive renal changes have time to develop. If a patient has complete obstruction of both ureters for a period of four to six days, death from postrenal uremia will result.

F. *The time required to produce irreversible functional damage to kidneys by obstruction to urine outflow is variable.*
   1. Studies performed in dogs in which total obstruction of one ureter was induced by ligation revealed that, in the presence of a normally functioning contralateral kidney:
      a. Permanent structural and functional alteration did not occur provided the obstruction was removed within six to seven days.
      b. If the obstruction was allowed to persist for two weeks prior to removal, the affected kidney regained only 50 to 60 per cent of its pre-obstruction functional capacity.
   2. Experimental studies in dogs have been interpreted to suggest that hydronephrotic kidneys regain greater functional capacity when there is urgent need for recovery. This concept is called the renal counterbalance theory.
      a. Studies in dogs in which complete unilateral ureteral obstruction was induced, and in which the contralateral kidney was removed at the time of release of ureteral obstruction, revealed that a two to three week period of ligation was followed by return of normal renal function.
      b. If nephrectomy of the contralateral kidney was not performed, the obstructed kidney regained only 33 per cent of its pre-obstruction functional capacity.
      c. An efficient compensatory mate diminishes, and an insufficient contralateral kidney enhances the potential of repair of unilateral hydronephrosis.

G. *Bacterial infection is a common complication of obstructive uropathy and may aggravate the rate of destruction of nephrons.*

H. *The predisposing cause may result in death of the patient before extensive renal changes have time to occur.*

IV. Pathology

A. *Pathologic changes in the urinary system are variable, being dependent on:*
   1. The location of the obstructing lesion.
   2. Involvement of one or both kidneys.
   3. The completeness (partial or total) of obstruction to urine flow.
   4. The duration of the disease.

B. *In mild cases, or early during the course of more severe cases, uncomplicated distention of the renal pelvis with minimal change in the renal parenchyma will occur (Fig. 22–6).*

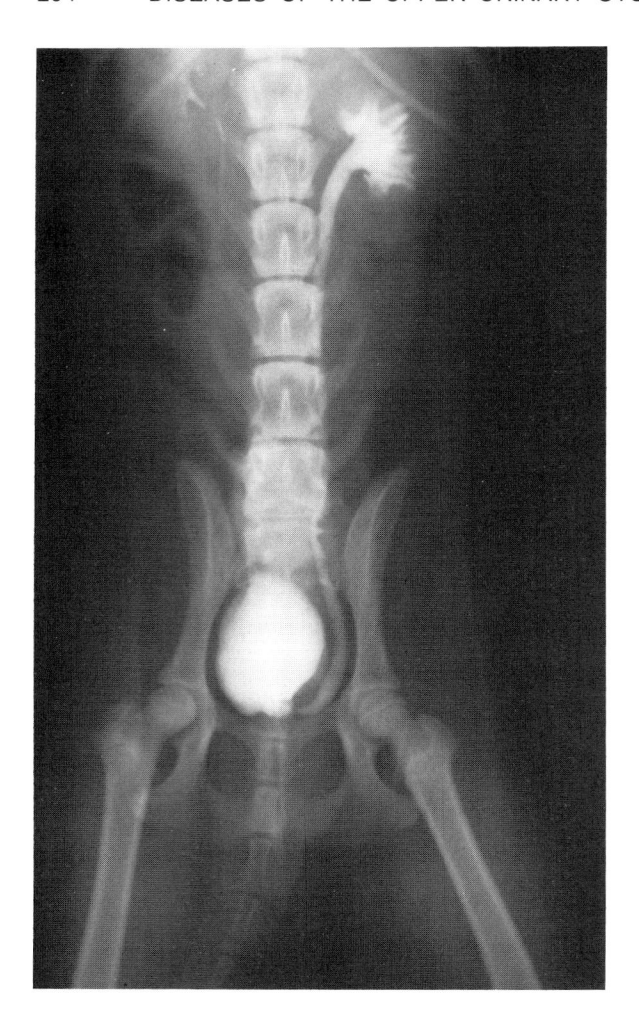

Figure 22-6. Postsurgical intravenous urogram of a 5-month-old male wire-haired fox terrier with urinary incontinence caused by an ectopic left ureter. Partial constriction of the left ureter at its junction with the urinary bladder has caused mild hydronephrosis. The constriction of the ureter developed following its transplantation into the bladder. The constriction had undergone spontaneous resolution when evaluated 10 days later.

C. *Unilateral hydronephrosis*
  1. Unilateral hydronephrosis has the potential of being associated with the greatest degree of renal change (Fig. 22–7).
     a. The kidney undergoes progressive pelvic distention and parenchymal atrophy and may be transformed into a large thin-walled sac with a rim of atrophic renal parenchyma.
     b. If the disease is not complicated by infection, fluid in hydronephrotic kidneys usually resembles urine.
     c. The fluid may be cloudy and viscous if infection is present.
  2. The contralateral kidney will increase in size and functional capacity as a result of compensatory hypertrophy and hyperplasia.
  3. The histopathologic changes are characterized by varying degrees of tubular dilatation, tubular atrophy, and fibrosis. The glomeruli often appear morphologically normal. These changes may be associated with suppurative inflammation (Figs. 22–4 and 22–5).

D. *Bilateral hydronephrosis*
  1. In general, the morphologic findings associated with bilateral hydronephrosis are similar to those associated with unilateral hydronephrosis,

HYDRONEPHROSIS

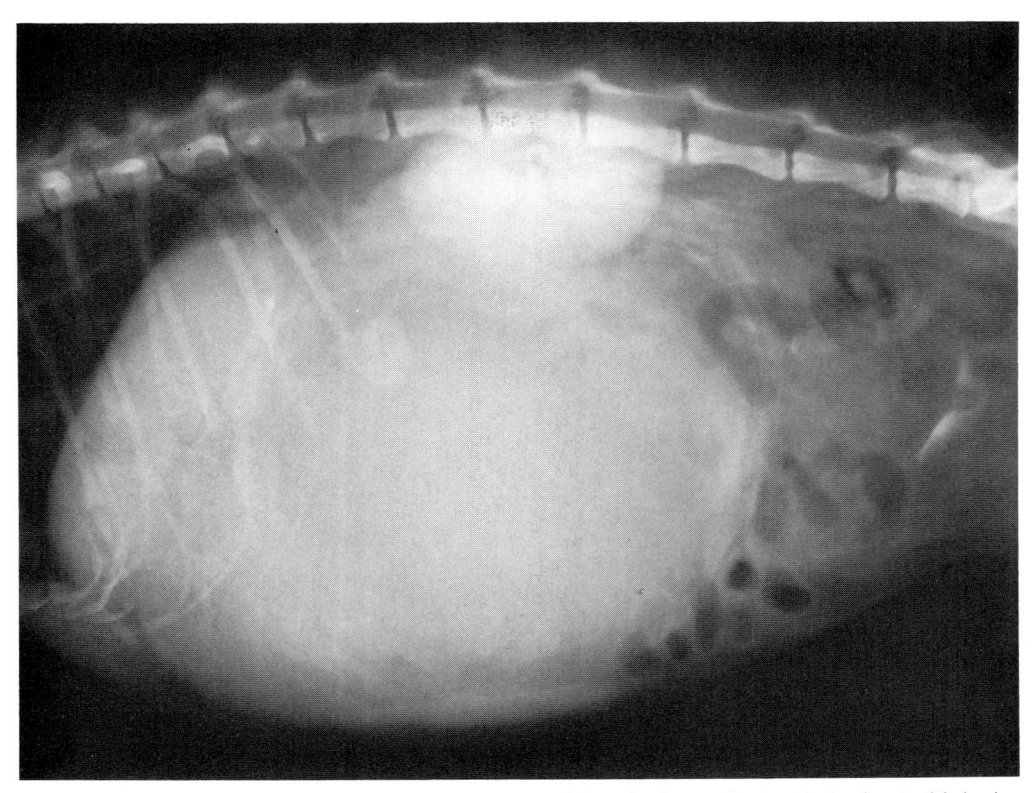

Figure 22-7. Intravenous urogram of a 3-year-old female domestic shorthaired cat with hydronephrosis of the left kidney. Radiopaque media has been excreted by the right kidney in normal fashion, but the left kidney did not excrete any. The radiopaque circular object in the dilated renal pelvis is composed of heteroplastic bone. (Courtesy of Dr. C. R. Jessen, College of Veterinary Medicine, University of Minnesota.)

but are less severe since the patient usually dies or is successfully treated before extensive changes have time to develop.
2. The degree of pathologic alteration in each kidney of patients with bilateral hydronephrosis may be unequal, depending on the location and nature of the primary cause (Fig. 22-3).

E. *Depending on the location and nature of the obstruction, hydronephrosis may be associated with:*
1. Pyonephrosis (i.e., hydronephrosis complicated by marked suppuration) (Fig. 22-8).
2. Hydroureter or pyoureter.
3. Overdistention of the urinary bladder.

F. *Heteroplastic bone formation has been reported in association with naturally occurring and experimentally induced hydronephrosis of canine and feline kidneys on several occasions.*

The bone contained marrow and haversian canals (Fig. 22-7).
1. Hydronephrosis is not an essential prerequisite to heteroplastic bone formation in the urinary system. It has been observed:
   a. Following transplantation of canine and feline transitional epithelium to various sites in the body.

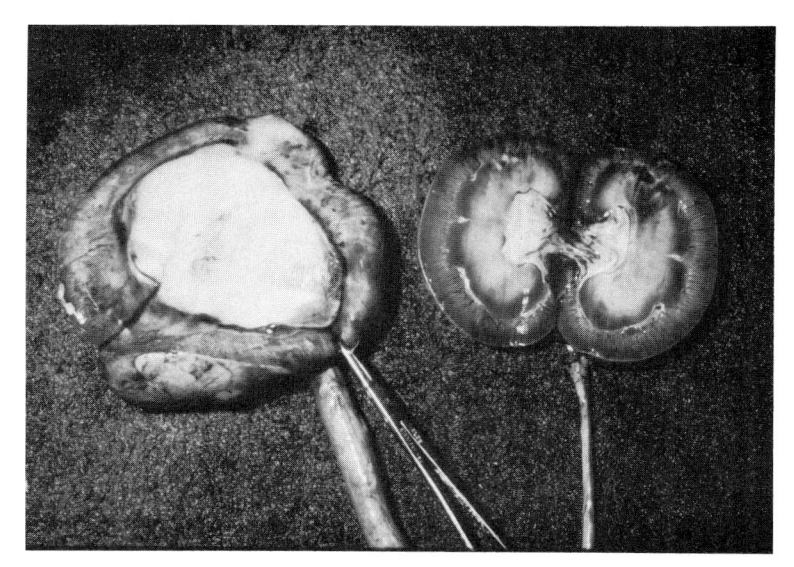

Figure 22–8. Unilateral pyonephrosis of the left kidney of an adult female mixed breed dog. Pyonephrosis occurred as a result of partial stricture of the left ureter. The right kidney has undergone compensatory hypertrophy.

      b. Following surgical operations on the urinary tract of dogs and man.
      c. In association with urinary neoplasms in man.
   2. The exact mechanism(s) by which heteroplastic bone develops in association with urinary tract tissues has not been established, but the consistent close relationship of bone to transitional epithelium has led to the hypothesis that normal urinary transitional epithelium has some relationship to osteogenesis. The results of one experimental study in dogs were interpreted to suggest that transitional epithelium stimulated transformation of certain fibroblasts to osteoblasts.

V. Clinical findings

   A. Hydronephrosis may remain asymptomatic for long periods of time, especially if it is unilateral and the unaffected kidney is capable of adequate renal function.

   B. Early signs are often produced by the underlying cause.

   C. Kidneys which are enlarged and distended with fluid may be palpated per abdomen.

      The lesion causing obstruction to urine flow may be palpated.

   D. Signs of uremia may be present if hydronephrosis is bilateral, or when hydronephrosis is unilateral and disease is present in the opposite kidney.

   E. Fever and leucocytosis may be detected if the involved kidney becomes secondarily infected with bacteria.

      If obstruction to urine outflow is not complete, hematuria, proteinuria, pyuria, and bacteriuria may also be detected.

   F. Radiography may reveal both obstruction to urine outflow and abnormalities related to the primary cause.

      High dosage urography should be considered since it may enhance visualization of the excretory pathway of the urinary system.

VI. Diagnosis

The following may be of value in establishing an ante mortem diagnosis of hydronephrosis:

A. *History, physical examination, and pertinent laboratory data.*

B. *High dose excretory urography.*

C. *Double contrast cystography.*

D. *Percutaneous aspiration of hydronephrotic fluid with a 22 to 25 gauge needle and syringe.*

E. *Exploratory laparotomy.*

VII. Treatment

A. *The primary objective of treatment should be to eliminate the underlying cause before irreversible renal changes have time to develop (see pathogenesis of hydronephrosis in this chapter).*

B. *Unilateral obstruction of a ureter may be corrected by segmental ureterectomy and ureteral anastomosis.*

C. *Attempts to dilate obstructed ureters in experimental dogs have been unsuccessful.*

D. *Nephrectomy may be indicated in cases of unilateral hydronephrosis, provided adequate function is present in the opposite kidney.*

E. *No cure is available for advanced bilateral hydronephrosis (except renal transplantation) because the damage to renal parenchyma is irreversible.*
   1. Conservative medical management may permit comfortable survival for a period of months (see Chapter 31, Treatment of Renal Failure).
   2. If infection is present, appropriate antibiotic therapy should be considered (see Chapter 33, Drug Therapy in Renal Failure).

VIII. Prognosis

A. *Prognosis is dependent on the likelihood of successful treatment of the primary cause and on the potential for recovery of sufficient renal function to maintain life.*

B. *If the cause of obstruction is removed prior to development of structural renal damage, a good prognosis is justified.*

C. *If the obstructive lesion has been present for a sufficient period of time to cause severe bilateral hydronephrosis, the prognosis will be guarded to poor in most instances.*

D. *The biological behavior of the underlying cause (i.e., malignant neoplasm) may become the limiting factor with respect to survival.*

REFERENCES

Abbott, A. C., Goodwin, A. M., and Stephenson, E.: Heterotropic bone formation produced by epithelial transplants from urogenital tract of dogs, rabbits, guinea pigs and cats. J. Urol., *40*:294–311, 1938.

Berlyne, G. M., and Macken, A.: On the mechanism of renal inability to produce a concentrated urine in chronic hydronephrosis. Clin. Sci., *22*:315–324, 1962.

Boyarsky, S., and Martinez, J.: Pathophysiology of the ureter: Partial ligation of the ureter in dogs. Invest. Urol., 2:173–180, 1964.

Copher, G. M.: Effects of urinary bladder transplants and extracts on formation of bone: A further experimental study. Ann. Surg., 108:934–940, 1938.

Damadian, R. V., Shwayri, E., and Bricker, N. S.: On the existence of non-urine forming nephrons in the diseased kidney of the dog. J. Lab. Clin. Med., 65:26–39, 1965.

Damjanov, I.: Heterotropic ossification in implantation metastasis from a carcinoma of the bladder. J. Urol., 101:863–865, 1969.

Draper, J. W., Pearce, J. M., and Lavengood, R. W.: Bone formation in experimental pyeloureteroneostomy. J. Urol., 78:730–737, 1957.

Finkle, A. L., and Smith, D. R.: Parameters of renal functional capacity in reversible hydroureteronephrosis in dogs. V. Effect of 7 to 10 days of ureteral constriction on RBF-Kr, C-In, T_c-H_2O, C-PAH, osmolality, and sodium reabsorption. Invest. Urol., 8:319–323, 1970.

Friedland, G. W., and Dale, R. L.: Minature kidneys due to obstructive atrophy. Experimental observations in dogs. Radiology, 99:273–277, 1971.

Gilbert, G. H., and Gorman, H. A.: Transplantation of urinary bladder mucosa for osteogenic effect. J.A.V.M.A., 158:77–81, 1971.

Harrington, S. W.: The effect on the kidney of various surgical procedures on the blood supply, capsule, and on the ureters. Arch. Surg., 2:547–592, 1921.

Hinman, F.: The pathogenesis of hydronephrosis. Surg. Gynec. Obst., 58:356–376, 1934.

Huggins, C. B.: Formation of bone under the influence of epithelium of the urinary tract. Arch. Surg., 22:377–408, 1951.

Huggins, C. B., McCarroll, H. R., and Blacksom, B. H.: Experiments on the theory of osteogenesis. Arch. Surg., 32:915, 1936.

Hurov, L., Ellett, E. W., and O'Harra, P. J.: Bilateral hydronephrosis resulting from a transitional epithelial carcinoma in a dog. J.A.V.M.A., 149:412–417, 1966.

Joelson, J. J., Beck, C. S., and Moritz, A. R.: Renal counterbalance. Arch. Surg., 19:673–711, 1929.

Katal, M. J., and Wax, S. H.: Evaluation of renal function during experimental hydronephrosis by means of radioisotope renogram. Surg. Gynec. Obstet., 126:563–571, 1968.

Kerr, W. S.: Effects of complete ureteral obstruction in dogs on kidney function. Amer. J. Physiol., 184:521–526, 1956.

Klinger, M. E.: Bone formation in the ureter. A case report. J. Urol., 75:793–795, 1956.

Malvin, R. L.: Partial ureteral obstruction and renal function. In Urodynamics: Hydrodynamics of the Ureter and Renal Pelvis. Edited by S. Boyarski, C. W. Gottshalk, E. A. Tanagho, and P. D. Zimskind. New York, N.Y., Academic Press, 1970.

Navar, L. G., and Baer, P. G.: Renal autoregulatory and glomerular filtration responses to graded ureteral obstruction. Nephron, 7:301–316, 1970.

Nielsen, S. W., and Medway, W.: Canine renal disorders. I. Hydronephrosis. No. Amer. Vet., 35:849–852, 1954.

Olesen, S., and Madsen, P. O.: Renal function during experimental hydronephrosis: Function during partial obstruction following contralateral nephrectomy in the dog. J. Urol., 99:692–699, 1968.

Olson, C.: Spontaneous hydronephrosis in the dog with osteoid tissue in the renal pelvis. J.A.V.M.A., 87:74–80, 1935.

Pridgin, W. P., Woodhead, D. M., and Younger, R. K.: Alterations in renal function produced by ureteral obstruction. Determination of critical obstruction time in terms of renal survival. J.A.M.A., 178:563–564, 1961.

Rawlings, C. A.: Bilateral hydronephrosis and hydroureter in a young dog. J.A.V.M.A., 155:26–29, 1969.

Schirmer, H. K. A., and Marshall, K. E.: Metabolism of atrophic renal tissue following removal of complete ureteral obstruction. J. Urol., 100:596–597, 1968.

Sheehan, H. L., and Davis, J. C.: Experimental hydronephrosis. Arch. Path., 68:185–225, 1959.

Suki, W., Eknoyan, G., Rector, F. C., and Seldin, D. W.: Patterns of nephron perfusion in acute and chronic hydronephrosis. J. Clin. Invest., 45:122–131, 1966.

Ticer, J. W.: Capsulogenic renal cyst in a cat. J.A.V.M.A., 143:613–614, 1963.

Weaver, R. G.: Mechanical factors in production of hydronephrosis. J. Urol., 94:514–519, 1965.

Chapter 23
DIOCTOPHYMA RENALE

I. Dioctophyma renale is the largest known species of nematode and is commonly referred to as the "giant kidney worm."

It has been reported from all over the world in man and many different species of animals including dogs, coyotes, foxes, wolves, jackals, cats, weasels, muskrats, coatimundies, and pigs.

II. Morphologic characteristics

A. These parasites are variable in size, depending on the species of mammal they parasitize.

1. Females are 20 to 103 cm. in length and 5 to 12 mm. in diameter in dogs.
2. Males are 14 to 45 cm. in length and 4 to 6 mm. in diameter in dogs.

B. The eggs of D. renale *are thick shelled and oval in shape and have characteristic surface mammilations, except at their poles (Fig. 23–1).*

III. Life cycle

A. The kidneys are sites of predilection of D. renale.

Gravid females shed ova which escape from the definitive host via the urine.

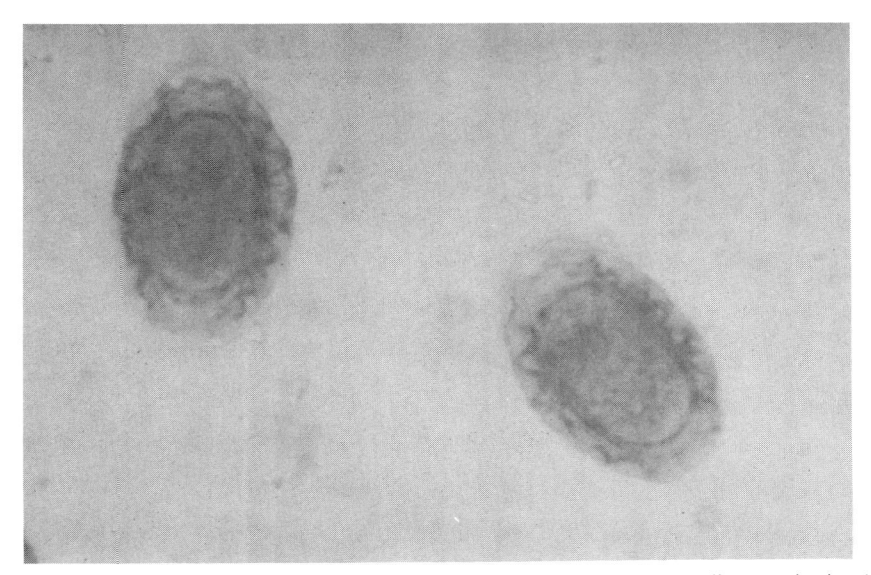

Figure 23–1. Photomicrograph of *Dioctophyma renale* ova in urine sediment obtained from a 15-month-old female golden retriever dog. ×560. (Courtesy of Dr. J. B. Stevens, College of Veterinary Medicine, University of Minnesota.)

B. *Fertile eggs voided in water require one to seven months to embryonate.*

C. *When eggs containing first stage larvae are ingested by annelid worms that are parasitic on crayfish, they develop into second-stage larvae and encyst.*

D. *When northern black bullhead fish ingest infected annelid worms, the larvae encyst and develop into an infective stage in the liver and mesentery of the fish.*

E. *The definitive host becomes infected by eating uncooked fish, especially fish entrails.*

F. *The larvae then excyst in the stomach or intestines of the definitive host and migrate to the renal pelves via the liver and peritoneal cavity.*

G. *The entire life cycle from egg to adult may take as long as two years.*

H. *Currently available data suggest that the time required for infective larvae to become mature gravid females in dogs is three and one half to six months.*

I. *Infected dogs have been reported to harbor as few as one or as many as 27 adult parasites.*

J. *Available data suggest that adult parasites may survive for one to three years or longer in dogs.*

IV. **Although infrequent, this parasite continues to be encountered on a sporadic basis in the peritoneal cavity and kidneys of dogs.**

In 1971, *D. renale* were found in 2 dogs evaluated at the University of Minnesota.

V. **Pathology**

A. Adult D. renale *are most commonly found in the peritoneal cavity in dogs.*

Less commonly, they are found in the renal pelvis, especially of the right kidney.

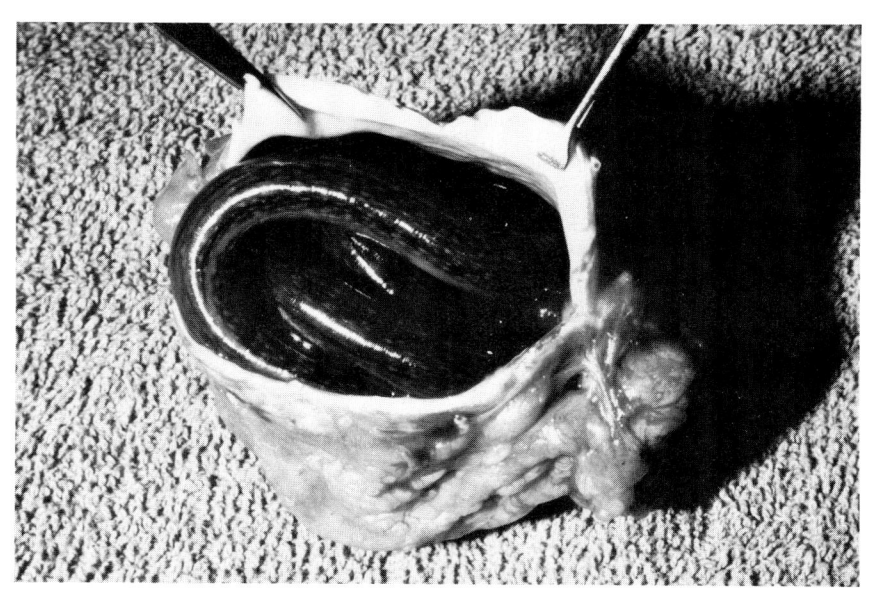

Figure 23–2. Adult male and female *Dioctophyma renale* in the right kidney of the dog described in Figure 23–1. Advanced hydronephrosis has reduced the renal parenchyma to a fibrous sac. (J.A.V.M.A., *155*:605–620, 1969.)

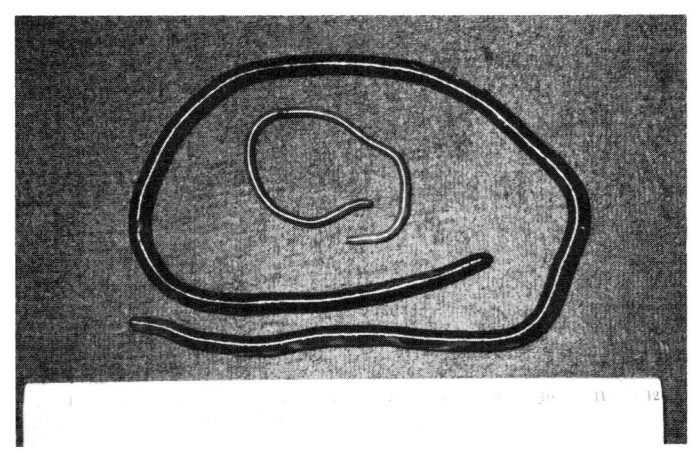

Figure 23-3. Male and female *Dioctophyma renale* obtained from the right kidney of the dog described in Figure 23-1. (J.A.V.M.A., *155*:605-620, 1969.)

B. D. renale *located in the peritoneal cavity may cause varying degrees of peritonitis, adhesions, and destruction of liver parenchyma.*

C. D. renale *located within the renal pelves usually cause destruction of the renal parenchyma by obstruction of urine flow and secondary hydronephrosis.*
   1. The degree of renal dysfunction is dependent upon the number of parasites in the kidney, the duration of infection, the number of kidneys parasitized, and the presence or absence of concomitant renal disease.
   2. If only one kidney is parasitized, severe hydronephrosis or pyonephrosis may develop, with the result that the kidney is converted to a large fibrous sac containing sanguinopurulent fluid and adult parasites (Figs. 23-2 and 23-3).
   3. If both kidneys are parasitized, or if the nonparasitized kidney has marginal renal function and is unable to compensate, the animal may die of renal failure before extensive pathologic changes have time to develop.

VI. Clinical signs

A. *If neither or only one kidney is parasitized, affected dogs are usually asymptomatic.*

B. *If both kidneys are parasitized, or if only one kidney is parasitized and the other has concomitant generalized renal disease, clinical signs of renal failure may be seen (see Chapter 13, Extrarenal Manifestations of Uremia).*

C. *Gross hematuria has been reported in dogs with* D. renale *infection, but it is not a constant finding.*

D. *Enlarged hydronephrotic kidneys may be palpated per abdomen.*

VII. Laboratory findings

A. *Urinalysis will reveal the presence of the characteristic ova of* D. renale, *provided a gravid female is present in a portion of the urinary system that communicates with the exterior of the body (Fig. 23-1).*

B. *Urinalysis may reveal findings characteristic of inflammation (i.e., RBC, WBC, proteinuria).*

C. *In dogs with renal insufficiency, renal function tests will reveal glomerular and tubular dysfunction (see Chapter 7, Tests of Renal Function).*

D. *An intravenous urogram may reveal that affected kidneys cannot properly excrete radiopaque media.*

VIII. Diagnosis

A. *A definitive diagnosis must be based on identification of adult parasites, larvae, or ova.*

B. *History, physical findings, and pertinent laboratory data provide supportive diagnostic evidence.*

IX. Treatment

A. *Nephrectomy is indicated for patients with severe unilateral kidney lesions.*

B. *In dogs with parasitism of both kidneys, nephrotomy and removal of the parasites from the renal pelvis may be of value if irreversible renal insufficiency has not occurred.*

X. Control

Susceptible hosts should be prevented from consuming raw or improperly cooked fish.

REFERENCE

Osborne, C. A., Stevens, J. B., Hanlon, G. H., Rosin, E., and Bemrick, W.: Dioctophyma renale in the dog. J.A.V.M.A., *155*:605–620, 1969.

Chapter 24
MISCELLANEOUS PARASITES OF THE URINARY SYSTEM

I. Toxocara canis

Focal areas of inflammation and scarring which occur in response to the presence of the second-stage larvae of *Toxocara canis* are occasionally encountered as incidental necropsy findings in the kidneys of dogs over six months of age. The larvae localize in the kidneys and other viscera during the somatic phase of their migration. Disturbance of renal function is rarely if ever attributable to the larvae of *T. canis*, even when numerous parasitic lesions are present.

II. Dirofilaria immitis

Proteinuria may occur in dogs with dirofilariasis as a result of congestive heart failure, or as a result of the presence of microfilaria in the glomerular capillaries. On rare occasions, microfilaria have been observed in the urine sediment. When microfilaria become trapped in the kidneys of a living animal, they often provoke a chronic inflammatory response. Clinical signs attributed to renal lesions induced by microfilaria have not been reported.

III. Spirocerca lupi

Although adult *Spirocerca lupi* are characteristically found in the wall of the esophagus posterior to the aortic arch, they have been encountered in the stomach wall, trachea, and urinary bladder on rare occasions. On one occasion, an adult *S. lupi* was found in the renal artery.

REFERENCES

Soulsby, E. J. L.: Textbook of Veterinary Clinical Parasitology. Vol. I—Helminths. Philadelphia, Pa., F. A. Davis Co., 1965.
Sprent, J. F. A.: Observations on the development of Toxocara canis in the dog. Parasitology, *48*:184–209, 1958.

Chapter 25

PRIMARY DISEASES OF THE GLOMERULI

I. **Glomerulonephritis**

A. *Definition*

Glomerulonephritis is characterized by inflammation of the glomeruli, which in later stages may be associated with secondary changes in the renal tubules, interstitial tissue, and sometimes blood vessels (see Chapter 12, Pathophysiology of Renal Failure). Glomerulonephritis is differentiated from other forms of renal disease by changes that are initially and predominantly glomerular.

B. *The term glomerulonephritis is commonly used in reference to several different forms of focal or diffuse inflammatory diseases which involve the glomeruli.*

Because of basic similarities of glomerulonephritis in dogs to glomerulonephritis in man, and because of the paucity of information in the veterinary literature concerning the clinicopathologic aspects of glomerulonephritis, comparative aspects of the disease are discussed.

1. In man, several different types of glomerulonephritis have been described including:
    a. Acute and subacute proliferative glomerulonephritis.
        (1) The etiology is thought to be related to an immunologic response to certain species of bacteria, including streptococci.
        (2) This type of glomerulonephritis is characterized by varying degrees of exudation of inflammatory cells into glomeruli, and swelling and proliferation of glomerular mesangial cells, glomerular endothelial cells and glomerular epithelial cells (Fig. 25–1). The functional effect of these changes is to impair renal function by reduction of glomerular filtration.
        (3) The disease process usually undergoes complete resolution, but may result in uremic death of the patient, or progress to chronic glomerulonephritis.
        (4) Clinical signs of glomerulonephritis include various combinations of oliguria secondary to reduced GFR, hematuria, proteinuria, and the presence of hyaline, granular or red cell casts. Early in the course of the disease the renal tubules retain the ability to concentrate urine. If a sufficient number of glomeruli lose their function (approximately 75 per cent or more), clinical signs of renal failure will be present.

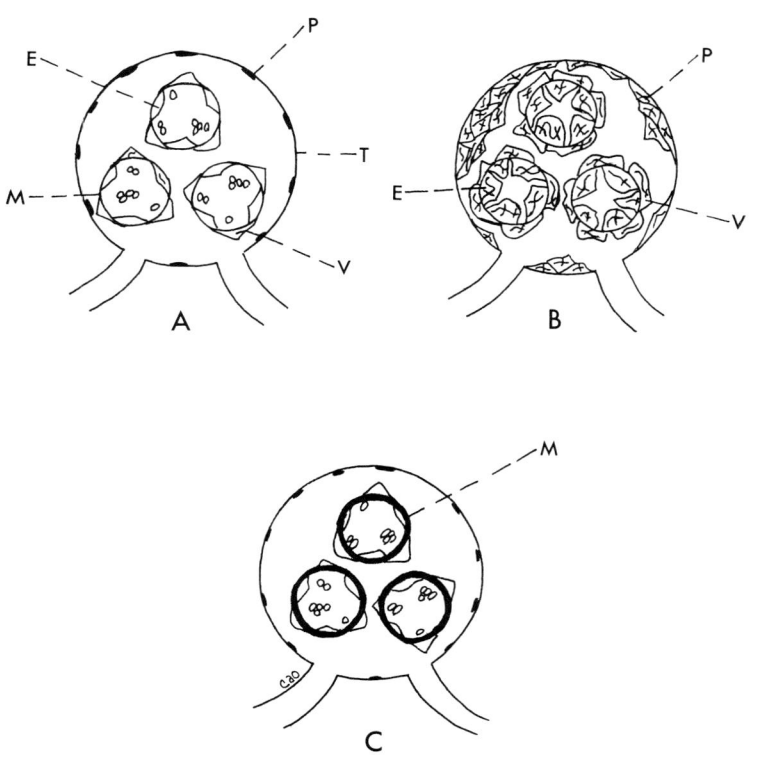

Figure 25-1. Schematic drawings of different types of glomerulonephritis. A. Normal glomerulus. B. Proliferative glomerulonephritis. C. Membranous glomerulonephritis. M, glomerular capillary basement membrane; E, endothelial cell of glomerular capillary; P, parietal epithelium; T, Bowman's capsule; V, visceral epithelium.

    b. Membranous glomerulonephritis.
       (1) The etiology of this type of glomerulonephritis is thought to be related to a poorly understood immunologic response.
       (2) It is usually associated with profound proteinuria, and may be associated with the nephrotic syndrome (see Chapter 27, nephrotic syndrome).
       (3) Early stages and mild cases are not associated with glomerular lesions which are detectable by light microscopy, but are associated with fusion of the foot processes of glomerular epithelial cells as seen by electron microscopy. More severe cases are associated with generalized and marked thickening of glomerular basement membranes which can be detected by light microscopy (Fig. 25-1). The epithelial cells of the proximal tubules are usually laden with lipid throughout the course of the disease (thus the name lipoid nephrosis).
       (4) This disease process may undergo spontaneous resolution, cause the death of the patient, or progress to chronic glomerulonephritis.
    c. Mixed glomerulonephritis refers to glomerular disease characterized by changes of proliferative glomerulonephritis and membranous glomerulonephritis.
    d. Chronic glomerulonephritis.
       (1) Both proliferative glomerulonephritis and membranous glomerulonephritis may progress to chronic glomerulonephritis.

(2) Some patients develop chronic glomerulonephritis, but have no clinical history of having acute or subacute proliferative, or membranous glomerulonephritis.

(3) Generalized chronic glomerulonephritis is characterized grossly by a shrunken end-stage kidney which is very similar in appearance to the end-stage kidneys of renal amyloidosis, pyelonephritis, or chronic interstitial nephritis. Many glomeruli and renal tubules undergo atrophic and ischemic necrosis and are replaced with connective tissue. Marked hypercellularity may be seen in some glomeruli. Viable nephrons undergo compensatory hypertrophy and hyperplasia (see Chapter 20, End-Stage Kidneys).

(4) The clinical signs of chronic generalized glomerulonephritis are the same as those caused by any chronic progressive irreversible renal disease (see Chapter 12, Pathophysiology of Renal Failure and Chapter 13, Extrarenal Manifestations of Uremia).

2. In the past the reported incidence of spontaneously occurring glomerulonephritis in dogs and cats has been infrequent.

   a. Glomerular lesions are often seen in association with polysystemic diseases such as systemic lupus erythematosus, pyometra, and diabetes mellitus.

   b. Glomerular lesions characteristic of acute, subacute, and chronic glomerulonephritis have been reported in a few dogs with naturally occurring renal disease by several authorities.

      (1) Because the diagnosis was established at necropsy, the clinical features were not well documented.

      (2) In a few cases in which the clinical findings were evaluated in retrospect, the clinical signs and laboratory findings were essentially the same as those observed in man.

   c. Glomerulonephritis has been experimentally produced in dogs with toxic bacterial products, anti-kidney serum and foreign protein. The pathologic changes were characterized by varying degrees of inflammatory changes in glomeruli, endothelial cell and epithelial cell swelling and proliferation, thickening of glomerular basement membranes, and attempts of the body to repair severe lesions by replacement fibrosis. Damage to tubules was less extensive.

   d. Two well documented cases of membranous glomerulonephritis have recently been observed in dogs.

      (1) In one reported case in an 8-year-old, female Rhodesian ridgeback, proteinuria and hypoproteinemia were observed. Light and electron microscopic evaluation of sections of renal tissue revealed generalized thickening of the basement membranes of glomerular capillaries. Ultrastructural changes were characterized by the presence of electron dense deposits in glomerular basement membranes, and generalized fusion of the foot processes of epithelial podocytes.

      (2) Membranous glomerulonephritis was diagnosed in a one-and-one-half-year-old, male golden retriever at the University of Minnesota. The dog had a nephrotic syndrome characterized by subcutaneous edema and ascites, severe proteinuria (17 grams of protein lost in the urine per 24 hours), hypoproteinemia, hypoalbuminemia, and hypercholesterolemia. Abnormalities in renal function tests were not observed. Evaluation of renal tissue obtained by percutaneous

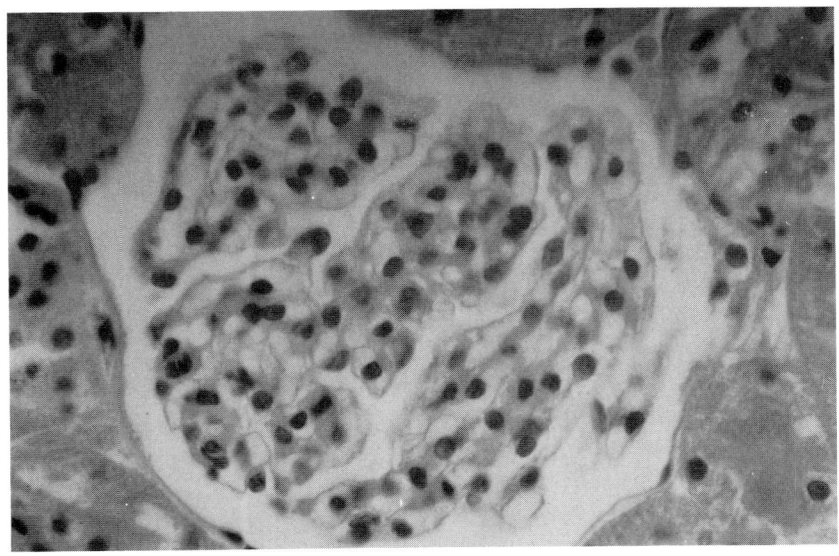

Figure 25–2. Photomicrograph of a normal glomerulus obtained by needle biopsy from an adult male dog. H&E stain; × 450.

        biopsy revealed the presence of generalized thickening of glomerular capillary basement membranes (Figs. 25–2 and 25–3).
   e. Recently, several well documented cases of spontaneous glomerulonephritis have been described in cats.
      (1) Diffuse membranous glomerulonephritis was reported in a cat and was characterized by diffuse thickening of the basement membranes of all glomeruli. A nephrotic syndrome was also present.
      (2) Diffuse membranous glomerulonephritis was reported in another cat in which LE cells were demonstrated in peripheral blood (see

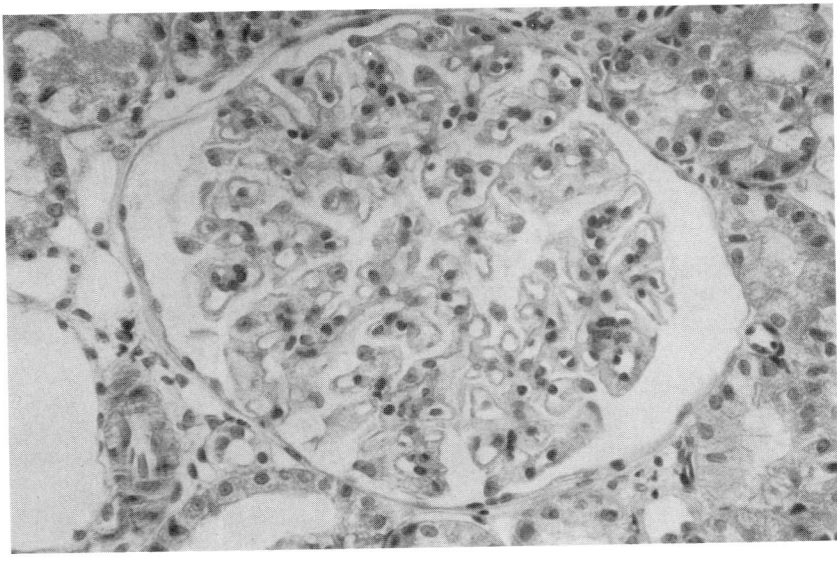

Figure 25–3. Photomicrograph of a renal biopsy specimen obtained from a 1.5-year-old male golden retriever dog with membranous glomerulonephritis. Generalized thickening of the glomerular capillary walls was observed in all glomeruli. H&E stain; × 400. (Courtesy of Dr. J. B. Stevens, College of Veterinary Medicine, University of Minnesota.)

Systemic lupus erythematosus, in Chapter 28). Sections of kidney stained with hematoxylin and eosin revealed diffuse thickening of glomerular capillary walls. Epithelial crescents were not observed. Fluorescence microscopic and electron microscopic examination of sections of kidney suggested localization of soluble antigen-antibody complexes in glomerular capillary walls.

(3) Diffuse membranous glomerulonephritis was reported in three cats that also had lymphocytic leukemia.

(4) Diffuse membranous glomerulonephritis was reported in one cat that also had myelogenous leukemia.

3. The etiology and pathogenesis of spontaneous glomerulonephritis in dogs and cats have not been established.
   a. The etiopathogenesis of glomerulonephritis in man and laboratory animals appears to be related to at least two distinct abnormalities.
      (1) Autoantibodies against glomerular basement membrane antigens may be produced by the host.
      (2) Antigen-antibody complexes, which are produced as a result of antibody formation against nonglomerular antigens, may be trapped in glomeruli.
   b. Electron microscopic and fluorescence microscopic evaluation of sections of kidney obtained from a cat with spontaneous membranous glomerulonephritis revealed findings consistent with an immune disturbance.

4. Clinical findings associated with spontaneously occurring membranous glomerulonephritis in dogs and cats have been associated with one or more of the following:
   a. Subcutaneous edema of the dependent portions of the body, and ascites in some cases.
   b. Persistent proteinuria.
   c. Hyaline or granular casts in urine sediment.
   d. Hypoproteinemia and hypoalbuminemia.
   e. Hypercholesterolemia.
   f. Abnormalities in renal function tests (i.e., low specific gravity, abnormal increase in the serum concentration of BUN or creatinine, abnormal decrease in urinary excretion of PSP dye). The latter were not consistent findings in all cases.

5. Diagnosis.
   a. Clinical findings provide supportive evidence.
   b. Renal biopsy may provide a definitive morphologic diagnosis.

6. Treatment and Prognosis. Well documented clinical cases of spontaneous glomerulonephritis in dogs and cats have been too few in number to allow meaningful generalizations to be made regarding specific treatment and prognosis. Corticosteroid therapy is sometimes of benefit to human patients with membranous glomerulonephritis, and should be considered for dogs and cats with this disease. Corticosteroids must be administered with caution to azotemic or uremic patients since steroids may aggravate uremic signs as a result of gluconeogenesis. Symptomatic and supportive treatment of uremia may be of value.

II. Sclerosing glomerular disease

A sclerosing glomerular disease characterized by generalized pericapillary sclerosis is a common lesion in old dogs. The degree of individual glomerular involvement is variable. This lesion has not been reported in association with clinical signs of renal disease.

III. Glomerular lipoidosis

Glomerular lipoidosis in dogs is characterized by the presence of large foam cells which contain sudanophilic droplets in one or more lobules of the glomerular tuft. The unaffected portion of the glomerulus appears histologically normal. The number of glomeruli involved is variable. The etiopathogenesis of this lesion is unknown. Clinical signs attributed to glomerular lipoidosis have not been reported in dogs or cats.

IV. Infarction

A. Definition

An infarct is an area of coagulation necrosis which occurs as a result of rapid and total occlusion of circulation.

B. Arterial infarcts are commonly observed in the kidney because of the large renal blood flow, and because the kidneys contain end arteries without significant collateral blood supply.

C. The sequelae of renal infarction is dependent upon the number and the size of the involved vessels, and whether the obstructing material is nonseptic or septic.

D. Renal infarcts are most commonly encountered in association with embolism (see Bacterial endocarditis, in Chapter 28).

V. Renal amyloidosis—In dogs, renal amyloidosis is primarily a disease of glomeruli (see Chapter 26, Renal Amyloidosis).

REFERENCES

Anderson, L. J.: The glomeruli in canine interstitial nephritis. J. Path. Bact., 95:59–65, 1968.
Anderson, L. J., and Jarrett, W. F. H.: Membranous glomerulonephritis associated with leukemia in cats. Res. Vet. Sci., 12:179–180, 1971.
Brown, P.: A case of feline membranous glomerulonephritis. Vet. Rec., 89:557–558, 1971.
Carr, B. R., Lim, V. S., and Greene, J. A.: Glomerular and tubular changes during the development of acute antiserum nephritis in dogs. J. Lab. Clin. Med., 72:863, 1968.
Dhar, S., and Pathak, R. C.: Immune nephritis in dogs. Indian J. Exp. Biol., 8:281–285, 1970.
DiDomizio, G., and Minoccheri, F.: Ultrastructural aspects of diffuse glomerulosclerosis in the dog. Pathogenesis and lesions. Archo. Vet. Ital., 18:29–48, 1967.
Farrow, B. R. H., Huxtable, C. R., and McGovern, V. J.: Nephrotic syndrome in the cat due to diffuse membranous glomerulonephritis. Pathology, 1:67–72, 1969.
Fisher, E. R., and Fisher, B.: Glomerular lipoidosis in the dog. Amer. J. Vet. Res., 15:285–286, 1954.
Highman, B., Altland, P. D., and Roshe, J.: Staphylococcal endocarditis and glomerulonephritis in dogs. Circulation Res., 7:982–987, 1959.
Margolis, G., Forbus, W. D., Kuby, G. P., and Lide, T. N.: Glomerulonephritis occurring in experimental brucellosis in dogs. Amer. J. Path., 23:983–993, 1947.
Monlux, A. W.: The histopathology of nephritis in the dog. III. Inflammatory vascular diseases of the kidney. Amer. J. Vet. Res., 14:440–447, 1953.
Murray, M., Pirie, H. M., Thompson, H., and Jarrett, W. F. H.: Glomerulonephritis in a dog. A histologic and electron microscopical study. Res. Vet. Sci., 12:493–495, 1971.
Rosen, S.: Membranous glomerulonephritis: Current status. Human Pathology, 2:209–231, June 1971.
Slauson, D. O., Russell, S. W., and Schechter, R.: Naturally occurring immune-complex glomerulonephritis in the cat. J. Path., 103:131–133, 1971.
Ward, J. M., Sodikoff, C. H., and Schalm, O. W.: Myeloproliferative disease and abnormal erythrogenesis in the cat. J.A.V.M.A., 155:879–888, 1969.
Yamauchi, H., Cheu, D., Rooney, P., and Hopper, J.: Renal lesions induced by aminonucleoside in dogs. Arch. Path., 77:20–26, 1964.

Chapter 26
RENAL AMYLOIDOSIS

I. Amyloid is a glycoprotein of varied composition which is deposited in an intracellular location.

II. No concept of the pathogenesis of amyloidosis has been uniformly accepted since none correlate all of the available clinical, pathologic, and experimental data.

   A. Although it is generally accepted that the genesis of amyloid is related to an immunologic disturbance, the formation of amyloid does not occur as a result of a specific immune response since it can be experimentally induced in a variety of animals following administration of diverse and apparently unrelated antigens.

   B. The hypothesis that amyloid forms as a result of deposition of antigen-antibody complexes has not been supported by a large volume of clinical and experimental evidence.

   C. Recent observations in man, dogs, and laboratory animals have provided strong evidence suggesting that the genesis of amyloid is intimately related to local production by cells.

   A variety of cells, including reticuloendothelial cells, fibroblasts, histiocytes, mesangial cells, renal glomerular endothelial and epithelial cells, and plasma cells have been incriminated in the production of amyloid. It has been hypothesized that an insoluble glycoprotein is deposited intercellularly at the site of its production.

   D. Amyloid formation in cats may be associated with hypervitaminosis A.

III. Classically amyloidosis has been divided into primary and secondary categories.

   A. Primary amyloidosis is characterized by amyloid deposition without evidence of any predisposing disease.

   B. Secondary amyloidosis is characterized by amyloid deposition associated with chronic suppuration, necrosis, or neoplasia.

   C. These categories of amyloidosis are probably different manifestations of one fundamental disturbance.

   Amyloid deposits associated with each category have a similar electron microscopic appearance and a similar biochemical composition.

IV. **Significance of amyloid deposition**

   A. Amyloid may be deposited in any organ or tissue of the body in a focal or generalized fashion.

B. *Alteration of organ functions is probably related to the physical presence of amyloid.*
   1. Amyloid does not provoke an inflammatory response.
   2. Amyloid is commonly found in perivascular areas of capillaries, arterioles, and venules.
      a. Progressive perivascular deposits of amyloid encroach on vascular lumens and result in decreased blood flow. As a result the tissues supplied by the altered vessels undergo ischemic atrophy and necrosis.
      b. Amyloid deposition may depress cellular function by restriction of fluid and gas exchange across vessel walls.

V. Renal Pathology

   A. Dogs
   1. The kidneys are the sites where amyloid deposition assumes major clinical significance in dogs. This observation may be related to the large blood supply and numerous capillaries characteristic of the kidneys.
   2. Renal amyloidosis is primarily a glomerular disease in dogs since signs referrable to renal dysfunction occur as the result of amyloid deposition in glomeruli. Although amyloid may be deposited in blood vessels, tubular basement membranes, and renal interstitial tissue, these locations are usually not affected until late in the course of the disease process, and are rarely as seriously affected as the glomeruli. Renal amyloidosis may be associated with variable degrees of amyloid deposition in other tissues and organs of the body, but, in general, they are not as severely affected as the kidneys, and they are uncommonly associated with the development of clinical signs.
   3. Gross Pathology. The size of the kidneys may be normal, increased, or decreased depending on the duration of the disease process.

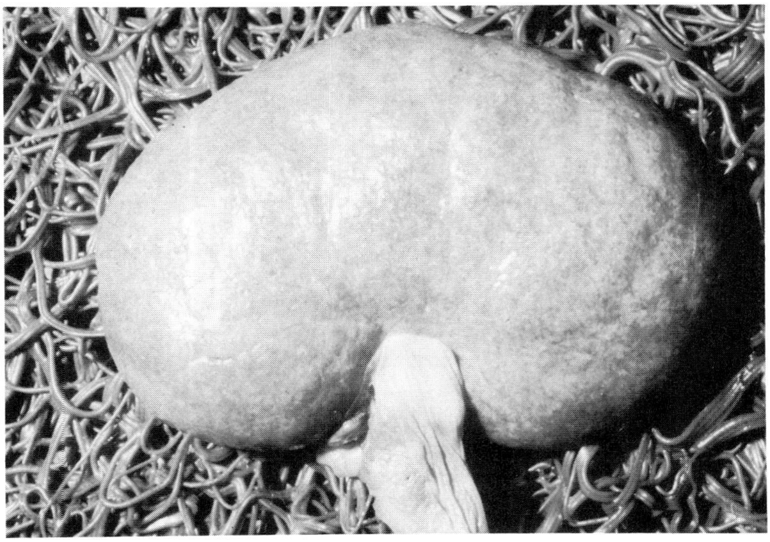

Figure 26-1. End-stage amyloid contracted kidney of a 12-year-old male cocker spaniel. The surface of the renal cortex is pitted and irregular (see Figs. 26-3 and 26-4).

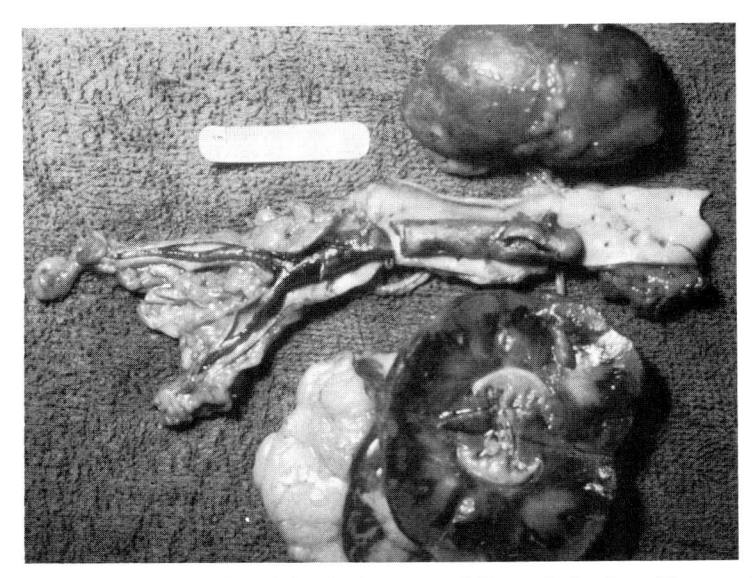

Figure 26–2. Thrombosis of the abdominal aorta and iliac arteries in a 12-year-old male mixed breed dog. Death from uremia occurred as a result of occlusion of the renal arteries. Microscopic examination of the kidneys revealed amyloidosis, and infarction of all of the renal parenchyma.

    a. Kidney size is not significantly altered during the early course of the disease when relatively little amyloid has accumulated in the kidneys.
    b. Increased kidney size occurs in association with rapid and massive accumulations of amyloid, but prior to the occurrence of a significant degree of ischemic atrophy, necrosis, and connective tissue replacement of involved nephrons.
    c. The development of amyloid contracted kidneys is dependent upon a sufficiently slow rate of progression of the disease to allow the patient

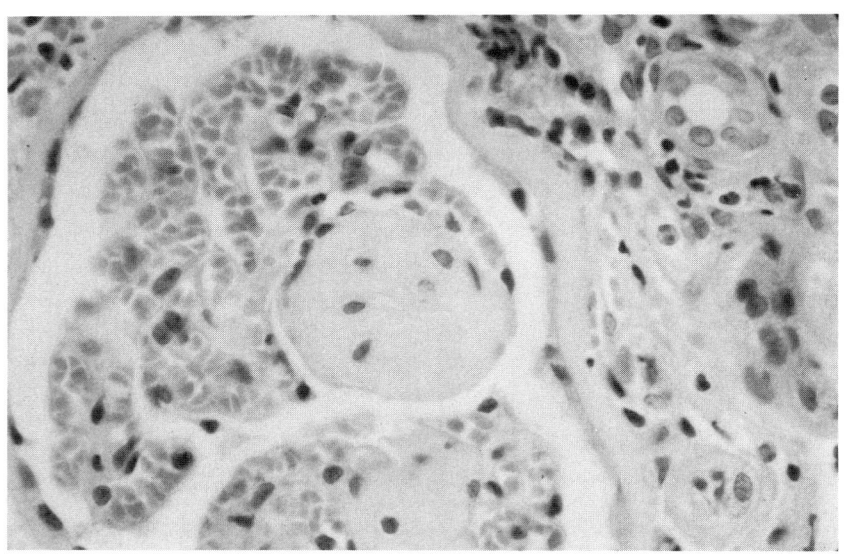

Figure 26–3. Photomicrograph of a renal biopsy specimen obtained from the dog described in Figure 26–1. At the time of biopsy, clinical findings were absent except for persistent proteinuria. Portions of the glomerulus contain lobular deposits of amyloid. H&E stain; × 450. (J.A.V.M.A., *157*: 203–219, 1970.)

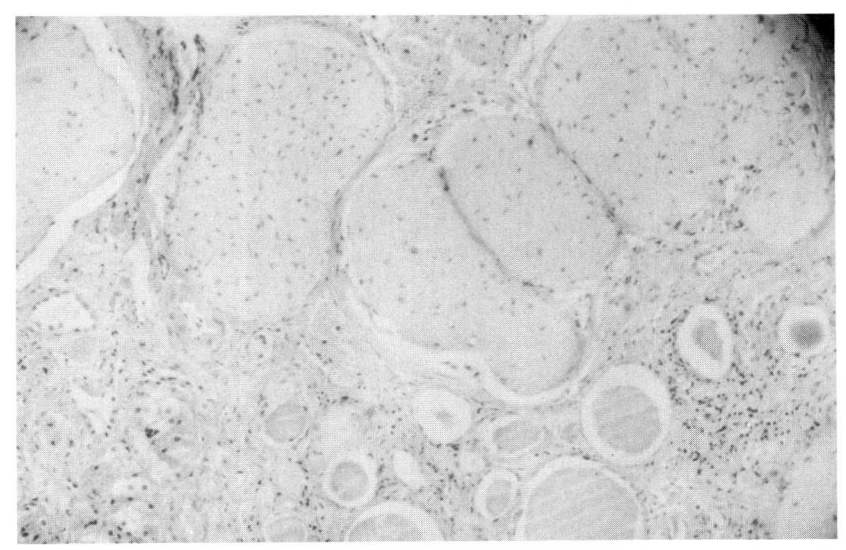

Figure 26-4. Photomicrograph of a renal biopsy specimen obtained from the right kidney of the dog described in Figure 26-1. This biopsy sample was obtained approximately 13 months following procurement of the biopsy sample described in Figure 26-3. Amyloid deposits have almost completely obliterated the glomerular capillaries. Many of the renal tubules are distorted and shrunken, and others have been obliterated by connective tissue. Some dilated tubules lined by flattened epithelium contain amorphous, eosinophilic proteinaceous casts. The dog died of chronic renal failure. H&E stain; × 450. (J.A.V.M.A., *157*:203–219, 1970.)

      to survive by adaptation to progressive renal failure (see Chapter 12, Pathophysiology of Renal Failure). Kidneys which are decreased in size are small and have an irregular "pitted" surface contour as a result of ischemic atrophy and necrosis of renal parenchyma associated with replacement by fibrous connective tissue.
    d. Amyloid contracted kidneys cannot be distinguished grossly from the end-stage kidneys caused by chronic generalized pyelonephritis or chronic interstitial nephritis (Fig. 26-1).
    e. Thrombosis and infarction of many organs including the renal veins has been reported in association with renal amyloidosis in dogs (Fig. 26-2).
4. Histopathology.
    a. The glomeruli show the earliest and most consistent alterations. Characteristically all of the glomeruli in the kidneys are involved in a similar fashion (Fig. 26-3).
    b. As amyloid deposits accumulate, the glomeruli become large, bloodless, homogenous, hyaline appearing structures (Fig. 26-4).
    c. Generalized and progressive destruction of glomerular capillaries is responsible for:
       (1) Proteinuria which is a consistent finding in this disease.
       (2) Renal insufficiency.
       (3) Ischemic atrophy and necrosis of renal tubules.
    d. The body responds to severe damage of nephrons by replacement of them with connective tissue.
       (1) Nephrons have a very limited ability to regenerate following injury.
       (2) Contraction of fibrous tissue leads to the formation of amyloid contracted kidneys.

B. *Cats*
1. Unlike the disease in dogs, renal amyloidosis in cats is usually characterized by accumulation of amyloid in the papilla and outer medulla.
    a. Glomerular amyloidosis is not a consistent finding, and when present it is usually mild in character.
    b. Capillary and tubular basement membranes in the medulla become thickened.
        (1) Occlusion of capillaries may result in papillary necrosis.
        (2) Occlusion of collecting ducts may result in atrophy and fibrosis of affected nephrons.
2. The paucity of reported cases of renal amyloidosis in cats may be associated with the unusual location of amyloid in the kidney of this species. Because of the common occurrence of amyloid in glomeruli of most other species, cat kidneys may have been erroneously assumed to be free of amyloid on the basis of unaffected glomeruli.
3. Proteinuria may not be a significant clinical finding associated with amyloidosis in cats since glomerular involvement is not an important lesion. If this hypothesis is valid, the clinical nature of chronic generalized amyloidosis in cats would be similar or identical to that associated with other types of chronic generalized renal diseases.

VI. Clinical findings

A. *Clinical manifestations related to amyloidosis are dependent upon the organs or tissues of the body which are affected, the severity and extent of amyloid deposition, and the length of time amyloid has been present.*

The following discussion applies to renal amyloidosis in dogs. Evaluation of the clinical and laboratory findings of amyloidosis in cats has been too meager to establish any meaningful generalizations.

B. *The owner's complaint may be related to predisposing illnesses if present (i.e. suppurative processes or neoplasia).*

C. *Signs of renal dysfunction may provide the first and only clinical clue.*
1. Persistent and severe proteinuria is the *hallmark* of renal amyloidosis. Persistent proteinuria is not pathognomonic of amyloidosis, however, since it may be caused by other types of glomerular disease.
2. Signs related to relatively rapid and generalized glomerular replacement with amyloid (amyloid enlarged kidneys) are usually associated with abnormalities referable to decreased glomerular perfusion, including:
    a. Decreased glomerular filtration rate.
    b. Retention of nonprotein nitrogen (BUN, creatinine).
    c. Retention of phosphorus.
    d. Metabolic acidosis.
3. In spite of the decrease in glomerular filtration, a disproportionate degree of tubular function may persist early in the course of the disease.
    a. Urinary PSP excretion may be normal or slightly depressed.
    b. The kidneys may retain the ability to concentrate urine.
    c. Even if the kidneys lose the ability to concentrate or dilute urine due to nephron damage, and the specific gravity approaches that of glomerular filtrate, extensive intrinsic tubular damage is not necessarily present. Obligatory osmotic diuresis, loss of the counter-current

osmotic gradient, and rapid flow of filtrate through renal tubules may cause impairment of urine concentration and dilution, and associated polyuria and polydipsia, even though the renal tubules retain a significant degree of function (see Chapter 12, Pathophysiology of Renal Failure).
   d. Administration of antidiuretic hormone may reveal that the kidneys can still concentrate urine.
4. Urinalysis.
   a. An acid pH will be present in patients with metabolic acidosis associated with renal failure.
   b. Proteinuria (primarily albumin) is a consistent finding.
   c. Hyaline, granular, or waxy casts may be present in the urine sediment, but they are not a consistent finding. Waxy casts were not observed in 20 dogs with renal amyloidosis at the University of Minnesota, and, contrary to earlier reports, are not pathognomonic of amyloidosis.
5. Signs referable to amyloid contracted kidneys include those related to tubular disease in addition to those related to glomerular disease.
   a. Urinary excretion of PSP dye is decreased.
   b. Tubular disease contributes to the inability to concentrate or dilute urine although the presence of tubular disease cannot be consistently established on the basis of specific gravity (see 3b above).
   c. Administration of antidiuretic hormone will not be associated with a significant increase in urine specific gravity.
6. Serum protein.
   a. The concentration of serum protein may be normal.
   b. In some cases hypoproteinemia occurs.
      (1) It is primarily related to the loss of albumin in urine.
      (2) It may be associated with a nephrotic syndrome (see Chapter 27, Nephrotic Syndrome).
   c. The serum concentration of globulins is variable. They may be normal, increased, or decreased.
7. Hypercholesterolemia is a consistent finding. The percentage of cholesterol as esters is usually normal (60 to 80 per cent).
8. The results of other laboratory tests are dependent on the presence or absence of predisposing disease(s).

VII. Diagnosis. Diagnostically significant information includes:

A. *A typical history characterized by signs of renal failure. Suppuration, severe necrosis, and/or neoplasia may also be present, but are not consistent findings.*

Clinical signs of progressive renal disease due to amyloidosis may occur without clinical manifestations of a predisposing disease.

B. *Physical examination findings, including:*
   1. Signs of generalized renal disease (see Chapter 13, Extrarenal Manifestations of Uremia).
   2. Chronic suppuration or neoplasia.
   3. Palpation of an enlarged spleen or liver. Clinical experience has revealed that these are extremely uncommon findings in dogs and cats.

C. *Laboratory findings including:*
   1. Proteinuria (primarily albumin). Severe and persistent proteinuria of renal origin which occurs in association with chronic suppuration,

necrosis, or malignant neoplasia should be considered as renal amyloidosis until proven otherwise.
2. Hyposthenuria (i.e., decreased ability to concentrate or dilute urine).
3. Elevated BUN or serum creatinine concentration.
4. Nonregenerative anemia if the condition is chronic and generalized.

D. *Congo red dye test*

Because more accurate diagnostic tests are available, this test is not recommended.

E. *Renal biopsy findings*

Microscopic demonstration of amyloid in biopsy samples is the only method by which an ante mortem diagnosis can be conclusively established.
1. Special stains such as congo red, crystal violet, or thioflavine-T may be required to demonstrate amyloid in some cases.
2. Hematoxylin and eosin stain is usually satisfactory in most cases associated with clinical manifestations of renal disease (Figs. 26–3 and 26–4).

VIII. Treatment

A specific therapeutic approach for the elimination of amyloid deposits is not available since the exact cause is unknown. No known regimen of therapy will consistently result in a cure, and, as a generality, most patients ultimately succumb to progressive renal failure, or to a predisposing disease.

A. *Treatment and elimination of predisposing diseases have been reported to halt or reverse amyloid deposition in human beings on rare occasions.*

Unfortunately, by the time renal amyloidosis manifests itself clinically, it may be too far advanced for treatment of the predisposing cause to have significant effect on the course of the disease.

B. *Corticosteroids*

Steroids are contraindicated in the treatment of renal amyloidosis because:
1. Steroid therapy has been of no benefit to human patients with amyloidosis.
2. Steroids enhance experimental production of amyloid in laboratory animals.
3. Steroids may aggravate the severity of clinical signs associated with renal failure because they induce gluconeogenesis. Deamination of protein during conversion to carbohydrate increases the quantity of protein metabolic waste products which must be excreted by the kidneys.

C. *Symptomatic and supportive treatment of progressive renal failure is often beneficial as it may prolong the patient's life.*

At the University of Minnesota, two dogs receiving such treatment lived for more than a year after the diagnosis of renal amyloidosis was established by renal biopsy (see Chapter 31, Treatment of Renal Failure).

IX. Prognosis. Patients with renal amyloidosis should receive a guarded to poor prognosis.

A. *Generally, renal amyloidosis in dogs is progressive and irreversible.*

B. *Specific treatment which will eliminate the primary abnormality is not available.*

C. Following establishment of a specific diagnosis, the patient may succumb in a matter of weeks or survive for several months.

REFERENCES

Clark, L., and Seawright, A. A.: Amyloidosis associated with chronic hypervitaminosis A in cats. Aust. Vet. J., *44*:584, 1968.

Clark, L., and Seawright, A. A.: Generalized amyloidosis in seven cats. Path. Vet., *6*:117–134, 1969.

Lucke, V. M., and Hunt, A. C.: Interstitial nephropathy and papillary necrosis in the domestic cat. J. Path. Bact., *89*:723–728, 1965.

Osborne, C. A., Johnson, K. H., Perman, V., Fangmann, G. M., and Riis, R.: Clinicopathologic progression of renal amyloidosis in a dog. J.A.V.M.A., *157*:203–219, 1970.

Osborne, C. A., Johnson, K. H., Perman, V., and Schall, W. D.: Renal amyloidosis in the dog. J.A.V.M.A., *153*:669–688, 1968.

Slauson, D. O., Gribble, D. H., and Russell, S. W.: A clinicopathological study of renal amyloidosis in dogs. J. Comp. Path., *80*:335–343, 1970.

Chapter 27
NEPHROTIC SYNDROME

I. **Definition**

   The nephrotic syndrome is a renal disease complex characterized by proteinuria, hypoproteinemia, hypercholesterolemia, and edema.

II. **Etiology**

   A. *Although the kidneys are involved in the pathogenesis of most types of generalized fluid retention, primary renal disease is an uncommon cause of edema in the dog and cat.*

   Nephrotic edema is apparently much more common in man. These differences between species may be related to the following:
   1. Generalized glomerular diseases are more prevalent in the human being than in the dog and cat.
   2. Species differences in susceptibility to formation of generalized edema exist.

   B. *Renal diseases which cause generalized alteration of the permeability of glomerular capillaries to plasma proteins, especially albumin, may result in the nephrotic syndrome.*

   C. *Renal amyloidosis is a known cause of the nephrotic syndrome in dogs; however, renal amyloidosis is not consistently associated with the nephrotic syndrome.*

   D. *A nephrotic syndrome has been reported in a cat with glomerulonephritis.*

   E. *The nephrotic syndrome has been reported in some dogs in which the specific underlying renal disease responsible for this symptom complex was not determined.*

   F. *Diseases known to cause the nephrotic syndrome in man include:*
   1. Membranous glomerulonephritis.
   2. Proliferative glomerulonephritis.
   3. Diabetic glomerulosclerosis.
   4. Systemic lupus erythematosus.
   5. Renal vein thrombosis.
   6. Constrictive pericarditis.
   7. Various inorganic and organic toxic agents.

III. **Pathogenesis**

   A. *The common denominator of diseases associated with the nephrotic syndrome is abnormal glomerular permeability to plasma proteins and associated severe proteinuria.*

   B. *Severe albuminuria contributes to hypoalbuminemia and a decrease in colloidal osmotic pressure.*

   In uremic patients, increased rate of endogenous catabolism of albumin, and decreased dietary intake of protein may also contribute to hypoalbuminemia.

C. *Edema is initiated by the decrease in colloidal osmotic pressure caused by hypoalbuminemia.*

The latter results in an abnormal shift of fluid from the vascular compartment to extravascular compartments.
1. Serum albumin levels below 1 Gm. per 100 ml. are usually associated with generalized edema of the body tissues.
2. As a result of contraction of the vascular fluid compartment, there is a compensatory release of aldosterone, and possibly antidiuretic hormone, in order to restore plasma volume. These compensatory mechanisms enhance and perpetuate the edema.

D. *The pathogenesis of hypercholesterolemia is unknown.*
1. The percentage of cholesterol esters is normal (60 to 80 per cent).
2. Although as yet unproven, it has been hypothesized that hypercholesterolemia may be in some way linked to hypoalbuminemia.
   a. This hypothesis was based on evidence obtained from plasmapheresis and experimentally induced nephrosis in dogs and cats.
   b. Clinical investigation of the nephrotic syndrome in man has revealed that serum lipid and serum albumin concentrations often have an inverse relationship. The fact that the concentration of serum lipids in human patients with the nephrotic syndrome decreases following parenteral administration of albumin has been used as additional support for this hypothesis.

IV. Clinical Findings

A. *Marked and persistent proteinuria (albuminuria) is a consistent finding.*

B. *Edema is a consistent finding.*
1. The severity of the edema is variable.
2. Generalized, dependent, pitting, nonpainful, subcutaneous edema occurs

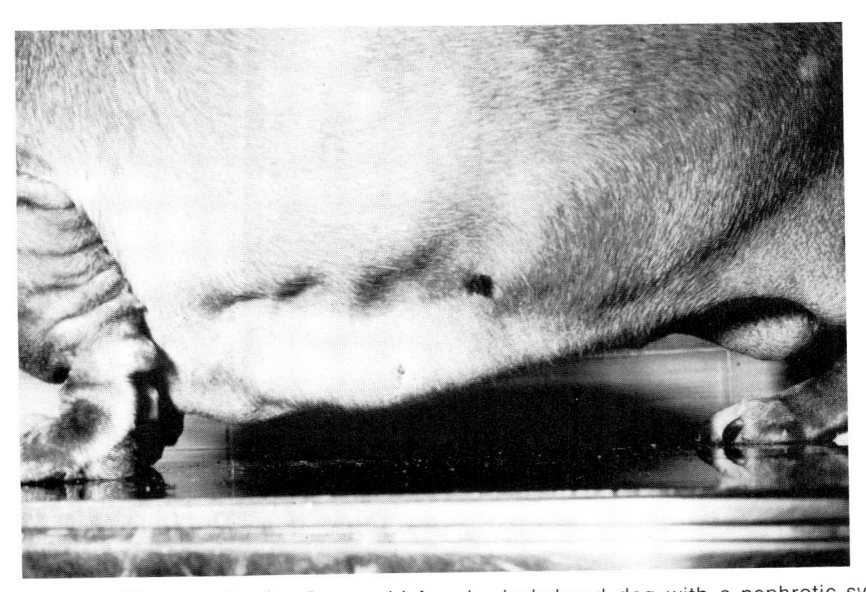

Figure 27–1. Photograph of a 5-year-old female dachshund dog with a nephrotic syndrome caused by renal amyloidosis. Edematous subcutaneous tissue has retained imprints created by digital pressure.

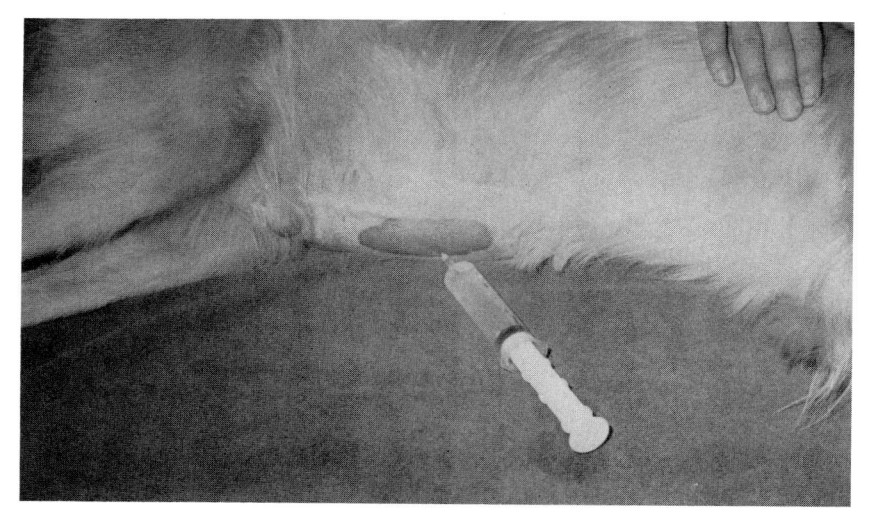

Figure 27–2. Transudative ascites in a 1.5-year-old male golden retriever dog with a nephrotic syndrome caused by membranous glomerulonephritis (see Fig. 25–3). The dog was losing approximately 17.5 grams of protein in the urine each 24 hours.

initially (Fig. 27–1). It may be associated with ascites or hydrothorax, or both, in severe cases (Fig. 27–2).

C. *Serum proteins*
1. Hypoalbuminemia is a consistent finding.
2. Serum globulin concentrations are variable. They may be normal, increased, or decreased.
3. Total serum protein concentration is variable, being dependent on the concentrations of albumin and globulin. Generally, the serum concentration of protein in patients with clinical evidence of the nephrotic syndrome is abnormally decreased.

D. *Hypercholesterolemia is a consistent finding.*

E. *Signs referable to the underlying renal disease*
1. Signs related to renal failure may occur as a result of progressive destruction of nephrons.
2. Chronic diseases characterized by suppuration, necrosis, or malignant neoplasia may be found in nephrotic dogs with renal amyloidosis.

V. Diagnosis

A. *A diagnosis of the nephrotic syndrome may be established on the basis of clinical findings and laboratory data.*

However, since the nephrotic syndrome may be caused by more than one disease entity, such a diagnosis lacks specificity.

B. *The nephrotic syndrome must be differentiated from other causes of hypoproteinemia and edema (e.g., malabsorption syndrome).*

C. *Renal biopsies must be employed in order to determine the specific renal disease which is responsible for the nephrotic syndrome.*

VI. Treatment

A. *Specific treatment of the nephrotic syndrome must be based on a specific diagnosis, and should be directed toward elimination or modification of the underlying glomerular lesion.*
   1. Corticosteroids are of proved benefit in causing remission of clinical signs in human patients with the nephrotic syndrome caused by membranous glomerulonephritis, disseminated lupus erythematosus, and selected cases of proliferative glomerulonephritis. Corticosteroids have been ineffective in treatment of human patients with the nephrotic syndrome secondary to renal amyloidosis (see Chapter 26, Renal Amyloidosis).
   2. Corticosteroids have not been employed as treatment for the nephrotic syndrome in dogs and cats in a sufficient number of clinical cases to make meaningful generalizations.
   3. Injudicious use of corticosteroids in patients with renal failure is contraindicated since they stimulate gluconeogenesis. The latter may aggravate the severity of uremic signs.

B. *In most instances, treatment of patients with the nephrotic syndrome must be directed toward elimination of edema.*
   1. Diuretics, aldosterone antagonists, serum albumin, dextrans, cation exchange resins, and high protein diets have been used with variable success in treatment of nephrotic edema in man.
   2. Daily administration of furosemide has been successfully used to control nephrotic edema in nonazotemic dogs with renal amyloidosis.

C. *Additional quantities of high quality dietary protein may be required to balance protein loss in patients with severe proteinuria (see Chapter 31, Treatment of Renal Failure).*

D. *Patients with the nephrotic syndrome caused by progressive irreversible renal diseases should receive symptomatic and supportive therapy for progressive renal insufficiency (see Chapter 31, Treatment of Renal Failure). The use of oral sodium chloride and sodium bicarbonate is often beneficial in the treatment of uremia in dogs with marked renal insufficiency, but may enhance the severity of edema in nephrotic patients. Calcium lactate may be beneficial in the treatment of acidosis of uremic patients with less danger of additional fluid retention.*

VII. Prognosis

A. *The prognosis is dependent on the biological behavior of the specific renal disease responsible for the nephrotic syndrome (see Chapter 25, Primary Diseases of Glomeruli).*

B. *Patients with renal amyloidosis should receive a guarded to poor prognosis since specific treatment is not available.*

REFERENCES

Farrow, B. R. H., Huxtable, C. R., and McGovern, V. J.: Nephrotic syndrome in the cat due to diffuse membranous glomerulonephritis. Pathology, *1*:67–72, 1969.

Osborne, C. A., Johnson, K. H., and Perman, V.: Amyloid nephrotic syndrome in the dog. J.A.V.M.A., *154*:1545–1560, 1969.

Watson, A. D. J.: The nephrotic syndrome due to renal amyloidosis in a dog. Aust. Vet. J., *47*:398–401, 1971.

Chapter 28

RENAL DISEASES ASSOCIATED WITH POLYSYSTEMIC DISEASES

Bacterial Endocarditis

I. **Definition**

   Bacterial endocarditis is an acute or subacute febrile systemic disease characterized by bacterial infection of the heart valves and endocardium and formation of vegetations (thrombi) containing many bacteria.

II. **Hearts with pre-existing congenital anomalies (patent ductus arteriosus, atrial septal defect, ventricular septal defect) or acquired lesions are predisposed to the development of bacterial endocarditis.**

III. **Vegetations may form on valve leaflets (valvular) or on the lining of the atrium or ventricles, or both (mural).**

   A. *Vegetations are composed of fibrin, platelets, cellular debris, calcium, and bacteria.*
      1. They are very friable.
      2. They may break and form emboli which escape into the general circulation.
   B. *Location*
      1. Vegetations are more common on the left side of the heart.
      2. The mitral valve is more often involved than the aortic valve.

IV. **Clinical syndrome**

   Patients with bacterial endocarditis may have any combination of the following:

   A. *Systemic infection characterized by:*
      1. Depression.
      2. Chronic, recurrent fever.
      3. Progressive weight loss.
      4. Concomitant infectious processes such as abscesses or pyorrhea.

B. *Cardiac abnormalities*
 1. Murmurs may be auscultated and are especially significant if associated with signs of systemic infection.
 2. Valvular insufficiency or stenosis may lead to varying degrees of decreased cardiac output and associated clinical manifestations.

C. *Embolic phenomena*
 1. Musculoskeletal. Embolism of the aorta, iliac, or femoral arteries may be associated with lameness, paresis, paraplegia, no femoral pulse, and cold extremities.
 2. Embolism of the myocardium may be associated with myocarditis and conduction disturbances.
 3. Embolism of the brain may be associated with CNS dysfunction.
 4. Embolism of the gastrointestinal tract may cause infarction of the intestinal wall and result in peritonitis.
 5. Although other organs such as the spleen are frequent sites of embolism, they usually are not associated with clinical signs.
 6. Kidneys (see below).

V. **Associated renal disease**

A. *The kidneys are predisposed to embolism because of their anatomy.*
 1. They receive 10 to 20 per cent of the cardiac output.
 2. They have a system of end arteries which do not have a significant collateral blood supply.

B. *The degree of renal dysfunction is variable.*
 1. It is dependent on the size and number of emboli.
  a. Embolism of the renal artery or a major branch produces total or subtotal necrosis.
  b. Smaller emboli produce small infarcts.
 2. Aseptic vs. septic emboli.
  a. Aseptic emboli produce infarcts.
  b. Septic emboli produce suppurative lesions.

C. *Renal pathology*
 1. Embolism of large and medium sized arteries typically produces conical shaped infarcts in the kidneys.
  a. The base of the infarct is usually located at the capsular surface of the cortex while the apex points toward the medulla.
  b. Recent infarcts are pale with a surrounding zone of hyperemia.
  c. Infarcts appear as depressed gray scars when they heal by progressive fibrosis.
 2. Emboli of small arterioles produce linear infarcts.
 3. Septic emboli may produce single or multiple abscesses instead of pale infarcts.
 4. Recurrent episodes of infarction are indicated by infarcts and/or abscesses or varying stages of healing.

D. *Laboratory findings*
 1. Findings in the urinalysis suggest an inflammatory lesion of the kidneys (i.e., casts, proteinuria, pyuria, and hematuria).

234 DISEASES OF THE UPPER URINARY SYSTEM

2. When infarction or infection or both are massive, abnormalities in renal function tests may be detected,
3. Leucocytosis associated with immature neutrophils (i.e., a shift to the left) and a nonregenerative anemia (anemia of infection) may be present.

VI. Diagnosis

A. *Establishment of a specific ante mortem diagnosis of bacterial endocarditis is sometimes difficult because of the polysystemic nature of the disease.*

B. *The history, physical examination, and laboratory findings provide supportive evidence.*

C. Blood culture
  1. The site of venipuncture must be aseptically prepared.
  2. Blood to be cultured should be obtained prior to antimicrobial therapy.
  3. The organisms most commonly incriminated are hemolytic and nonhemolytic streptococci, staphylococci, *Pseudomonas* and *Escherichia* spp.

VII. Treatment

A. *Antimicrobial therapy*
  1. Withhold antibiotic therapy until blood samples for culture have been obtained.
  2. Choose antibiotics on the basis of antibiotic sensitivity when possible.
  3. Administer high doses of antibiotics (see Chapter 33, Drug Therapy in Renal Failure).
  4. Because bacteria in vegetative lesions are difficult to eradicate, antibiotics should be given for prolonged periods.

B. *It may be necessary to surgically remove an embolus if a major vital blood supply is occluded.*

Surgical correction is frequently unsuccessful, however, and does not eliminate the predisposing disease process.

C. *Prophylaxis*

Use the proper dosage of antimicrobials, especially when patients with pre-existing cardiac lesions are exposed to potential bacteremias from any source such as:
  1. Surgical manipulation of an infected area.
  2. Severe dental disease.
  3. Localized infections.

Diabetes Mellitus

I. Definition

Diabetes mellitus is a syndrome characterized by polyuria, polydipsia, polyphagia, hyperglycemia, and glucosuria which occurs because of an inability of the pancreas to secrete an adequate quantity of insulin.

II. Etiology

Insufficient output of insulin by the beta cells in the islets of Langerhans of the pancreas may occur secondary to progressive chronic pancreatitis, or as a result of idiopathic alteration of the beta cells. Other factors, including diabetogenic hormones, may contribute to the development of this disease. Regardless of the initiating cause(s), the basic abnormality in diabetes mellitus is the inability of the beta cells to secrete enough insulin to satisfy the body's requirements.

III. Abnormalities of diabetes mellitus related to the urinary system

A. *The osmotic diuresis created by hyperglycemia and glucosuria results in obligatory polyuria and compensatory polydipsia.*

Although it is often stated that dogs with diabetes mellitus have a large urine output with a high specific gravity, this generality must be kept in proper perspective. The specific gravity of the urine in patients with diabetes is dependent on:
1. The volume of urine excreted. A specific gravity of 1.020 in a patient excreting a large volume of urine is high when interpreted in the light of urine volume.
2. The quantity of glucose in the urine.
3. The functional integrity of the nephrons.
4. Urine specific gravities of random urine samples obtained from diabetic patients are variable (1.015 to 1.060+) and may be in the 1.015 to 1.020 range.

B. *Diabetes mellitus is sometimes mistaken for generalized renal failure because polyuria and polydipsia are encountered in both situations.*

This error is sometimes further compounded by the frequent occurrence of azotemia in diabetic dogs. Evaluation of a complete urinalysis to confirm or eliminate the presence of glucose and acetone usually eliminates this confusion.

C. *Pathogenesis of uremia in diabetes mellitus*
1. Development of renal failure in diabetes is related to prerenal and primary renal factors.
2. Prerenal factors.
   a. Lack of renal perfusion may be associated with dehydration caused by osmotic diuresis and vomiting.
   b. Increased catabolism of body stores of protein may increase the quantity of metabolic waste to be excreted by the kidneys.
3. Renal Factors.
   a. Abnormal metabolism of lipid and carbohydrate predisposes the patient to extensive fatty degeneration of tubular epithelial cells. The degree to which fatty change in tubular cells contributes to impaired renal function has not been established.
   b. Diffuse involvement of the glomerular basement membranes (diabetic glomerulosclerosis) has been observed in some dogs with long standing (two to 10 years) experimental and spontaneous diabetes mellitus. Sufficient glomerular destruction may occur to cause secondary tubular disease (see Chapter 12, Pathophysiology of Renal Failure).
   c. Deposits of spherical, homogeneous, hyaline appearing material in

DISEASES OF THE UPPER URINARY SYSTEM

the periphery of glomerular tufts (Kimmelsteil-Wilson disease) has been observed in dogs with experimentally induced and spontaneously occurring diabetes.

IV. Clinical findings are dependent on the stage of the disease process.

  A. *Diabetes mellitus is often seen in middle aged and older female dogs.*

  B. *Signs associated with the uncomplicated form of diabetes mellitus include:*
   1. Polyuria, polydipsia, and nocturia.
   2. Polyphagia and weight loss.
   3. Sudden onset of bilateral cataracts. Cataracts have been reported to occur in approximately 10 to 15 per cent of the cases in dogs. Diabetic retinopathy, a common manifestation of diabetes in man, is apparently uncommon in dogs.
   4. Palpable enlargement of the liver. Hepatomegaly occurs as a result of excessive lipid accumulation in liver cells.

  C. *Signs associated with the complicated (acidotic) form of diabetes include:*
   1. Signs mentioned for the uncomplicated form.
   2. Anorexia, depression, and weakness.
   3. Vomiting and dehydration.

  D. *Signs referable to recurrent acute pancreatitis may be present, including fever, anorexia, depression, weakness, vomiting, and abdominal pain.*

  E. *Signs referable to pancreatic fibrosis (i.e., the end stage of recurrent pancreatitis) may be present and are referable to a deficiency of pancreatic enzymes (i.e., voluminous feces, steatorrhea, and weight loss).*

V. Laboratory Data

  A. *Uncomplicated form*
   1. Urinalysis.
      a. The specific gravity is variable (1.015 to 1.060+). The presence of glucose in large quantities causes a significant increase in the S.G. Each 0.27 Gm. of glucose per 100 ml. of urine increases the S.G. by 0.001.
      b. Glucosuria.
      c. Ketonuria.
      d. Evidence of cystitis may be detected, although the latter is not a consistent finding.
   2. Blood chemistry.
      a. Hyperglycemia.
      b. Hypercholesterolemia and hyperlipemia.
   3. There may be a decrease in the quantity of exogenous pancreatic enzymes in the feces if the patient has chronic generalized pancreatitis.

  B. *Complicated (acidotic) form*
   1. Urinalysis.
      a. Same as above.
      b. The urine pH will be acid (pH = 5.5 or less).

2. Blood chemistry.
   a. Same as above.
   b. The concentration of BUN and creatinine may be increased. The uremia associated with diabetes mellitus is usually of prerenal origin and is thus reversible if abnormalities in fluid balance are corrected. In cases of several years' duration, uremia may occur as a result of primary renal disease associated with diabetes mellitus.
   c. Blood pH and bicarbonate concentration are often decreased. The latter is a consequence of metabolic acidosis caused by abnormal accumulations of organic acids associated with fat metabolism.
   d. Increased serum amylase.
      (1) Hyperamylasemia may occur as a result of pancreatic cellular necrosis in patients with acute or recurrent pancreatitis.
      (2) Hyperamylasemia may also occur as a result of inadequate renal clearance in dogs with renal insufficiency.
3. Hemogram. Leucocytosis may occur as a result of pancreatitis, secondary bacterial infection, or the stress phenomenon. In the latter instance, the leucocytosis will be characterized by mature neutrophilia. In the first two diseases, leucocytosis is usually associated with an abnormal increase in the quantity of immature WBC.

VI. Diagnosis

A. *Characteristic history, physical findings, and pertinent laboratory data are usually sufficient to establish a diagnosis of diabetes mellitus.*

B. *Differentiation between prerenal renal failure and primary renal failure may be determined by one or more of the following:*
   1. Response to treatment.
   2. Serially performed urinalyses and renal function tests.
   3. Renal biopsy.

VII. Treatment

A. *Consult standard veterinary text books for treatment of diabetes mellitus.*

B. *See treatment of renal failure.*

VIII. Prognosis

A. *A guarded to good prognosis is usually justified for patients with uncomplicated diabetes, provided they receive appropriate therapy.*

B. *Patients with severe pancreatic disease or severe primary renal disease should receive a guarded to poor prognosis.*

REFERENCES

Bloodworth, J. M. B.: Experimental diabetic glomerulosclerosis. II. The dog. Arch. Path., 79:113–125, 1965.
Meier, H.: Diabetes mellitus in animals. A review. Diabetes, 9:485–489, 1960.
Ricketts, H. T., Petersen, E. S., Steiner, P. E., and Tupikova, N.: Spontaneous diabetes mellitus in dogs: An account of eight cases. Diabetes, 2:288–294, 1953.

Infectious Canine Hepatitis

I. Varying degrees of interstitial nephritis have been reported in dogs with experimentally induced and spontaneously occurring infectious canine hepatitis (ICH).

Recovered dogs may be one of the main reservoirs of infection as ICH virus has been found in the urine more than five months following inoculation of the virus into susceptible dogs. Characteristic basophilic intranuclear inclusions have been observed in the endothelial cells of renal vessels and glomerular capillaries, in the epithelial cells of the renal tubules and collecting ducts, in the transitional epithelium of the renal pelvis, and in inflammatory interstitial lesions. Currently there are conflicting opinions concerning the relationship of ICH virus to chronic interstitial nephritis in dogs, and meaningful generalizations cannot be made without further investigation. On the basis of currently available information, it appears that ICH does not play an important role in the development of the chronic, generalized, progressive, irreversible renal disease of dogs.

REFERENCES

Persson, F., Persson, S., and Sibalm, M.: The etiological role of hepatitis contagiosa canis (HCC) in chronic nephritis in dogs. Acta Vet. Scand., 2:137–150, 1961.

Wright, N. G.: The relationship between the virus of infectious canine hepatitis and interstitial nephritis. J. Sm. Anim. Pract., 8:67–70, 1967.

Wright, N. G.: Interstitial nephritis in a dog associated with infectious canine hepatitis. Vet. Rec., 86:92–93, 1970.

Leptospirosis

I. Etiology

   A. *Canine leptospirosis is a polysystemic disease usually caused by* Leptospira canicola *or* L. icterohemorrhagiae.

   B. *Many other serotypes of leptospiras exist, however, and infections with some of these have also been reported in the dog.*

   C. *Leptospirosis in the cat is not commonly encountered.*

II. History

   A. *Clinical signs may be very mild or very severe.*

   Subclinical and mild forms of the disease are common. Peracute and subacute forms have been described. Infections due to *L. canicola* and *L. icterohemorrhagiae* can only be distinguished by serological means. Clinical signs and laboratory findings are similar for both organisms.

   B. *Owners may observe any combination of the following:*
   1. Vomiting.
   2. Diarrhea, often bloody.
   3. Anorexia.
   4. Weight loss.
   5. Depression.

6. Coughing.
7. Nasal discharge, sometimes bile stained or sanguineous.
8. Dark-colored urine.

III. Physical examination

A. *Fever (103 to 106° F.) is sometimes present, but it may be transient.*

B. *Jaundice may be present.*

C. *Tonsillitis frequently occurs.*

D. *Hemorrhage may be observed in mucous membranes, in the feces, in the sclera, or in the anterior chamber of the eye.*

E. *Marked dehydration may occur.*

F. *Scleral injection is common.*

G. *Secondary pneumonia may occur.*

H. *Intussusceptions may be detected by abdominal palpation.*

IV. Laboratory findings

A. *Hemogram*
   1. Blood loss may be reflected by an abnormally low PCV and Hb. concentration.
   2. WBC.
      a. Early in the course of the disease, a leucopenia often exists.
      b. Later in the course of the disease, a leucocytosis develops.

B. *Urinalysis*
   1. Proteinuria is usually present.
   2. Bilirubinuria may be present.
   3. The specific gravity usually is in the normal range.
   4. Microscopic examination of urine sediment may reveal:
      a. An increased number of WBC and RBC.
      b. Abnormal number of casts.

C. *Blood chemistry values*
   1. The concentration of BUN and creatinine are dependent on the severity of renal damage. They may be normal or markedly elevated.
   2. Evaluation of serum electrolytes usually reveals changes typical of renal disease (see Chapter 6, Laboratory Findings in Diseases of the Urinary System).

D. *Tests of liver function (SGPT, alkaline phosphatase, serum bilirubin, sulfobromophthalein excretion) may indicate the presence of liver damage.*

E. *Microscopic agglutination test*
   1. Samples of serum should be obtained during the acute phase of the disease and during convalescence.
   2. A fourfold increase in titer in the convalescent sample provides strong evidence of leptospiral infection.

V. Renal alterations during leptospiral infection

A. The pathogenesis of leptospirosis is poorly understood, and the mechanisms responsible for the development of renal failure have not been elucidated.

B. Morphologically, the kidneys are often swollen and appear congested. Microscopic examination of renal tissue will reveal an acute or subacute interstitial nephritis.

C. Available evidence suggests that leptospiral infection is not followed by chronic generalized nephritis and that most, if not all, cases of chronic generalized nephritis have a different etiology.

  1. Following experimental leptospiral infection of dogs, survivors regained normal renal function (as measured by glomerular filtration rate, renal plasma flow, and tubular excretion) in approximately three months. Function remained normal for periods of study up to four and one half years following the date of infection.
  2. Chronic generalized nephritis is commonly observed in areas (Sweden, North-central United States) where clinical cases of leptospirosis are rarely observed, and where serologic surveys have indicated a very low prevalence of infection.
  3. Many dogs with a significant titer against leptospirosis have normal renal function.

VI. Diagnosis

A. The history and clinical signs provide supportive diagnostic evidence.

B. Hemograms, urinalyses, and blood chemistries provide additional diagnostic evidence, and may aid in establishing a prognosis.

C. Confirmation

  1. Although isolation and identification of leptospiral organisms in blood or urine confirms the diagnosis of leptospirosis, it is technically difficult and time consuming. The use of this technique is usually limited to special laboratories.
  2. Demonstration of a fourfold increase in antibody titer between acute and convalescent samples is good evidence of leptospirosis.
  3. The diagnosis may be confirmed by identification of leptospires in tissues using silver stains. Tissues may be obtained by:
     a. Renal biopsy.
     b. Necropsy.

VII. Treatment

A. Parenteral penicillin and streptomycin therapy of at least seven days duration is recommended.

  1. Administer 50,000 I.U. of aqueous procaine penicillin per lb. of body weight once daily.
  2. Administer 7.5 mg. of streptomycin per lb. of body weight every 12 hours.

B. Supportive therapy

  1. Combat dehydration if present.
  2. Blood transfusions may be indicated if hemorrhage is severe.

VIII. Prognosis is variable.

    A. In acute disease the prognosis is fair to poor, and is dependent on:

        1. The interval between appearance of signs and initiation of treatment. To be of benefit, antibiotic therapy must be instituted early in the course of the disease.

        2. The severity of the disease in each individual case.

    B. Recovery from the acute disease warrants a good prognosis since chronic nephritis is an uncommon complication.

REFERENCES

Finco, D. R., and Low, D. G.: Water, electrolyte, and acid-base alterations in experimental canine leptospirosis. Amer. J. Vet. Res., 29:1799–1807, 1968.

Low, D. G., Hiatt, C. W., Gieiser, C. A., and Bergman, E. N.: Experimental canine leptospirosis. I. Leptospira icterohemorrhagiae infections in immature dogs. J. Inf. Dis., 98:249–259, 1956.

Low, D. G., Mather, G. W., Finco, D. R., and Anderson, N. V.: Longterm studies of renal function in canine leptospirosis. Amer. J. Vet. Res., 28:731–739, 1967.

McIntyre, W. I. M., and Montgomery, G. L.: Renal lesions in Leptospira canicola infection in dogs. J. Path. Bact., 44:145–160, 1952.

Taylor, P. L., Hanson, L. E., and Simon, J.: Serologic, pathologic, and immunologic factors of experimentally induced leptospiral nephritis in dogs. Amer. J. Vet. Res., 31:1033–1049, 1970.

Malignant Lymphoma

I. Prevalence

    A. Malignant lymphoma is the most common renal tumor of cats, but is less frequently encountered in the kidneys of dogs.

        1. Dogs with malignant lymphoma have renal involvement in less than 50 per cent of the cases.

        2. The abdominal form of malignant lymphoma in cats is usually associated with neoplasia of the kidneys.

    B. Malignant lymphoma may be encountered at any age in dogs or cats.

        1. In dogs, the disease is more prevalent after four to five years of age.

        2. In cats, the abdominal form of malignant lymphoma is more prevalent in middle-aged and old cats, whereas the mediastinal form is more prevalent in young cats.

II. Etiology

    A. Malignant lymphoma in the cat is caused by ribonucleic acid C-type leucoviruses.

    B. Although viruses have never been proved to cause malignant lymphoma in the dog, they have been incriminated.

III. Pathophysiology

    A. Unless malignant lymphoma is detected early in the course of development, it is unusual to encounter it confined to a single organ or system of the body.

    B. Generally the distribution throughout the body is different in dogs than in cats.

1. Dogs.
    a. In dogs, peripheral lymphadenopathy occurs in the majority of cases, and is frequently associated with varying degrees of neoplastic involvement of internal lymph nodes and the spleen.
    b. Although severe extranodal involvement has been encountered in dogs, it occurs less frequently and is usually less severe than in cats.
    c. Renal neoplastic lesions usually appear as discrete areas in the renal cortex.
        (1) In one study, necropsy evaluation of 26 dogs revealed neoplastic lesions in the kidneys of 12 (46 per cent) of them.
        (2) Generalized renal neoplasia with uremia occurred in only one dog.
2. Cats.
    a. In cats, viscera that are not primary lymphoid tissue often are severely affected with neoplastic lesions, but the peripheral lymph nodes are not usually enlarged.
    b. On the basis of the severity of organ or tissue involvement, this disease complex has been arbitrarily divided into two forms in cats:
        (1) The mediastinal form is characterized by neoplasia of the mediastinal lymph nodes, thymus, or both, and is usually associated with hydrothorax and clinical signs referable to respiratory disease.
        (2) The abdominal form is usually associated with neoplasia of the kidneys and intestines, although the mesenteric lymph nodes, liver, spleen, and other abdominal organs may be neoplastic.
        (3) In contrast to dogs, cats with the abdominal form of malignant lymphoma usually have severe bilateral involvement of the kidneys.

C. *Multifocal neoplastic lesions that often are not distributed in a manner suggestive of metastasis have led to the hypothesis that malignant lymphomas may be of multicentric origin.*

The distribution of lesions in some patients, however, has been interpreted to suggest that the neoplasm may spread by metastasis.

D. *In both dogs and cats, neoplastic involvement of the kidneys may be focal or diffuse.*
    1. The extent of kidney destruction varies independently of involvement of other organs and body tissues.
    2. In many cases, renal involvement is not detected until necropsy.
    3. When renal neoplasia is one of the predominant lesions of malignant lymphoma, and is not characterized by focal lesions associated with more extensive lesions elsewhere, it is usually bilateral and generalized in dogs and cats (Figs. 28–1 and 28–2).
    4. Evaluation of tissues obtained at necropsy from dogs with naturally occurring and experimentally induced malignant lymphoma has revealed that:
        a. Early lesions are often confined to the renal cortex and are especially common at the corticomedullary junction.
        b. The lesions tend to coalesce and obliterate the cortex of each kidney as the disease progresses.
        c. The renal medulla usually remains unaffected, although it may contain neoplastic lesions in advanced cases.

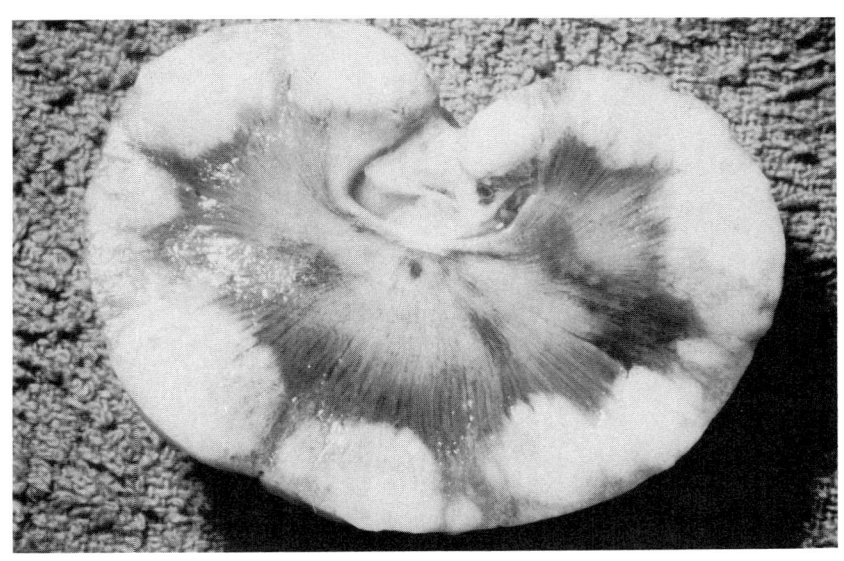

Figure 28–1. Neoplastic kidney obtained from a 14-year-old male mixed breed cat with malignant lymphoma. Multiple, large, white spherical nodules of malignant lymphocytes have replaced much of the renal parenchyma.

5. The apparent predilection of this neoplasm for the renal cortex may be related to the vascular anatomy of the kidney.
6. Microscopic examination of affected kidneys usually reveals variable degrees of neoplastic displacement, destruction, and replacement of renal parenchyma.

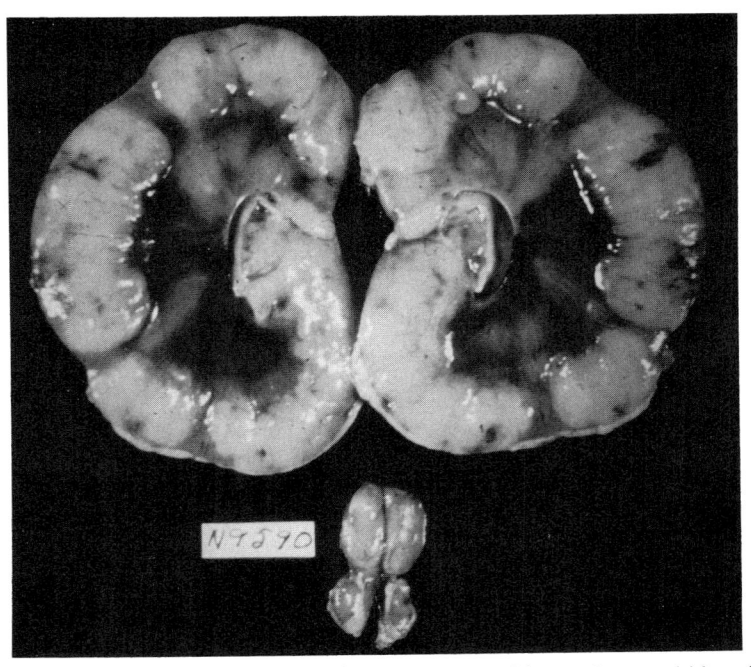

Figure 28–2. Neoplastic kidney and adrenal gland obtained from a 2-year-old female Basenji dog with malignant lymphoma. Lymphoid tissue has replaced most of the renal cortex and extended into the renal medulla. (J.A.V.M.A., *158*:2058–2070, 1971)

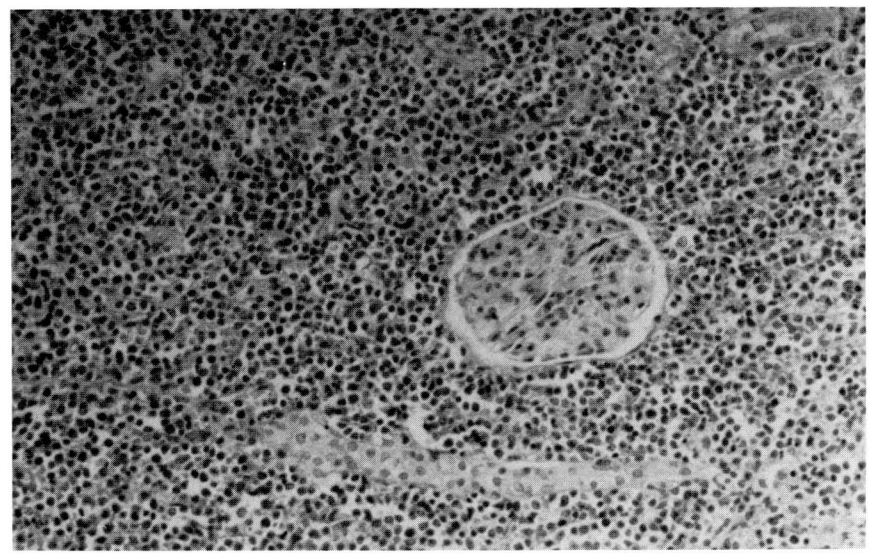

Figure 28–3. Photomicrograph of a section of the kidney described in Figure 28–2. A glomerulus, which appears morphologically normal, is surrounded by neoplastic lymphoid tissue. H&E stain; ×400. (J.A.V.M.A., *158*:2058–2070, 1971.)

    a. Because accumulations of neoplastic cells are most prominent in the interstitial tissue, it has been hypothesized that the neoplasm spreads, at least in part, by invasion along pathways of least resistance (i.e., loose connective tissue).

    b. The morphologic appearance of renal lesions suggests that the neoplasm destroys the kidneys by progressive infiltration into renal parenchyma located adjacent to the periphery of accumulations of neoplastic cells.

        (1) Progressive accumulation of neoplastic cells separates nephrons from each other.

        (2) As a result of destruction of interstitial tissue and peritubular capillaries, associated nephrons undergo progressive atrophy and necrosis.

    c. Glomeruli and blood vessels appear to be more resistant to the effects of neoplastic destruction of renal parenchyma (Fig. 28–3).

    d. Structures that are relatively dense in consistency, such as renal capsules, are usually not invaded by lymphoid cells.

IV. Clinical findings

    A. Malignant lymphomas often are associated with a wide variety of clinical manifestations that are dependent on:

        1. The site(s) of neoplasia.
        2. The extent to which normal structures have been destroyed.
        3. The duration of the disease process.
        4. The presence or absence of concomitant disease.

    B. Neoplasms at an early stage of development usually do not cause abnormalities that can be detected by physical examination.

        1. Painless enlargement of one or more peripheral lymph nodes is an early and frequently encountered clinical sign in dogs.

2. Nonspecific clinical signs such as progressive weight loss, depression, anorexia, coughing, dyspnea, vomiting, diarrhea, nonhealing wounds, and regional edema may be detected during various stages of the disease process, but are not consistent features of the disease complex.

C. *Cachexia, fever, anemia and secondary infections commonly occur during terminal phases of the disease.*

D. *Most patients with neoplastic renal lesions succumb as a result of neoplastic destruction of some other body organ or tissue before signs referable to renal disease have time to develop.*

When a sufficient number of nephrons have been incapacitated, however, signs and lesions characteristic of chronic progressive renal disease become manifest clinically (see Chapter 13, Extrarenal Manifestations of Uremia).
1. Abdominal palpation typically reveals enlarged and irregularly shaped kidneys.
2. In some cases, hydronephrosis may develop as a result of partial or total occlusion of ureters by neoplastic tissue.

E. *Because renal lymphomas usually are associated with neoplastic lesions in other organs, the intestines, mesenteric lymph nodes, liver, and spleen should be carefully palpated, and the thorax should be carefully auscultated.*

F. *Renal failure caused by bilateral lymphoma occurs more commonly in cats than in dogs.*

V. Laboratory findings

A. *As with the history and physical findings, the results of various laboratory procedures are dependent on:*
1. The organs or tissues involved with malignant lymphoma.
2. The duration and extent of neoplasia.
3. The presence or absence of concomitant renal disease.

B. *Evaluation of a hemogram may reveal:*
1. No abnormal findings.
2. Leucocytosis or leukopenia.
3. Thrombocytopenia.
4. Anemia. Anemia may occur as a result of decreased life span of RBC, myelophthisis, or decreased erythropoietin production by diseased kidneys.
5. Atypical or neoplastic lymphocytes. Examination of WBC concentrated in the buffy coat may enhance detection of abnormal cells in circulating blood.

C. *Urinalyses usually do not reveal specific diagnostic information.*
1. Signs indicative of renal disease, including hyposthenuria, proteinuria, and hematuria may be detected.
2. Depending on the nature and severity of renal pathologic changes induced by neoplastic tissue, pyuria or casts may be detected.
3. Although there have not been any reported instances of detection of malignant lymphocytes in the urine sediment of dogs or cats with renal lymphoma, the number of reported cases in which specific attempts were made to identify neoplastic cells in urine sediment have been too

few to make any valid generalizations as to the actual frequency with which they occur. In man, neoplastic cells have been infrequently encountered in urine sediment of patients with renal lymphoma although they have been reported.

D. *The results of renal function tests are not diagnostic of lymphoma, but may indicate the severity of renal parenchymal destruction by neoplastic tissue.*
   1. If both kidneys are not extensively involved, abnormalities of renal function are usually not detectable.
   2. As the quantity of functional renal tissue decreases, abnormalities referable to nephron destruction become evident (see Chapter 7, Tests of Renal Function).

E. *Evaluation of serum electrolytes is usually not of diagnostic significance but may be of value in the treatment of uremia.*

Detection of hypercalcemia and hypophosphatemia or normophosphatemia in dogs or cats with pseudohyperparathyroidism due to malignant lymphoma is a notable exception to this generality.

VI. Radiographic findings

A. *Because of the nonspecificity of radiographic changes that occur in dogs and cats with renal lymphoma, such changes must be considered in association with history, physical findings, laboratory data, and biopsy findings in order to be meaningful.*

B. *Survey radiographs and contrast urographs may reveal enlargement of one or both kidneys, abnormalities in surface contour related to localized renal masses, or loss of the ability to excrete a sufficient quantity of dye to outline the excretory pathway of the urinary system.*

C. *Detection of space-occupying lesions in other organs and tissues of the body provides supportive evidence of malignant neoplasia.*

D. *Renal osteodystrophy may be detected radiographically and is characterized by demineralization of the skeleton.*

VII. Diagnosis

A. *A tentative diagnosis of malignant lymphoma can usually be established on the basis of the history, physical findings, radiographic interpretation, and laboratory findings.*

B. *Establishment of a specific diagnosis must be based on detection of malignant cells in:*
   1. Circulating blood.
   2. Bone marrow.
   3. Biopsy specimens of affected tissues.
   4. Urine sediment.

C. *Ante-mortem confirmation of neoplastic involvement of the kidneys may be obtained by renal biopsy.*

VIII. Treatment

A. *Treatment of generalized malignant lymphoma of dogs and cats has been the subject of extensive clinical investigation.*

B. Because of the propensity of this neoplasm to affect multiple organs and tissues of the body and because many cases are at an advanced stage when they are first encountered, complete removal or destruction of neoplastic tissue with maintenance of normal structure and function of affected organs and tissues is usually not feasible.

C. Palliative treatment with immunosuppressive agents including alkylating agents, antimetabolites, corticosteroids, irradiation, or a combination of these agents may be considered for patients with inoperable neoplasms.
   1. These agents may induce varying degrees of temporary remission of clinical signs.
   2. The goal of this type of treatment should be to prolong the patient's life in such a manner as to provide a reasonable degree of comfort and activity.
   3. The use of antimetabolites and alkylating agents in human beings with renal failure has aggravated the uremic state as a result of increasing the quantity of metabolic by-products that the kidneys must excrete.

D. Symptomatic and supportive treatment of patients with progressive renal failure may be of benefit (see Chapter 31, Treatment of Renal Failure).

IX. Prognosis

A. With rare exception, the prognosis for survival of dogs and cats with malignant lymphoma is poor to grave.

B. Although the severity and rate of progression of malignant lymphomas is variable, no known regimen of therapy has been effective in curing this disease.

X. Renal failure, pseudohyperparathyroidism and malignant lymphoma

A. Dogs with lymphoma may develop pseudohyperparathyroidism characterized by renal failure.

This syndrome does not appear to be a consistent finding in every dog with lymphoma. Unlike secondary renal hyperparathyroidism which is characterized by hyperphosphatemia and varying degrees of hypocalcemia, renal failure associated with pseudohyperparathyroidism is characterized by hypercalcemia and varying degrees of hypophosphatemia. The latter is similar to phosphorus and calcium alterations associated with primary hyperparathyroidism.

B. In man, hypercalcemia has been a frequent complication of some neoplasms including renal cell carcinomas, bronchogenic carcinomas, and malignant lymphomas, even in the absence of detectable skeletal or parathyroid gland lesions.

It has been hypothesized that these neoplasms produce a parathormone-like substance, and immunologic assays of neoplastic tissue have revealed the presence of antigens that cannot be distinguished from parathormone. The marked elevation in the concentration of serum calcium causes calcium nephropathy and renal failure.

C. Affected dogs may develop signs consistent with uremia.
   1. Generalized peripheral lymphadenopathy is not usually present. The liver or spleen may be enlarged.
   2. Evaluation of renal function tests usually reveals findings consistent with renal failure.

3. Alterations in the serum concentration of calcium (increased) and phosphorus (decreased) provide strong supportive evidence of pseudohyperparathyroidism when detected in patients with renal failure.
4. Evaluation of a renal biopsy sample typically reveals findings consistent with calcium nephropathy.
5. Evaluation of a liver biopsy obtained at the same time as the kidney biopsy will often permit establishment of a diagnosis of malignant lymphoma since malignant lymphocytes may be detected in the periportal portions of the hepatic parenchyma.

D. *Signs of hypercalcemic nephropathy are sometimes so nonspecific that this condition is not suspected unless hypercalcemia is detected.*

REFERENCES

Osborne, C. A., Johnson, K. H., Kurtz, H. J., and Hanlon, G. F.: Renal lymphoma in the dog and cat. J.A.V.M.A., *158*:2058–2070, 1971.

Riggs, B. L., Arnaad, C. D., Reynolds, J. C., and Smith, L. H.: Immunologic differentiation of primary hyperparathyroidism from hyperparathyroidism due to nonparathyroid cancer. J. Clin. Invest., *50*:2079–2083, 1971.

Roof, B. S., Carpenter, B., Fink, D. J., and Gordon, G. S.: Some thoughts on the nature of ectopic parathyroid hormones. Amer. J. Med., *50*:686, 1971.

Polyarteritis Nodosa

I. Definition

Polyarteritis nodosa is a subacute or chronic recurrent vascular disease characterized by focal necrotizing inflammation of the walls of medium and small sized arteries and arterioles.

II. Etiology

The etiology of polyarteritis nodosa has not been established, but it has been hypothesized that the cause is related to an allergic or hypersensitivity reaction.

III. In man, polyarteritis nodosa is characterized by necrotizing vasculitis of small arteries and arterioles anywhere in the body.

Thrombosis is a frequent sequel to the vasculitis. The clinical signs are dependent on the organs or tissues involved, and the severity and duration of the lesions. Generally, the disease affects many body systems and is characterized by nonspecific systemic reactions including low grade fever, malaise, weakness, and leucocytosis. When the kidneys are involved, varying degrees of hematuria and albuminuria are usually observed.

IV. Polyarteritis nodosa has been reported in the kidneys of cats, but is apparently an uncommon disease in this species.

Because the diagnoses were established at necropsy, the clinical features of this disease in cats has not been well documented.

REFERENCES

Altera, K. P., and Bonash, H.: Polyarteritis nodosa in a cat. J.A.V.M.A., *149*:1307–1311, 1966.
Lucke, V. M.: Renal polyarteritis nodosa in the cat. Vet. Rec., *82*:622–624, 1968.

Pyometra

I. Definition

Pyometra is an acute or chronic suppurative disease of the uterus which is usually associated with accumulation of a large quantity of pus in the uterine lumen.

II. Pathogenesis of uterine lesions

The initial phase in the development of pyometra is related to hormonal dysfunction which causes endometrial hyperplasia. Subsequently, endometritis may develop, and bacteria may be demonstrated in the uterine contents. Bacterial invasion probably occurs at metestrus.

III. Pathogenesis of renal lesions

A. *Impairment of renal function associated with pyometra is related to:*
  1. Reduction in the ability of the kidneys to concentrate urine.
  2. Reduction in glomerular filtration.
  3. Dehydration. If the patient is dehydrated, renal function may be impaired by poor renal perfusion (prerenal uremia).

B. *The effect that each of these factors has on renal function is apparently unrelated.*

C. *Reduction in glomerular filtration rate (GFR).*
  1. Reduction in GFR is probably caused by primary lesions of glomeruli.
  2. The degree of reduction of GFR is dependent on the degree of pathological alteration of glomeruli.
  3. Glomerular changes observed with the light microscope are similar to changes seen in membranous or mixed membranous proliferative glomerulonephritis in man and experimentally induced nephrotoxic glomerulonephritis of dogs (see Glomerulonephritis, in Chapter 25). The glomerular lesions of pyometra are characterized by:
     a. Thickening of glomerular capillary walls.
     b. A moderate degree of swelling and proliferation of glomerular capillary endothelial cells.
     c. Varying degrees of periglomerular fibrosis associated with swelling and proliferation of glomerular capillary epithelium.
  4. Glomerular changes are usually accompanied by secondary changes in the proximal tubules (see Chapter 12, Pathophysiology of Renal Failure).
  5. The renal cortex is usually heavily infiltrated with plasma cells.
  6. The following observations have been used to support the hypothesis that the glomerular injury associated with pyometra may occur, at least in part, as a result of an immunological process.
     a. A morphologic similarity exists between glomerulonephritis associated with pyometra, experimentally induced nephrotoxic glo-

merulonephritis in dogs, and acute proliferative glomerulonephritis in man.
   b. Plasma cells may be observed in the renal cortex of kidneys with pyometra nephritis.
   c. Lesions in kidneys of dogs with pyometra develop in association with uterine disease, and often undergo resolution following ovariohysterectomy.
   d. A latent period occurs between the probable time of onset of pyometra and the development of significant renal lesions.

D. *Reduction in concentrating ability of the kidneys*
   1. Polydipsia is often observed in bitches with pyometra and occurs as a compensatory response to the impaired ability of the kidneys to concentrate urine.
   2. Abnormal renal function, polyuria, and polydipsia in bitches with pyometra differs from the isosthenuria associated with severe acute and chronic renal disease, in that dogs with pyometra have no impairment of the ability to dilute urine.
   3. Inability of the kidneys to concentrate urine is related to a decrease in the capacity of the distal tubules and collecting ducts to reabsorb water, and to a decrease in the concentration of sodium in the renal medulla. The specific cause of the reduced permeability of the distal tubules and collecting ducts to water, and the loss of the normal concentration of sodium in the renal medulla has not been established. They may be related to:
      a. Thickening of basement membranes at all levels of the nephron.
      b. *Escherichia coli* endotoxin absorbed from the uterus. Parenteral injection of large doses of *E. coli* endotoxin into normal dogs produced similar dysfunction which was reversible. To date, however, there is no proof that endotoxins from *E. coli* are responsible for the inability to concentrate urine associated with spontaneously occurring pyometra.

E. *Polydipsia, polyuria, and inability to concentrate urine are not related to:*
   1. Disturbances in the release of antidiuretic hormone.
   2. Endocrine dysfunctions associated with uterine lesions.
   3. Osmotic diuresis associated with destruction of the functional capacity of large numbers of nephrons.
   4. Abnormal potassium or calcium metabolism.

IV. Clinical findings

A. *History and physical findings*
   1. There is a higher incidence of pyometra in middle aged and older bitches that have not whelped in recent years.
   2. Pyometra occurs during metestrus.
   3. A purulent vaginal discharge of varying degrees of severity may be seen if the cervix is open.
   4. Progressive abdominal enlargement may be observed.
   5. An enlarged and abnormal uterus can often be palpated.
   6. Lethargy, depression, anorexia, and weight loss may be observed in severe cases.

7. Temperature is usually normal, but on occasion it may be subnormal, or slightly elevated.
8. Dehydration may be present.
9. Vomition may be observed, especially in uremic patients.
10. Pallor of mucous membranes may be present in anemic patients, but is not a consistent clinical finding.

B. *Laboratory findings*
1. Hemogram.
   a. A marked leucocytosis (20,000 to 100,000 or more WBC per cmm.) with immature neutrophils is a characteristic finding.
   b. A nonregenerative anemia may be present, but is not a consistent finding.
2. Urinalyses (when not contaminated with vaginal or uterine exudate) are usually characterized by:
   a. Low specific gravity (1.001 to 1.006).
   b. Mild to moderate proteinuria.
   c. Mild hematuria.
3. An increase in BUN or creatinine concentration may be detected by routine laboratory methods when glomerular filtration rate is less than 25 to 30 per cent of normal.
4. An increase in serum amylase may be seen in uremic dogs.
5. An elevation in the serum cholesterol concentration often occurs in dogs with pyometra and associated renal diseases.
6. Hyperproteinemia.
   a. A normal to low serum albumin concentration is often present.
   b. Elevated serum globulin concentrations often occur.

V. Diagnosis

A. *The history, physical findings, and pertinent laboratory data provide supportive diagnostic evidence.*

B. *Radiography usually confirms the presence of an abnormally enlarged uterus.*

C. *Typical laboratory data provide supportive evidence.*

D. *Exploratory laparotomy and visual examination of the uterus will confirm the diagnosis in most instances.*

E. *Carefully palpate the kidneys at the time of laparotomy to evaluate the presence or absence of significant concurrent renal disease.*
   1. The glomerular and tubular lesions of pyometra may be reversible provided the source of infection is eliminated.
   2. Dogs with chronic renal disease due to other causes, which develop renal lesions associated with pyometra, may develop a uremic crisis which is unresponsive to treatment.
   3. It may be advisable to perform a needle biopsy of the kidney(s) in some instances in order to eliminate or establish the presence of concurrent generalized renal disease unrelated to the renal lesions of pyometra. Such information may be of diagnostic, prognostic, and therapeutic significance.

VI. Treatment

A. Nonuremic dogs

1. Ovariohysterectomy is the treatment of choice.
2. Renal function should be evaluated prior to and immediately following surgery so that if renal failure develops it can be recognized and treated early in the course of development.

B. Azotemic or uremic dogs

1. Perform osmotic diuresis at the time of surgery and continue this therapy following surgery for as long as is necessary.
2. If osmotic diuresis is unsuccessful, furosemide or ethacrynic acid should be considered.
3. If the above are unsuccessful, peritoneal dialysis should be considered.
4. See treatment of renal failure.

C. Most patients regain the ability to concentrate urine following ovariohysterectomy.

VII. Prognosis

A. For dogs without evidence of glomerular disease, a guarded to good prognosis is justified, provided the patient is an acceptable surgical risk, and ovariohysterectomy is performed.

B. For dogs with evidence of glomerular disease caused by pyometra, the prognosis is variable.

Since the glomerular and tubular lesions which occur in association with pyometra are often reversible, a guarded to good prognosis is justified if the dog is an acceptable surgical risk, ovariohysterectomy is performed, and the patient responds to treatment of renal failure. Dogs which do not respond to osmotic diuresis (or other suitable treatment for uremia) should receive a poor prognosis.

C. For dogs with pyometra and associated renal lesions, and concomitant generalized renal disease, the prognosis is dependent on the severity and biological behavior of the concomitant renal disease in addition to the factors mentioned above.

Generally, the prognosis in such patients is guarded to poor.

REFERENCES

Asheim, A.: Renal function in dogs with pyometra. 1. Studies of the hypothalamic-neurohypophyseal system. Acta Vet. Scand., 4:281–291, 1963.

Asheim, A.: Renal function in dogs with pyometra. 2. Concentrating and diluting ability. Acta Vet. Scand., 4:293–306, 1963.

Asheim, A.: Renal function in dogs with pyometra. 3. Glomerular filtration rate, effective renal plasma flow and the relation between solute excretion rate and maximum urine osmolarity during dehydration. Acta Vet. Scand., 5:56–73, 1964.

Asheim, A.: Renal function in dogs with pyometra. 4. Maximum concentrating capacity during osmotic diuresis. Acta Vet. Scand., 5:74–87, 1964.

Asheim, A.: Renal function in dogs with pyometra. 5. Sodium content of the renal medulla in relation to concentrating ability. Acta Vet. Scand., 5:88–98, 1964.

Asheim, A.: Renal function in dogs with pyometra. 6. Sodium excretion during osmotic diuresis and its relation to the renal dysfunction. Acta Vet. Scand., 5:99–114, 1964.

Asheim, A.: Renal function in dogs with pyometra. 7. Calcium and potassium levels in dogs with pyometra and polyuria. Acta Vet. Scand., 5:115–127, 1964.

Asheim, A.: Renal function in dogs with pyometra. 8. Uterine infection and the pathogenesis of the renal dysfunction. Acta Path. Microbiol. Scand., 60:99–107, 1964.
Asheim, A.: Comparative pathophysiological aspects of the glomerulonephritis associated with pyometra in dogs. Acta Vet. Scand., 5:188–207, 1964.
Asheim, A.: Pathogenesis of renal damage and polydipsia in dogs with pyometra. J.A.V.M.A., 147:736–745, 1965.
Dicker, S. E.: Polydipsia in relation to pyometra. J. Sm. Anim. Pract., 10:479–489, 1969.
Lewis, R. M., Schwartz, R., and Henry, W. B.: Canine systemic lupus erythematosus. Blood, 25:143–160, 1965.
Low, D. G.: Pyometra in the bitch. Vet. Med., 49:527–530, Dec., 1954.
Marcato, P. S., and Sjaban, M.: Histopathology of the kidney in dogs with pyometra. Att: Soc. Ital. Sci. Vet., 21:650–655, 1967.
Obel, A. L., Nicander, L., and Asheim, A.: Light and electron microscopical studies on the renal lesions in dogs with pyometra. Acta Vet. Scand., 5:146–178, 1964.

Systemic Lupus Erythematosus

I. Definition

Systemic lupus erythematosus (SLE) is an acute or subacute polysystemic disease which may be caused by autoimmunization. It is characterized by the presence of lesions in many body organs and tissues. In dogs, it is often associated with autoimmune hemolytic anemia, thrombocytopenia, and membranous glomerulonephritis.

II. SLE has been reported in many breeds of dogs including German shepherds, poodles, cocker spaniels, wire haired fox terriers, and mixed breeds.

III. Diffuse membranous glomerulonephritis was reported in a cat in which LE cells were demonstrated in peripheral blood.

IV. Clinical findings

Any one of the following may be observed in dogs with SLE.

A. *Regenerative hemolytic anemia (reticulocytosis, normoblastosis, spherocytosis).*

B. *Thrombocytopenia and hemorrhage.*

C. *Positive direct Coomb's test.*

D. *Positive LE test.*

E. *Icterus.*

F. *Proteinuria.*

G. *Bilirubinuria.*

V. Associated renal disease

A. *Dogs with SLE frequently have focal or generalized membranous glomerulonephritis which is characterized by:*
   1. Thickening and hyalinization of the glomerular capillaries and Bowman's capsule.
   2. Acidophilic thickening of the basement membranes of the glomerular capillaries (wire loop lesions).
   3. Plasma cell accumulation in injured tissue.

254 DISEASES OF THE UPPER URINARY SYSTEM

    B. *These renal lesions are responsible for:*
        1. Slight to heavy proteinuria.
        2. Renal failure in severe cases.

VI. Diagnosis

    A. *Typical clinical and laboratory findings usually permit establishment of a specific diagnosis.*

    B. *The presence of glomerulonephritis may be suspected if persistent proteinuria occurs, but such a diagnosis may only be conclusively established ante-mortem by renal biopsy.*

VII. Treatment

    A. *The hemolytic anemia often responds to large doses of corticosteroids (1 to 10 mg. of dexamethasone per day, depending on size of patient).*
       Relapses are common.

    B. *The membranous glomerulonephritis is reportedly unresponsive to steroid therapy.*
       Further investigation is required before meaningful generalizations can be made.

VIII. Prognosis

Because of the unpredictability of the biological behavior of systemic lupus erythematosus in each patient, a guarded prognosis is justified.

REFERENCES

Lewis, R. M., Schwartz, R., and Henry, W. B.: Canine systemic lupus erythematosus. Blood., *25*:143–160, 1965.
Slauson, D. O., Russell, S. W., and Schecter, R. D.: Naturally occurring immune complex glomerulonephritis in the cat. J. Path., *103*:131–133, 1971.

Systemic Mycoses

I. The kidneys of dogs and cats are sporadically affected with granulomatous inflammatory lesions caused by histoplasmosis, blastomycosis, cryptococcosis, coccidioidomycosis, and mucormycosis.

Depending on the degree of destruction of the renal parenchyma, varying degrees of renal insufficiency may occur. In general, clinical signs related to involvement of other body systems and organs are also present and often overshadow signs related to renal disease (see standard veterinary texts for more detailed information about each mycotic disease).

Chapter 29

NEOPLASMS OF THE KIDNEY

I. **Benign renal tumors**

   A. *Benign renal tumors have been less commonly reported than malignant renal tumors.*

   B. *They are usually incidental necropsy findings and are not of clinical significance.*

   C. *Neoplasia of any tissue component is possible.*

   1. Adenomas:
      a. Are rare.
      b. Occur in the renal cortex.
      c. May be single or multiple.
      d. Are usually of small size (2 cm. in diameter or less).
   2. Lipomas are uncommon. When encountered, they usually have been subcapsular in location.
   3. Other benign tumors which could potentially occur include:
      a. Fibromas.
      b. Leiomyomas.
      c. Angiomas.
      d. Chondromas.
      e. Myxomas.
      f. Osteomas.
   4. Papillomas of the renal pelvis:
      a. Are uncommon.
      b. May occlude the ureter and result in hydronephrosis. (See Chapter 41, Neoplasms of the Urinary Bladder).

II. **Primary malignant renal tumors**

   A. *Neoplasia of any tissue component is possible.*

   1. Renal carcinoma (hypernephroma, clear cell carcinoma, malignant nephroma).
      a. The incidence of this neoplasm increases as age advances.
      b. Renal carcinomas are the most common primary malignant kidney tumors in dogs and cats.
      c. They originate from tubular epithelium, not adrenal rests.
      d. Their size is variable, ranging from microscopic dimensions to two or three times the normal size of the kidney.
      e. They are often located at one pole of the kidney and are usually well demarcated from adjacent compressed renal parenchyma (Fig. 29–1).
      f. They are often yellow, white, or gray in color.

256 DISEASES OF THE UPPER URINARY SYSTEM

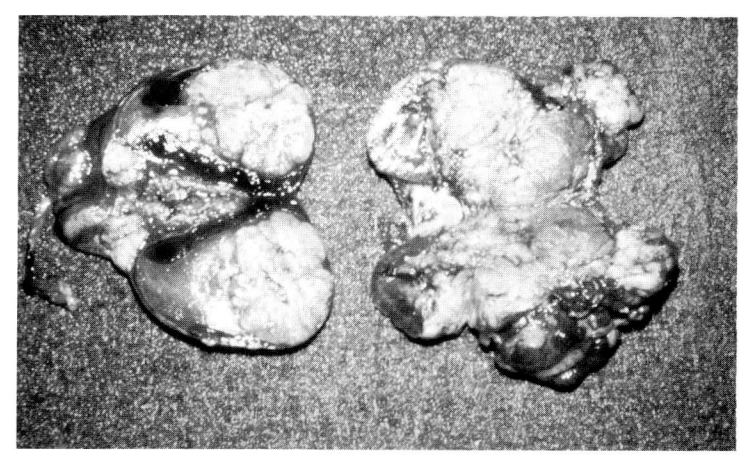

Figure 29–1. Neoplastic kidneys obtained from a 5-year-old male German shepherd dog. The only abnormalities noted by the owner were persistent hematuria and mild anorexia. Abdominal palpation revealed the presence of enlarged and asymmetrical kidneys. Evaluation of survey radiographs of the chest revealed findings consistent with metastatic neoplasia. Laboratory evaluation of the dog's renal functional capacity revealed no abnormalities. A diagnosis of renal cell carcinoma was established on the basis of microscopic examination of a renal biopsy sample.

    g. The microscopic appearance of neoplastic tubular cells is variable.
       (1) Some appear as small, dark, granular cells.
       (2) Others are characterized by the presence of cytoplasm which has a clear, homogeneous appearance. Detection of such cells in any

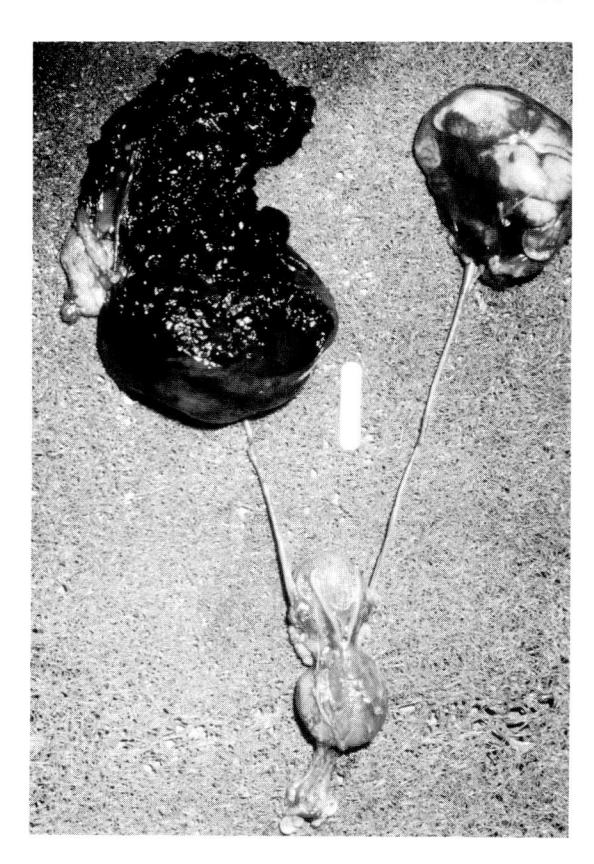

Figure 29–2. Bilateral renal cell carcinoma in the kidneys of a 10-year-old black Labrador retriever. The left kidney has ruptured. Metastatic lesions were found in the adrenal glands, lungs, liver, lymph nodes, prostate gland, and heart.

NEOPLASMS OF THE KIDNEY

part of the body is pathognomonic for renal cell carcinoma. Neoplasms containing this type of cell are commonly called clear cell carcinomas.
    (3) All variations of cytologic patterns of growth may be present in the same tumor.
  h. Renal cell carcinomas frequently metastasize.
    (1) They may metastasize prior to giving rise to any signs associated with the urinary system.
    (2) They may metastasize by direct extension, blood, or lymphatic channels. Metastatic lesions are often found in the opposite kidney, lungs, liver, and adrenals (Fig. 29-2). The bones and brain are less commonly affected with metastatic lesions.
  i. The clinical findings associated with renal cell carcinomas are not pathognomonic.
    (1) Persistent gross or microscopic, asymptomatic hematuria is a frequent finding.
    (2) If the tumor is of sufficient size, it may be palpated as an abnormality of the surface contour of the involved kidney(s).
    (3) If a sufficient quantity of renal parenchyma is destroyed, signs related to progressive renal insufficiency may be detected.
    (4) In advanced stages, anorexia, weakness and weight loss commonly occur.
    (5) Clinical signs may be related to metastatic lesions.
2. Nephroblastomas (Wilms' tumor, embryonic nephroma, adenosarcoma, congenital mixed tumor):
  a. Occur most frequently in young animals.
  b. Are derived from vestigial embryonic tissue which has persisted and retained its primitive characteristics.
  c. Have a variable size (microscopic to very large).
  d. Are usually unilateral, but may be bilateral.
  e. Have a variable microscopic appearance.
    (1) Some are primarily carcinomatous, some are primarily sarcomatous, and others have both types of neoplastic elements.
    (2) Tubule-like structures, fibrous tissue, fat, blood vessels, smooth and striated muscle, cartilage, and bone in varying degrees of differentiation may be observed.
  f. Frequently metastasize via blood and lymphatic channels to the liver, lungs, and regional lymph nodes.
  g. Are not associated with pathognomonic clinical findings.
    (1) They are usually encountered in young animals.
    (2) Clinical findings are similar to those observed in association with renal carcinomas.
    (3) Urinalyses may be normal since the renal collecting system may not be invaded by neoplastic tissue.
3. Other primary malignant tumors which could potentially occur in kidneys include:
  a. Fibrosarcomas.
  b. Liposarcomas.
  c. Myxosarcomas.
  d. Leiomyosarcomas.
  e. Rhabdomyosarcomas.

258   DISEASES OF THE UPPER URINARY SYSTEM

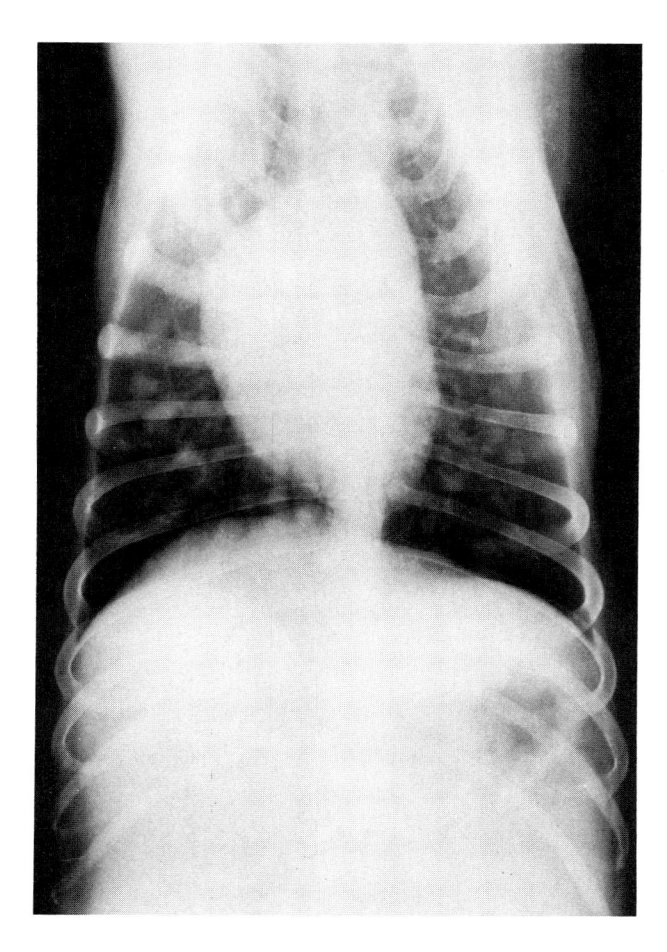

Figure 29-3. Survey radiograph of the ventrodorsal aspect of the chest of the dog described in Figure 29-1. Multiple focal areas of opacity are present in the lungs. Microscopic examination of these lesions revealed the presence of a metastatic renal cell carcinoma. (Courtesy of Dr. G. F. Hanlon, College of Veterinary Medicine, University of Minnesota.)

    4. Transitional cell carcinomas of the renal pelvis:
       a. Are much less common than the same type of tumor in the urinary bladder. They are rare in dogs and cats.
       b. May invade the kidney or ureter, or metastasize.
       c. May become clinically apparent in a relatively short period of time because of their location within the renal pelvis. They may cause secondary hydronephrosis before becoming very large.
       d. See Chapter 41, Neoplasms of the Urinary Bladder.
    5. Tumors of ureters are rarely encountered (see Chapter 35, Diseases of the Ureter, and Chapter 41, Neoplasms of the Urinary Bladder).

B. *Diagnosis of primary renal tumors*

    1. History, physical examination, and pertinent laboratory data provide supportive diagnostic evidence.
    2. Radiologic evidence of metastatic lesions provides supportive diagnostic evidence (Fig. 29-3).
    3. Polycythemia may be detected if the neoplastic tissue produces excessive quantities of erythropoietin.
       a. Two cases of polycythemia (PCV = 74 vol. % and 73 vol. %) have been diagnosed in dogs with renal carcinomas.*

---

*Scott, R. C., and Greene, R. W.: Personal communication, 1971. The Animal Medical Center, 510 East 62nd Street, New York, N.Y. 10021.

b. In one dog with a unilateral renal cell carcinoma of the left kidney, nephrectomy was followed by remission of the polycythemia (PCV = 48 vol. %).
4. Percutaneous renal biopsy.
   a. Histopathologic identification is the only method by which a definitive diagnosis may be established.
   b. Needle biopsy may be inadvisable if surgical extirpation is contemplated, since damage caused by the biopsy needle may induce metastasis.
5. Neoplastic cells that originate from renal tumors may be observed in urine sediment. This feature, however, is apparently uncommon.
6. Exploratory laparotomy followed by nephrectomy, needle biopsy, or surgical wedge biopsy may also be employed to establish a definitive diagnosis.

C. *Treatment*
1. Nephrectomy and ureterectomy is justified if the neoplasm has not metastasized and the opposite kidney has adequate function.
2. Palliative therapy may be used if the tumor has metastasized.
   a. Irradiation or chemotherapy, or both may be considered.
   b. See Chapter 31, Treatment of Renal Failure.

III. Metastatic tumors of the kidney

A. *The kidneys are commonly affected with metastatic neoplasms.*

This may be related, at least in part, to the large blood volume that the kidneys receive, and to their abundant supply of capillaries.

B. *Malignant lymphomas often affect the kidneys and are usually associated with neoplastic involvement of many body systems (see Malignant Lymphoma in Chapter 28).*

C. *Metastatic neoplasms may involve one or both kidneys.*

D. *The patient usually succumbs as a result of the primary neoplasm or as a result of other metastatic lesions, before signs referable to renal disease have a chance to develop.*

Malignant lymphomas are sometimes an exception to this generality.

E. *The presence of metastatic renal neoplasms is often difficult to establish ante mortem.*
1. Focal accumulations of malignant cells in the kidneys are not usually associated with clinical signs of renal disease.
2. When generalized bilateral renal involvement occurs, the clinical findings referable to the kidneys are similar to those associated with primary neoplasms of the kidney.
3. Recognition usually requires microscopic examination of renal tissue since gross changes are often inconstant and inconspicuous.

REFERENCES

Archibald, J., Putnam, R. W., and Sumner-Smith, G.: Partial nephrectomy—a technique. J. Sm. Anim. Pract., *10*:415–417, 1969.

Barron, C. N.: Spontaneous diseases in animals. *In* The Kidney. Edited by F. K. Mostofi and D. E. Smith. Baltimore, Md., The Williams and Wilkins Co., 1966.

Boyland, E.: Causes of cancer of the kidney. *In* Renal Neoplasia. Edited by J. S. King. Boston, Mass., Little Brown & Co., 1967.

Coleman, G. L., Gralla, E. J., Knirsh, A. K., and Stebbins, R. B.: Canine embryonal nephroma. A case report. Amer. J. Vet. Res., *31*:1315–1320, 1970.

Habermann, R. T., and Williams, F. P.: Papillary cystic adenocarcinoma of a kidney in a dog. J.A.V.M.A., *142*:1011–1014, 1963.

Jabara, A. G.: Three cases of primary malignant neoplasms arising in the canine urinary system. J. Comp. Path., *78*:335–339, 1968.

Jones, T. L.: Embryonal nephroma in a dog. Canad. J. Comp. Med., *16*:153–159, 1952.

Medway, W., and Nielsen, S. W.: Embryonal nephroma in a puppy. North Amer. Vet., *35*:920–923, 1954.

Moulton, J. E.: Tumors in Domestic Animals. Los Angeles, Calif., Univ. of Calif. Press, 1961.

Nielsen, S. W., and Archibald, J.: Canine renal disorders. III. Renal carcinoma in 3 dogs. No. Amer. Vet., *36*:36–40, 1955.

Osborne, C. A., Johnson, K. H., Kurtz, H. J., and Hanlon, G. F.: Renal lymphoma in the dog and cat. J.A.V.M.A., *158*:2058–2070 1971.

Osborne, C. A., Quast, J. F., Barnes, D. M., and Fitz, C. R.: Feline renal pelvic carcinoma. J.A.V.M.A., *159*:1238–1241, 1971.

Potkay, S., and Garman, R.: Nephroblastoma in a cat: The effects of nephrectomy and occlusion of the caudal vena cava. J. Sm. Anim. Pract., *10*:345–349, 1969.

Savage, A., and Isa, J. M.: Embryonal nephroma with metastasis in the dog. J.A.V.M.A., *124*:185, 1953.

Yang, Y. H.: The multicentric renal adenocarcinomas in situ of a dog. Pathol. Microbiol., *29*:181–185, 1966.

Zaruba, K.: Effect of local irradiation of the kidneys on the renal function of the dog. Radiat. Res., *35*:661–667, 1968.

Chapter 30
PROGNOSIS OF RENAL FAILURE

I. Definition

   A. *Prognosis of renal failure may be categorized as:*
      1. Prognosis concerning immediate survival (short-term prognosis).
      2. Prognosis concerning both relief of signs and elimination or resolution of the underlying morphologic and functional abnormalities (long-term prognosis).

   B. *Terminology*
      1. A guarded prognosis indicates that the chances of recovery are unpredictable.
      2. A fair, good, or excellent prognosis indicates that recovery is probable.
      3. A poor or grave prognosis indicates that recovery is improbable or hopeless.

II. Basis for prognosis

Prognosis of renal failure should not be based on a single observation or on a single laboratory determination performed on a patient. It should be based on a comprehensive consideration of history, physical examination, laboratory data, and frequently, renal biopsy findings. Prognosis should be formulated on the basis of the following questions:

   A. *What is the etiopathogenesis of the renal failure?*

   B. *What is the degree of renal dysfunction?*

   C. *What is the potential for reversibility of the lesions, and for improvement in renal function?*

III. Etiopathogenesis of renal failure

   A. *Prerenal and postrenal renal failure*
      1. Knowledge concerning the anatomic site of the renal failure is valuable, since early correction of prerenal and postrenal failure will prevent the development of significant kidney damage. Complete recovery from renal failure can then be expected (see Chapter 12, Pathophysiology of Renal Failure, and Chapter 2, Applied Physiology of the Urinary System).
      2. Numerous causes of prerenal and postrenal failure exist: the prognosis of the primary underlying disease is dependent on knowledge of the clinical characteristics of that disease. The overall prognosis should be based on the biological behavior of the primary disease, unless secondary damage to renal parenchyma has occurred.

3. Diagnosis of postrenal uremia can usually be made on the basis of history, physical examination, and special techniques which demonstrate either obstruction of urine outflow or rupture of a part of the urinary system with retention of urine in the body.
4. Prerenal uremia frequently can be suspected on the basis of history, physical examination, and laboratory aids which allow diagnosis of the causative disease. Difficulty in assessing renal blood flow by common diagnostic techniques may make confirmation of prerenal uremia more difficult. Renal biopsy frequently, but not invariably, is of value in differentiating between prerenal and primary renal uremia.

B. *Primary renal failure*
1. Prognosis of primary renal uremia is variable. A prognosis should not be made knowing only that failure is due to primary renal disease.
2. Knowledge of the action of a specific microbial or chemical agent provides the clinician with information that can be of value in prognosis.
3. For example:
   a. It is established that leptospiral serotypes cause an acute interstitial nephritis that does not progress to a chronic form. This knowledge makes it possible to give a good long-term prognosis for the disease, although the short-term prognosis is poor to fair, depending on the severity of the disease.
   b. Renal amyloidosis is a progressive, ultimately fatal disease. Knowledge that a patient has renal amyloidosis usually dictates a poor long-term prognosis, although the short-term prognosis may be good.

IV. Degree of renal dysfunction

A. *The degree of renal dysfunction can be estimated by certain common laboratory aids (see Chapter 7, Tests of Renal Function [BUN, serum creatinine, creatinine clearance, phenolsulfonphthalein excretion, water deprivation test]).*

B. *Renal function tests in which endogenous blood metabolites (i.e., creatinine, BUN) are evaluated do not always indicate the degree of renal dysfunction at the time the tests are performed because a variable period of time must elapse before a sufficient quantity of metabolites accumulate to be considered abnormal.*

For example, acute renal shutdown will not be associated with an abnormal increase in the concentration of BUN during very early stages of the disease. Serial determinations of the blood concentration of these metabolites provide more reliable information concerning the magnitude of dysfunction since the variable of elapsed time is minimized.

C. *Tests which measure a functional capacity of the kidney during a short period of time (20 minute phenolsulfonphthalein excretion, 20 minute creatinine clearance, water deprivation test) provide information that can be directly related to function at the time of the test.*

D. *Whereas estimation of the degree of renal dysfunction is valuable as one of several tools with which to formulate prognosis, it cannot be utilized as the only tool.*
1. Knowledge of the functional state of the kidneys provides no information concerning the etiology of the disease.
2. Knowledge of the functional state of the kidneys provides no information

concerning the potential reversibility of the morphologic lesions and functional insufficiency of the kidneys.
3. Methods of intensive supportive and symptomatic treatment make it possible to sustain life for short periods of time despite the presence of severe renal dysfunction. Because short-term prognosis is improved, long-term prognosis assumes more importance in formulating the overall prognosis. Long-term prognosis is more dependent on knowledge of the etiology and morphologic status of the kidney than it is on one assessment of renal function.

E. *Basing prognosis solely on a single determination of the blood concentration of a metabolite (BUN, creatinine, NPN) or on any other single function test (PSP, water deprivation test, creatinine clearance) has no logical or theoretical basis, and has been proved inadequate and unreliable in veterinary urologic practice.*

F. *Serial determinations of renal function may provide more valuable information since renal compensatory and regenerative processes, and response to therapy can be judged by comparison of results of function tests performed at different times.*

V. Potential for reversibility of renal lesions and improvement in renal function

A. *Reversibility of renal disease is dependent on the extent and severity of lesions, and on the rapidity and efficacy in eliminating the cause of the disease (see Chapter 12, Pathophysiology of Renal Failure).*

B. *In general, potential exists for reversibility of kidney lesions and improvement in kidney function in patients with acute primary renal failure.*

In acute disease, compensatory mechanisms have not been expended, and parenchymal regeneration has not had an opportunity to occur. The likelihood of regeneration is dependent on the severity of the lesions (see Chapter 12, Pathophysiology of Renal Failure).

C. *In general, the potential for reversibility of lesions present in chronic renal failure is poor since compensatory mechanisms have been exhausted, and since parenchymal regeneration has had an opportunity to occur.*

The fact that signs of renal dysfunction are present emphasizes the inadequacy of compensatory and regenerative efforts. Irreversibility of lesions of chronic renal disease, however, is not synonymous with irreversibility of signs of renal failure. Since extrarenal factors may contribute to the development of signs of uremia, correction of these factors may allow the patient to live a comfortable existence for months or years, despite the presence of renal disease (see Chapter 31, Treatment of Renal Failure).

D. *Differentiation of chronic from acute renal failure*
  1. History.
     a. The duration of clinical signs may aid in differentiating acute from chronic renal failure.
        (1) Acute onset of signs (days) is suggestive of acute renal failure.
        (2) Unfortunately the onset of uremic crises associated with chronic renal failure may be abrupt, and may be difficult to differentiate from the onset of acute renal failure.
        (3) Observation of polydipsia and polyuria for several months, com-

bined with evidence that renal disease is the etiology of the polyuria, is indicative of chronic renal disease.
  b. Known contact with nephrotoxic agents or contagious diseases may aid in differentiating acute from chronic renal disease.
2. Physical examination.
  a. Signs of uremia consistent with both acute and chronic renal failure include:
    (1) Depression.
    (2) Anorexia.
    (3) Vomiting.
    (4) Diarrhea.
    (5) Polydipsia.
    (6) Polyuria.
    (7) Oliguria.
    (8) Dehydration.
  b. Signs of uremia usually restricted to chronic renal failure include:
    (1) Mucosal ulceration.
    (2) Weight loss.
    (3) Mucosal pallor (anemia).
    (4) Skeletal changes caused by renal secondary hyperparathyroidism.
  c. Palpation of kidney size.
    (1) Determination of kidney size by palpation may aid in differentiating acute from chronic renal failure.
    (2) Knowledge that kidney size is normal is not informative, since acute or chronic changes are possible.
    (3) Increase in kidney size may occur in association with acute renal diseases, but it may also occur in association with hydronephrosis or with neoplasia.
    (4) Decrease in kidney size is usually associated with chronic generalized renal disease.
3. Radiography may aid in differentiating acute from chronic renal disease as follows:
  a. Kidney size may be estimated (see Chapter 8, Radiographic Evaluation of the Urinary System).
  b. Skeletal decalcification due to renal secondary hyperparathyroidism may be observed (see Chapter 8, Radiographic Evaluation of the Urinary System). Decalcification is not detectable in acute renal failure, but may be observed in association with chronic renal failure.
4. Laboratory aids in differentiation of acute from chronic renal failure.
  a. No test that measures renal function allows differentiation of acute from chronic renal disease.
  b. Urinalysis findings:
    (1) Contrary to some reports, single urine specific gravity determinations are of no value in differentiating acute and chronic renal disease since fixed specific gravity readings (1.008 to 1.012) occur with either category.
      (a) Urine specific gravity may be in the fixed range during acute renal failure due to impaired tubular function. If tubular function improves, the ability to concentrate urine may be regained.
      (b) The ability to concentrate urine is not regained with chronic renal failure.

(c) Care must be utilized in interpreting specific gravity of randomly collected samples of urine, since the kidney may or may not be elaborating urine representing maximal renal concentrating ability. (see Chapter 6, Laboratory Findings in Diseases of the Urinary System).
        (2) Inflammatory components (RBC, WBC, protein).
            (a) Evidence of acute inflammation in the urinary tract is more suggestive of an acute than of a chronic process.
            (b) Any part of the urinary tract, and portions of the genital tract, may be the source of the inflammatory components.
            (c) Acute renal disease may be superimposed on chronic renal disease; therefore, evidence of acute inflammation does not eliminate the possibility of chronic renal failure.
        (3) Casts may be detected in both acute and chronic renal disease.
5. Renal biopsy.
    a. Renal biopsy provides the only method for establishing the morphologic status of the kidney in the living patient.
    b. Knowledge of the morphologic status of the kidney provides the best single tool for determining the reversibility of kidney lesions.
    c. Correlation of biopsy results with history, physical examination, radiography, and laboratory aids allows the most precise prognosis of renal disease.
    d. See Chapter 9, Percutaneous Renal Biopsy, for technique and Chapter 12, Pathophysiology of Renal Failure, for interpretation of lesions regarding prognosis.

Chapter 31

TREATMENT OF RENAL FAILURE

I. **Specific and effective therapy can, in most instances, only follow an accurate diagnosis.**

   A. *Too frequently the diagnostic aspect of renal failure is overlooked and undue emphasis is placed on the relief of signs without enough consideration of eliminating the underlying cause.*

   B. *The treatment of renal failure should not be standardized, but rather should be based on findings of a careful and systematic search for primary and extrarenal causes of functional decompensation that can be partially or completely reversed by appropriate therapy.*

   1. In patients with prerenal uremia, rapid restoration of adequate renal blood flow may prevent the development of organic renal disease.
   2. Renal failure caused by obstructive uropathy or rents in the excretory pathway is potentially reversible provided the underlying cause is rapidly corrected or eliminated.
   3. In some instances, uremic crises may suddenly be precipitated by a combination of prerenal or postrenal factors which develop in patients with previously compensated primary renal failure. Correction of the extrarenal factors may permit such patients to return to a compensated state of renal failure.

   C. *Each patient should be evaluated and treated according to individual needs.*

II. **The type of treatment employed in patients with renal failure is variable, depending on the clinical status of the patient, the primary cause of the disease, and the specific objectives of treatment.**

   A distinction should be made between specific, supportive, symptomatic, and palliative types of treatment. Each type or combination of types may be indicated or contraindicated, depending on the circumstance in question. The value of each must be kept in perspective.

   A. *Specific treatment*
   1. Specific treatment is treatment given to modify, destroy, or eliminate the primary cause(s) of the disease process.
   2. Examples of specific treatments of renal disease include:
      a. Use of antibiotics to eliminate bacterial infections.
      b. Use of antidotes to counteract nephrotoxins.
      c. Removal of obstructive lesions which are causing postrenal uremia.

B. *Supportive treatment*
   1. Supportive treatment is that treatment which modifies or eliminates abnormalities that occur secondary to the primary disease.
   2. Successful specific therapy is often dependent on successful supportive therapy.
   3. Treatment of causes of uremic signs which occur as a result of generalized renal disease is an example of supportive therapy. For example:
      a. Dietary management is used to minimize accumulation of metabolic waste products of protein metabolism which cannot be excreted by diseased kidneys.
      b. Sodium chloride and sodium bicarbonate are often given to replace deficits which occur in chronic generalized nephron disease.

C. *Symptomatic treatment*
   1. Symptomatic treatment signifies therapy given to eliminate or suppress clinical signs.
   2. Examples of symptomatic treatment of renal disease include:
      a. Use of antiemetics to control vomiting.
      b. Use of diuretics to control edema associated with the nephrotic syndrome.
   3. Although symptomatic treatment is extremely important in some situations (e.g., hypovolemic shock), if chosen as the only method of therapy the signs being treated may not subside because of the continued presence of the underlying cause, or they may exacerbate following withdrawal of treatment.

D. *Palliative treatment signifies therapy chosen for situations in which the underlying disease cannot be cured, but in which the associated signs may be suppressed by therapy.*
   1. Palliative treatment is actually a combination of supportive and symptomatic treatment.
   2. If a disease is uncurable, and unless it is likely to cause undue discomfort to the patient or owner, the possibility of palliative treatment should be considered.
   3. Too often euthanasia is recommended by the veterinarian rather than being chosen by the owner.
   4. Symptomatic and supportive treatment of progressive renal failure which accompanies generalized irreversible renal diseases in dogs and cats may result in comfortable periods of survival for months or years.

III. From a prognostic and therapeutic point of view, it is useful to divide renal failure into prerenal, primary renal, and postrenal categories (see Chapter 12, Pathophysiology of Renal Failure).

A. *Prerenal uremia*
   1. Treatment of prerenal uremia should be:
      a. Specific. Eliminate the predisposing cause when possible.
      b. Supportive. In instances of fluid imbalance, reestablish renal perfusion by maintaining fluid balance (see Chapter 32, Fluid Therapy in Renal Failure and Chapter 17, Ischemic and Chemical Nephrosis).
   2. The prognosis of prerenal uremia is dependent on the primary cause.
      a. It is favorable for adequate renal function if perfusion is rapidly restored and maintained.

268   DISEASES OF THE UPPER URINARY SYSTEM

      b. Complete lack of renal perfusion in excess of two to four hours will result in generalized ischemic renal disease (see Chapter 17, Ischemic and Chemical Nephrosis).

B. *Postrenal uremia*
  1. Treatment of postrenal uremia should be:
    a. Specific. Eliminate the predisposing cause.
      (1) Surgically repair rents in the excretory pathway.
      (2) Remove lesions which obstruct outflow of urine.
    b. Supportive.
      (1) Maintain fluid, electrolyte, and acid-base balance.
      (2) Consider osmotic diuresis or peritoneal dialysis in patients with marked clinical signs of uremia.
  2. The prognosis of postrenal uremia is dependent on the primary cause.
    a. Obstructive uropathy.
      (1) Adequate renal function can be reestablished if the obstruction is rapidly removed (see Chapter 22, Hydronephrosis).
      (2) Prolonged obstruction will result in hydronephrosis and may result in death.
      (3) The cause of the obstruction may become the limiting factor with respect to survival (i.e., malignant neoplasm).
    b. Rent in excretory pathway.
      (1) Uremic patients in which a rent in the excretory pathway is rapidly and successfully repaired should receive a favorable prognosis since hydronephrosis is not a sequela.
      (2) Death is certain if the patient is uremic and the rent is not repaired.
      (3) Prognosis is dependent on the underlying cause (see Rupture of the urinary bladder, in Chapter 36).

C. *Primary uremia*
  1. Treatment of primary uremia should be:
    a. Specific. For details of specific therapy, consult sections on specific diseases of the kidneys.
    b. Supportive and symptomatic.
      (1) Once organic renal failure has developed, no regimen of therapy will eliminate the renal lesions.
      (2) Although the precipitating causes must be eliminated if life is to be maintained, the renal damage which has occurred must heal spontaneously over a period of days to weeks, and remaining viable nephrons must undergo compensatory adaptation.
      (3) If patients with primary renal failure are in need of extensive supportive and symptomatic therapy, every effort must be made to determine the potential reversibility of the underlying lesion. The detection of potentially reversible renal diseases is justification for vigorous application of available therapeutic techniques, whereas irreversible renal failure may not warrant such effort and expense.
      (4) The objective of therapy for patients with reversible renal failure must be to keep the patient alive until the processes of regeneration, repair, and compensatory adaptation allow the kidneys to regain sufficient function to reestablish homeostasis. This may be

accomplished by minimizing changes in fluid, electrolyte, and acid-base balance with various combinations of:
- (a) Conservative medical management.
- (b) Fluid therapy.
- (c) Intensive diuresis.
- (d) Peritoneal dialysis or hemodialysis.

(5) The objective of therapy for patients with generalized irreversible renal disease must be to reestablish and maintain biochemical homeostasis. The therapeutic principles are the same as those required to treat reversible primary renal failure, but therapy must be continued for the life of the patient since cure is not possible.

2. Depending on the regimen of symptomatic and supportive therapy, bilaterally nephrectomized dogs may be kept alive for variable periods of time. Death from uremia may be caused by any one or a combination of a variety of causes including hyperkalemia, acidosis, dehydration, and hypocalcemia (see Chapter 13, Extrarenal Manifestations of Uremia). By correcting these abnormalities, life may be sustained.
   a. When bilaterally nephrectomized dogs were provided with no treatment, they survived for approximately four days.
   b. When bilaterally nephrectomized dogs were provided with maintenance quantities of fluid (isotonic saline) and calories (10 per cent dextrose) orally, they survived for approximately five days.
   c. When bilaterally nephrectomized dogs were given a high nonprotein-calorie, electrolyte-free diet (corn oil 40 per cent, starch 35 per cent, and glucose 25 per cent), they survived for seven and a half days.
   d. When bilaterally nephrectomized dogs were given a high nonprotein-calorie, electrolyte-free diet and a cation exchange resin, they survived for nine days.
   e. Bilaterally nephrectomized dogs have been kept alive for as long as 111 days following surgery by intermittent peritoneal dialysis.

3. Because there are significant differences in the type and magnitude of excesses and deficits of fluids and electrolytes that develop in patients with oliguric and nonoliguric primary renal failure, it is imperative to divide candidates for therapy of renal failure into two groups: those with oliguria and those with polyuria (see Chapter 32, Fluid Therapy in Renal Failure).

4. Conservative medical management of renal failure.
   a. Treatment should be directed toward maintaining fluid, electrolyte, and acid-base balance by providing unlimited access to water, reducing the excretory load of metabolic waste products presented to the kidneys, and providing metabolites that diseased kidneys do not efficiently conserve.
   b. Conservative medical management of renal failure consists of various combinations of the following items:
      (1) Oral sodium chloride.
      (2) Oral sodium bicarbonate.
      (3) Dietary restrictions.
      (4) Vitamin supplements.
      (5) Anabolic steroids.
      (6) Access to water.
      (7) Avoiding stress.

c. Conservative medical management of renal failure is indicated when the clinical signs of uremia are not severe enough to require more intensive forms of therapy. Conservative medical management should be utilized:
  (1) In instances of symptomatic renal failure, but in which a uremic crisis is not present.
  (2) Following successful treatment of a uremic crisis by more intensive forms of therapy (e.g., diuresis, peritoneal dialysis).
d. Sodium chloride.
  (1) Rationale of therapy.
    (a) Administration of sodium chloride will help correct the negative balances of sodium and chloride, and as a result will maintain or increase extracellular fluid volume. The latter may augment renal blood flow and glomerular filtration rate.
    (b) By increasing plasma osmolality, sodium chloride will stimulate thirst. The resulting compensatory polyuria will augment water and solute turnover.
    (c) Administration of sodium chloride and sodium bicarbonate to human patients resulted in:
      [1] Increased urea clearance due to increased urine flow.
      [2] Decreased production of urea.
      [3] Expansion of extracellular fluid volume.
    (d) Administration of oral sodium chloride to normal dogs:
      [1] Caused a transient but significant increase in glomerular filtration rate and renal blood flow.
      [2] Did not result in formation of edema or significant increase in body weight, even when administered in doses of 4 Gm. per Kg. per day.
  (2) Oral dosage of sodium chloride.
    (a) As a generality, as much salt should be given as the patient will tolerate without vomiting or gaining weight due to accumulation of fluid. In some patients, serial determinations of the concentration of BUN or serum creatinine may be a useful index of response. Salt should be given until there is no further decrease in concentration of these substances.
      [1] In dogs, this may require a total of 1 to 15 grams per day divided into three doses.
      [2] A precise dosage schedule has not been established for cats, but, in general, a total of ½ to 3 grams per day divided into three doses has been adequate.
    (b) Salt may be provided:
      [1] As enteric coated tablets.
      [2] In gelatin capsules. A number 4 (human) capsule holds approximately 0.25 gram of sodium chloride.
      [3] In drinking water (¼ teaspoon per 500 ml.). Do not allow the patient access to any other source of water.
      [4] In food.
  (3) Duration of therapy.
    (a) Patients with reversible renal failure should be given sodium chloride until they have recovered, as determined by appropriate laboratory tests.

(b) Patients with irreversible renal failure should receive sodium chloride for life.
(4) Precautions:
 (a) An adequate water supply must be available at all times.
 (b) Sodium may increase the excess of fluid associated with oliguria, the nephrotic syndrome, or congestive heart failure. The presence of a cardiac murmur that is not associated with signs of heart failure (i.e., rapid heart rate, weak pulse, edema) is not a contraindication for salt therapy of renal failure.
 (c) Some dogs are unable to digest the enteric coating of salt tablets and pass partially digested and undigested tablets in their feces. In the latter instance, dosage should be increased or an alternative method of oral administration should be employed.
 (d) The onset of vomiting or rapid gains in body weight are signs indicating that the dosage should be decreased or temporarily discontinued.
e. Sodium bicarbonate.
 (1) Rationale for therapy. Administration of sodium bicarbonate will help correct the negative balances of sodium and bicarbonate and, as a result, will:
  (a) Minimize metabolic acidosis.
  (b) Maintain or expand extracellular fluid volume.
 (2) Oral dosage of sodium bicarbonate.
  (a) Urine pH should be used as an index for dosage. A sufficient quantity of sodium bicarbonate (15 to 90 grains per day divided into three doses) should be given to maintain urine pH between 6.0 and 7.5.
  (b) Sodium bicarbonate may be given as either 5 or 10 grain compressed tablets.
 (3) Duration of therapy and precautions.
  (a) See Sodium chloride above.
f. Dietary restrictions.
 (1) Complete aerobic metabolism of carbohydrates and fats for energy results in the production of carbon dioxide and water. The metabolism of proteins for energy, however, is associated with the production of metabolic by-products (urea, other nonprotein nitrogen substances, strong acids) in addition to carbon dioxide and water. These by-products are normally eliminated from the body in urine. Because they are osmotically active, these solutes require an obligatory urine volume for excretion.
 (2) Although the precise mechanisms have not been established, it is an accepted fact that protein by-products contribute significantly to the production of uremic signs in patients with severe renal failure. By providing diets that contain a minimum quantity of protein of high biological value and adequate nonprotein calories, many of the signs associated with uremia may be alleviated. For this reason, low protein diets are routinely used in treatment of renal failure.
 (3) The objective of dietary restriction should be to reduce protein intake while providing adequate quantities of total calories and essential amino acids to maintain nitrogen balance.

(a) An adequate nonprotein caloric intake is critical for optimum protein anabolism at low levels of protein intake.
(b) If protein is utilized for energy, the severity of uremic signs may be aggravated.
(4) In addition to decreasing the quantity of protein by-products for renal excretion and decreasing obligatory urine volume, feeding a low protein diet has the following advantages:
  (a) Meats contain a large quantity of intracellular potassium. Dietary restriction of protein tends to minimize accumulation of potassium in the patient.
  (b) Because most metabolic acids are derived from protein metabolism (phosphoric and sulfuric acid), restricting intake of dietary protein may help to combat metabolic acidosis associated with renal failure.
  (c) Because proteins are rich in phosphorus, restriction of dietary protein helps to minimize excessive accumulation of phosphorus in the body.
(5) Dietary therapy:
  (a) Is of value in minimizing signs of uremia.
  (b) Does not prevent the occurrence of renal disease.
  (c) Is of no significant therapeutic value in nonazotemic or nonuremic patients since such patients have sufficient renal function to excrete metabolic end-products of protein metabolism, and to maintain acid-base and electrolyte balance.
(6) Available diets.
  (a) Veterinary.
    [1] K/D, Hills Division, Riviana Foods Inc., Topeka, Kansas.
    [2] Clinicare N. Pfizer Inc., New York, N.Y.
    [3] Nephro Diet, Atlas Canine Products Inc., Glendale, Long Island, New York.
  (b) Medical (Human).
    [1] Resource Baking Mix, Doyle Pharmaceutical Co., Minneapolis, Minnesota 55410.
    [2] Controlyte Powder, Doyle Pharmaceutical Co.
  (c) Homemade.
    [1] All dietary proteins are not of equivalent nutritive value because they differ in quantity and types of amino acids.
    [2] Digestibility and palatability are not necessarily related to biological value.
    [3] Proteins of high biological value include lean meats, chicken, eggs, cottage cheese, milk, cream.
    [4] Sources of nonprotein calories include wheat starch bread, vegetable oils, high carbohydrate and fat desserts, and Lipomul (Upjohn Co., Kalamazoo, Mich.).
    [5] Proteins of poor biological value which should be avoided include plant proteins, meat scraps, tankage, gelatin, and fish meal.
(7) Recommendations for feeding.
  (a) The degree of dietary restriction is related to the degree of functional renal impairment.
  (b) It is suggested that homemade diets be composed of:

[1] One-half high quality meat-type foods (16 per cent protein).
[2] One-half carbohydrate and fat.
[3] Sufficient calcium supplementation to avoid problems associated with the feeding of all meat diets.
  (c) Diets must be fed on an individual basis.
    [1] Provide as many calories as the patient will tolerate without becoming obese.
    [2] Steady weight over a period of weeks or months is a reliable index of adequate caloric intake.
    [3] Additional quantities of high quality protein may be required to balance protein loss in patients with severe proteinuria.
g. Vitamin supplements. Since it is doubtful that B-complex vitamins and vitamin C are efficiently conserved by diseased kidneys, and since restricted diets may be deficient in these vitamins, it is recommended that therapeutic dosages of these vitamins be orally administered on a daily basis to patients with renal failure.
h. Anabolic steroids.
  (1) Commercially available anabolic steroids are testosterone or synthetic derivatives of testosterone.
  (2) They may be of benefit to patients with renal failure for the following reasons:
    (a) They promote positive nitrogen balance by stimulating appetite and stimulating protein synthesis. Anabolic steroids *do not* produce positive nitrogen balance unless caloric intake is adequate.
    (b) They promote production of red blood cells.
    (c) They decrease protein catabolism and thus production of nitrogenous waste products.
    (d) They enhance calcium deposition in bones.
  (3) Although anabolic agents are known to have a renotropic effect (i.e., they enhance compensatory hypertrophy of renal tubular cells), the functional effect of this phenomenon has not been documented. Recent investigations have been interpreted to suggest that the renotropic effect occurs as a result of water retention in renal tubular cells, and therefore is of no functional significance.
  (4) Available products include:
    (a) Winstrol-V, Winthrop Labs., New York, N.Y.
    (b) Delatestryl, E. R. Squibb and Sons, New York, N.Y.
  (5) Dosage.
    (a) These products may be given orally or parenterally.
    (b) They must be repeated at appropriate intervals.
    (c) Follow manufacturer's recommendations for specific dosage.
i. Access to water.
  (1) Because patients with renal failure lose the ability to concentrate urine, and because destruction of large numbers of nephrons impair renal excretion of metabolic by-products, excretion of solute loads through remaining viable nephrons requires a large obligatory urine volume.
  (2) Compensatory polydipsia develops in order to maintain fluid balance.
  (3) Except in instances of significant vomiting, dogs and cats with renal

failure should have an unrestricted water supply available at all times.
　j. Avoiding stress.
　　(1) Severely damaged kidneys have diminished ability to compensate for stresses imposed by change in external environment, dietary indiscretion, or disease states.
　　(2) In addition to progressive destruction of nephrons by progressive renal disease, uremic crises may be precipitated in patients with previously compensated renal disease by a variety of extrarenal factors (or stresses).
　　(3) Postulated mechanisms of "acute on chronic" uremic crises include the following:
　　　(a) Factors (anorexia, infection, extensive tissue necrosis) which accelerate endogenous protein catabolism increase the quantity of metabolic by-products in the body.
　　　(b) Stress states (change of environment, fever, infection) are associated with endogenous release of steroids. Steroids stimulate conversion of proteins to carbohydrates (gluconeogenesis) and thus increase the quantity of protein waste products in the body.
　　　(c) Any factor (decreased water consumption, vomiting, diarrhea, shock, cardiac decompensation) which decreases renal perfusion promotes prerenal uremia.
　　(4) As a generality, sudden deterioration in a patient with previously compensated renal failure should be viewed with a high index of suspicion as an "acute on chronic" uremic crisis. Differentiation of renal decompensation caused by potentially reversible extrarenal complications from renal decompensation caused by progressive destruction of the renal parenchyma is of prognostic and therapeutic significance.
　　(5) Recommendations.
　　　(a) Prevention is the best cure. Strive to keep stresses within the capacity of the kidneys to maintain homeostasis.
　　　　[1] Discourage change in external environment.
　　　　[2] Administer anabolic steroids to stimulate appetite.
　　　　[3] Provide adequate preoperative therapy.
　　　(b) Correct or eliminate reversible extrarenal factors.
　　　　[1] Treat infections with antibiotics (see Chapter 33, Drug Therapy in Renal Failure).
　　　　[2] Replace fluid deficits by oral or parenteral therapy.
　　　　[3] Restore caloric balance in anorexic patients by stomach tube or parenteral alimentation (see Chapter 32, Fluid Therapy in Renal Failure).
　　　　[4] Eliminate vomiting and diarrhea by eliminating the primary cause and by providing antiemetic or antidiarrheal therapy, or both.
　　　　[5] Restore cardiac decompensation with cardiac glycosides and rest (see Chapter 33, Drug Therapy in Renal Failure).
　　　(c) Correction of reversible extrarenal factors which precipitated the uremic crisis may result in restabilization of the patient.

5. Intensive diuresis.
    a. The objectives of intensive diuresis may be one or both of the following:
        (1) To establish and maintain adequate renal perfusion and glomerular filtration rate. The latter is particularly important in "high risk" surgical patients and patients with early stages of ischemic or nephrotoxic nephrosis.
        (2) To augment turnover of water in order to enhance renal excretion of metabolic waste products. Intensive diuresis of patients with renal disease is indicated when a uremic crisis occurs. Uremic crises are usually associated with anorexia, dehydration, vomiting, and diarrhea. Since the oral route of therapy cannot be used, maintenance of a high rate of water turnover by parenteral routes of therapy is essential.
    b. Osmotic diuresis.
        (1) Mechanism of action.
            (a) Therapy with osmotic diuretics causes a slight increase in renal blood flow and glomerular filtration rate by expanding extracellular fluid volume.
            (b) Osmotic diuretics cause a marked decrease in tubular reabsorption of solute.
                [1] Decreased water reabsorption initiated by the osmotic diuretic dilutes sodium concentration in tubules.
                [2] An unfavorable sodium gradient hinders sodium reabsorption by tubules.
                [3] The net increase in sodium excretion augments diuresis.
            (c) Osmotic diuretics may prevent the formation of tubular casts and interstitial edema by increasing tubular flow of fluid.
        (2) Equipment and materials.
            (a) Ten or 20% dextrose or 20% mannitol.*
            (b) Polyionic, isotonic electrolyte solution such as lactated Ringer's solution.
            (c) Intravenous catheter.**
            (d) Bandage for intravenous catheter.†
            (e) Flexible urinary catheter.
            (f) Colorimetric test paper for glucose.††
        (3) Procedure for 10 to 20% dextrose.
            (a) Aseptically place an intravenous catheter in the jugular vein and secure it in place with bandage material. The catheter must be rinsed with heparin solution to prevent coagulation of blood in its lumen.
            (b) Correct deficits in fluid and electrolyte balance prior to performing osmotic diuresis (see Chapter 32, Fluid Therapy in Renal Failure). Due to the critical condition of the patient, deficit therapy is provided over a period of a few hours rather than 24 to 48 hours.

---

*Osmitrol, Travenol Laboratories Inc., Morton Grove, Illinois 60053. 20% Mannitol in distilled water. McGaw Laboratories, Glendale, California 91201.
**Bardic inside needle catheter with stylet, C. R. Bard Inc., Murray Hill, N.J. 07974.
†Kling, Johnson and Johnson, New Brunswick, N.J.
††Tes-Tape, Eli Lilly, Indianapolis, Indiana 46206.

(c) Following rehydration, accurately determine the patient's body weight. This will serve as a baseline for future comparisons of gains or losses of body weight due to fluid.
(d) Catheterize the bladder and remove residual urine. Check urine for the presence of glucose with colorimetric test paper prior to intravenous glucose therapy.
(e) Administer 10 to 30 ml. per lb. of dextrose solution intravenously. In order to rapidly induce a hyperglycemia of sufficient magnitude to exceed the renal threshold for glucose, the dextrose should be administered at a rate of 2 to 10 ml. per minute for the first 10 to 20 minutes.
(f) After the first 10 to 20 minutes, check the urine for the presence of glucose with colorimetric test paper. A positive reaction provides a qualitative index of diuretic response.
(g) If following 10 to 20 minutes of dextrose administration dextrose is detected in the urine, the administration rate should be reduced and maintained at 1 to 5 ml. per minute.
(h) If therapy is to be considered effective, a significant diuresis should develop by the time one-half the calculated dose has been administered. To date, an adequate response has been defined as the production of slightly less than 1 ml. to more than 3 ml. of urine per minute.
(i) If significant diuresis does not occur, therapy should be discontinued at once in order to prevent the occurrence of overhydration. Other alternatives such as the use of furosemide or ethacrynic acid, peritoneal dialysis, or hemodialysis should be considered.
(j) Therapeutic agents may be added to the osmotic diuretic solution, including:
  [1] B-complex vitamins (1 ml. per liter of diuretic solution).
  [2] Sodium lactate or sodium bicarbonate (see Chapter 32, Fluid Therapy in Renal Failure).
  [3] Small doses of tranquilizers such as promazine or acepromazine. Tranquilizers may be effective in quieting restless patients and controlling vomiting.
(k) Osmotic diuresis should be repeated as necessary. Alternating the use of dextrose solution with lactated Ringer's solution is recommended. The necessity for continued therapy should be based on:
  [1] The clinical response of the patient.
  [2] The serum concentration of BUN or creatinine.
  [3] The ability of the patient to sustain an adequate urine output without diuretic therapy.
(l) Throughout the procedure the quantity of fluid administered should be recorded, and the output of urine should be periodically monitored. By correlating this information with body weight, dehydration or overhydration can be avoided.
  [1] The quantity of fluid given should be adjusted so that body weight remains stable at the original rehydration value.
  [2] If the patient is not consuming calories, a slight but con-

tinuous loss of body weight will occur due to body catabolism.
- [3] Significant increases in body weight indicate overhydration.
- [4] Significant decreases in body weight indicate dehydration.

(m) Since hypokalemia has been known to develop in patients receiving sustained or prolonged therapy, the development of signs characteristic of hypokalemia (skeletal muscle weakness and decreased gastrointestinal motility) should be considered suggestive of this abnormality. If hypokalemia does occur, replacement therapy with potassium should be administered (see Chapter 32, Fluid Therapy in Renal Failure).

(4) Procedure for 20% mannitol.
  (a) Mannitol is a 6 carbon alcohol closely related to mannose. Following a single intravenous injection, mannitol:
    - [1] Is not metabolized by the body.
    - [2] Equilibrates rapidly in the extracellular fluid space.
    - [3] Does not enter cells or cerebrospinal fluid.
    - [4] Increases renal blood flow and decreases vascular resistance.
    - [5] Is freely filtered by glomeruli.
    - [6] Is not reabsorbed or secreted by renal tubules.
    - [7] Creates high osmotic pressure in the renal tubular system.
  (b) The technique for performing osmotic diuresis with mannitol is identical to that described for hypertonic dextrose. It is emphasized that deficits in fluid and electrolyte balance must be corrected prior to performing osmotic diuresis (see Chapter 32, Fluid Therapy in Renal Failure).
    - [1] Since no simple qualitative test is available to detect the presence of mannitol in urine, urine output is the best guide with which to evaluate dosage and response to therapy.
    - [2] Dosages of mannitol suggested to induce osmotic diuresis are variable, but most investigators recommend an intravenous test dose of 0.25 to 0.5 Gm. of mannitol per Kg. of body weight.
    - [3] The diuretic should be given as a 20 to 25% solution over a three to five minute period.
    - [4] Provided satisfactory diuresis develops following test trials with mannitol, more prolonged therapy may be slowly administered (2 to 5 ml. per min.) as a 5 to 10% solution with the objective of sustaining urine output. Some investigators state that the daily dosage of mannitol should not exceed approximately 2 Gm. per Kg. body weight per 24 hours.
    - [5] Since osmotic diuresis induced by mannitol is accompanied by the loss of significant quantities of electrolytes in addition to water, many individuals prefer to give mannitol in a vehicle of physiologic saline solution or lactated Ringer's solution rather than in water.
    - [6] As was the situation with dextrose, if significant diuresis does not develop approximately 30 minutes after administration of the test dose, therapy with this agent should

be immediately discontinued in order to prevent hydremia. Unlike water intoxication associated with overdosage of dextrose solution, overhydration with mannitol is characterized by a state of vascular overload due to hyperosmolality and cellular dehydration. The latter occurs because mannitol is not metabolized by the body and does not enter cells.
- (5) Indications for osmotic diuresis. Osmotic diuresis may be useful in:
  - (a) Prophylaxis of surgical or traumatic oliguria (see Chapter 17, Ischemic and Chemical Nephrosis).
  - (b) Adjunctive therapy of oliguria or anuria.
- (6) Contraindications for osmotic diuresis include:
  - (a) Impaired renal function that fails to respond to a test trial of osmotic therapy.
  - (b) Patients with severe cardiovascular failure.
- (7) Advantages of dextrose over mannitol include:
  - (a) Metabolism of glucose for energy and production of glycogen provides a protein sparing effect.
  - (b) Colorimetric test paper can be used as a qualitative index of diuresis.
- (8) Advantages of mannitol over dextrose include the fact that mannitol is inert and is not metabolized by the body.
- (9) Overhydration due to dextrose or mannitol therapy.
  - (a) Clinical signs may include any combination of the following:
    - [1] Increase in body weight.
    - [2] Engorgement of superficial veins.
    - [3] Edema.
    - [4] Respiratory distress (dyspnea, moist rales).
    - [5] Signs related to interstitial cerebral edema.
  - (b) Laboratory signs of overhydration include hemodilution characterized by a decrease in PCV and the serum concentration of total protein.
  - (c) Treatment.
    - [1] Prevent its occurrence.
    - [2] Discontinue oral and parenteral administration of fluids.
    - [3] Consider oxygen therapy if the patient has difficulty breathing.
    - [4] Consider peritoneal dialysis using hyperosmotic (7% dextrose) dialysate solutions (see Peritoneal Dialysis in this chapter).
    - [5] Consider ethacrynic acid or furosemide as diuretic agents.
- c. Miscellaneous diuretic agents.
  - (1) In instances in which patients do not respond to osmotic diuretic therapy with mannitol or dextrose, treatment with ethacrynic acid* or furosemide** should be considered.
    - (a) A large volume of evidence obtained from clinical trials in man and experimental investigations in dogs has revealed that these agents may induce diuresis in some patients unresponsive to mannitol or dextrose therapy.

---

*Edecrin, Merck, Sharp, and Dohme, West Point, Pa. 19486.
**Lasix, National Labs Corp., Kansas City, Mo. 64108

(b) Administration of high doses (8 mg. per Kg.) of furosemide during early stages of experimentally induced acute renal failure in dogs improved renal function.

(c) The clinical use of these agents in dogs and cats has been too meager to permit establishment of any generalizations, but preliminary evaluation is encouraging. Continued use of these diuretics in the prevention and management of uremic crises in dogs and cats warrants further clinical trials.

(2) Mechanism of action. Both of these agents induce diuresis by inhibiting tubular reabsorption of sodium. Both are capable of inducing diuresis despite low glomerular filtration rate.

(3) Procedure.

(a) Deficits in fluid and electrolyte balance must be corrected prior to administration of these diuretics (see Chapter 32, Fluid Therapy in Renal Failure). If patients are already hydrated as a result of trial therapy with osmotic diuretics, additional fluid and electrolyte replacement prior to their use may be unnecessary.

(b) Either diuretic may be administered orally or intravenously. Calculate dosage on the basis of the manufacturer's recommendations.

(c) If significant diuresis is not achieved after a period of approximately two hours, the manufacturer's recommended dosage should be doubled or tripled and the drug should be administered again.

(d) Depending on patient response and the objectives of treatment, either drug may be repeated every eight hours, or the next dose may be scheduled the following day.

(e) Because ethacrynic acid and furosemide are extremely potent diuretics, the fluid and electrolyte balance of patients receiving them should be closely monitored in order to prevent dehydration. Periodic parenteral replacement therapy with polyionic solutions may be necessary.

(f) If significant diuresis does not develop, therapy with ethacrynic acid or furosemide should be discontinued.

(g) Ethacrynic acid has been reported to cause ototoxicity in human beings with renal failure. Experimental use of ethacrynic acid has also caused ototoxic lesions in cats. There is no information about the relationship, if any, of ototoxicity and ethacrynic acid in dogs.

d. If patients do not promptly develop a diuresis in response to test trials with the diuretics mentioned above, it can be concluded that primary generalized renal dysfunction has occurred.

(1) Continued use of diuretics in attempts to reestablish urine flow in such instances is probably of no value. Osmotic diuretics are contraindicated since such therapy will be ineffective and may cause severe overhydration.

(2) Other modes of therapy such as peritoneal dialysis or hemodialysis should be considered.

e. As soon as the patient can tolerate oral therapy, conservative medical management should be initiated.

6. Peritoneal dialysis.

a. Peritoneal dialysis provides an alternative means for eliminating waste products of protein metabolism and for regulating the volume and composition of body fluids.
b. Mechanism of action.
   (1) The peritoneum is a semipermeable membrane with a large surface area.
   (2) The rate of diffusion of low molecular weight substances across the peritoneal membrane is approximately proportional to the concentration gradient of each. Diffusion of these substances may therefore be altered by varying their concentration in dialysate solutions.
   (3) The absorption of fluid from the peritoneal cavity can be delayed for a significant period of time by adding glucose to the solution.
      (a) Although the peritoneum is permeable to glucose, glucose molecules have a slower diffusion rate than water and electrolytes.
      (b) Addition of glucose to an isotonic solution will result in formation of a hypertonic solution, and the latter will promote movement of fluid from extracellular spaces into the peritoneal cavity.
      (c) By increasing the glucose concentration of dialysate fluid, it is possible to remove a substantial volume of fluid from the body.
      (d) Commercial dialysate solutions contain either 1.5, 4.25, or 7 per cent glucose. As a generality, dialysate solutions with high glucose concentrations (4.25 and 7 per cent) should be used only when it is desirable to remove fluid from the body.
   (4) Diffusion rates of solutes across the peritoneum are affected by:
      (a) Tonicity. Solutions with a high glucose concentration promote a more rapid movement of diffusible solutes than solutions with a low glucose concentration.
      (b) Temperature. In one study, increasing the temperature of the dialysate solution from 20° C. to 37° C. prior to administration increased the clearance rate of urea by approximately 35 per cent.
      (c) Time permitted for diffusion. Almost complete equilibrium between peritoneal fluid and extracellular fluid is attained after the dialysate has been in the peritoneal cavity for approximately two hours. The greatest increase in the concentration of urea and potassium in the dialysate fluid occurs in the first 30 minutes. Depending on its original concentration, glucose will ultimately be absorbed from the peritoneal cavity in approximately two to six hours. In clinical practice, equilibration periods of 30 minutes to one hour are most efficient.
   (5) The peritoneal membrane is relatively impermeable to plasma proteins, but not completely so.
c. Equipment for peritoneal dialysis.
   (1) Commercial dialysate solutions:*
      (a) Contain 1.5, 4.25, or 7 per cent dextrose.

---

*Inpersol, Abbott Laboratories, North Chicago, Ill. 60064; Dianeal, Baxter Laboratories, Morton Grove, Ill. 60053; Peridial, Cutter Laboratories, Berkeley, Calif. 94710; Chronodial, Cutter Laboratories, Berkeley, Calif. 94710.

(b) Contain other electrolytes (Na, Cl, Ca, Mg) in concentrations similar to that of extracellular fluid.
(c) May or may not contain potassium.
   [1] Potassium free solutions should be used in patients with hyperkalemia.
   [2] Potassium fortified (4 mEq. per liter) solutions should be used in patients with normal serum potassium concentrations.
(d) Contain lactate. They do not contain bicarbonate because of stability problems. If necessary, bicarbonate may be added immediately prior to use of dialysate solutions.
  (2) Commercial administration sets are also available from companies that manufacture dialysate solutions. They perform well and are convenient.
  (3) Commercial peritoneal dialysis catheters. Catheters that contain stylets* are designed to permit their insertion into the peritoneal cavity without the need of a trocar or surgery.
d. Technique for peritoneal dialysis.
  (1) Accurately determine the patient's body weight. This will serve as a baseline to compare future gains or losses of body weight due to fluid.
  (2) If the urinary bladder is distended, empty it by manual compression or catheterization.
  (3) Aseptically prepare the skin over the midline.
  (4) Instill a small quantity of local anesthetic on the midline a few centimeters posterior to the umbilicus. In very small patients, it may be necessary to go cranial to the umbilicus.
  (5) Insert the catheter. (see Commercial peritoneal dialysis catheters, above).
    (a) Use strict asepsis.
    (b) Moisten the catheter with heparin. This will help to prevent occlusion of the catheter with fibrin.
    (c) Direct the catheter to the caudal quadrant of the abdomen. Although the exact placement of the catheter is not critical, directing it toward the iliac fossa on the right or left side usually provides the best results. The cranial quadrant of the abdomen should be avoided in order to minimize the risk of damaging viscera such as the liver and spleen. The midline of the caudal portion of the abdomen should be avoided in order to prevent damage to the urinary bladder.
    (d) Since the presence of intra-abdominal adhesions increases the risk of hemorrhage or damage to restricted viscera, catheters should be directed away from sites of previous surgery.
    (e) Tape or suture the catheter to the skin.
  (6) Instill the dialysate solution into the peritoneal cavity.
    (a) Warm the dialysate solution to body temperature prior to use. This step will enhance efficiency of solute exchange.
    (b) Administration of the dialysate solution into the peritoneal

---
*Stylocath, Abbott Laboratories, North Chicago, Ill. 60064; Diacath, Travenol Laboratories Inc., Morton Grove, Ill. 60053.

cavity may be performed prior to insertion of the catheter in order to:
- [1] Decrease the risk of catheter penetration of abdominal viscera.
- [2] Reduce the likelihood of fibrin occlusion of the catheter.

(c) Instill a sufficient volume of dialysate solution to mildly distend the abdomen.
- [1] The quantity of fluid required to distend the abdomen will vary from several hundred to several thousand ml. depending on the size of the patient.
- [2] Instillation usually requires 10 to 20 minutes. If flow is too slow, the catheter should be repositioned.
- [3] Avoid hindering movement of the diaphragm by over-distention of the abdomen.

(7) Allow the dialysate solution to equilibrate for 30 to 60 minutes.

(8) Remove the dialysate solution by siphoning it back into the original container.
- (a) To insist that the quantity of fluid removed be equal or greater in quantity than fluid administered may unnecessarily prolong the procedure. A priming volume is usually unrecoverable following the first exchange, but is not required during subsequent exchanges. Proceed to the next exchange when outflow slows to an intermittent drip, provided positive patient fluid balance is not progressive.
- (b) Recovery of fluid usually requires about 15 to 25 minutes.

(9) Repeat exchanges as necessary.
- (a) Record volumes of fluid administered and recovered.
- (b) Weigh the patient frequently.
- (c) Monitor clinical response of the patient and the serum concentration of BUN or creatinine.

(10) The number of exchanges required per unit of time will be variable depending on:
- (a) The severity of renal failure.
- (b) Patient response to therapy.
- (c) Patients with severe uremia may require five or more exchanges per day in order to control signs.
- (d) Following stabilization patients may be maintained with fewer exchanges. Bilaterally nephrectomized dogs have been maintained for months by two or three 1-liter exchanges per day.
- (e) It is not necessary to reduce the concentration of BUN or creatinine to normal in order to achieve significant clinical response. Since the goal of therapy is to ameliorate signs of renal failure until the kidneys heal or until a diagnosis can be established, the actual concentration that BUN or creatinine attain should not be overemphasized. In one study with bilaterally nephrectomized dogs, it was possible to reduce the plasma concentration of BUN to normal but exchanges had to be repeated every one and a half to three hours.

e. Technical complications. Recovery of dialysate solution from the peritoneal cavity may be impaired as a result of:
(1) Fibrin occlusion of the catheter. To minimize the likelihood of this complication:

(a) Rinse the catheter with heparin prior to use.
(b) Add 250 units of heparin to each liter of dialysate solution.
(c) Delay insertion of the catheter into the peritoneal cavity until the dialysate solution is to be removed.
(d) Reposition or replace the catheter if necessary.
(2) Occlusion of the catheter with omentum. To correct this complication:
(a) Reposition the catheter.
(b) Replace the catheter if necessary.
(3) Loss of the siphon effect due to the presence of a large pocket of air in the peritoneal cavity. This may be avoided by using a catheter with a stylet or by making abdominal incisions to accommodate catheters as small as possible.
f. Patient complications.
(1) Peritonitis.
(a) The likelihood of infection is greater if catheters are kept in place for more than two or three days.
(b) With good technique and short-term therapy, infection is usually not a problem.
(c) Use of a closed drainage system is desirable since it will minimize the likelihood of contamination of the peritoneal cavity (see commercial administration sets, in this chapter).
(d) Development of turbidity in fluid removed from the peritoneal cavity suggests the presence of peritonitis.
[1] Following centrifugation and staining, evaluate such fluid with a microscope and determine antibiotic sensitivity of bacteria if peritonitis is confirmed.
[2] The presence of leucocytes in dialysate solution is not pathognomonic of infection since they commonly occur in association with hydroperitoneum.
(2) Dehydration. The use of hypertonic dialysate solutions (4.25 or 7% dextrose) will induce a negative fluid balance. This complication may be prevented by parenteral fluid replacement therapy, or by using solutions containing 1.5 per cent dextrose.
(3) Hypokalemia. This complication may be avoided by using potassium free dialysate solutions only in patients with hyperkalemia.
(4) Hypoproteinemia.
(a) Peritoneal dialysis may result in loss of substantial quantities of plasma protein. The severity is dependent on the duration of dialysis, the presence or absence of peritonitis, and the tonicity of dialysate fluid.
(b) In an experimental study in normal dogs, approximately 35 grams of protein were recovered from four exchanges during a 24 hour period. Five hundred ml. of dialysate containing 1.5% glucose were used in each exchange.
(c) Depending on the status of the patient and the duration of therapy, replacement therapy with proteins may be required (see Chapter 32, Fluid Therapy in Renal Failure).
(5) Damage to viscera. This is an uncommon complication in patients with a normal peritoneal cavity.
(a) Since the presence of intra-abdominal adhesions increases the

risk of damage to viscera, catheters should be directed away from sites of previous surgery.
- (b) In problem cases, administration of the dialysate solution prior to insertion of the catheter may minimize the risk of iatrogenic damage to abdominal organs.
- g. Indications for peritoneal dialysis include:
  - (1) Acute renal failure; keep the patient alive until the kidneys regain adequate function.
  - (2) Chronic renal failure; restabilize decompensated renal failure.
  - (3) Overhydration.
  - (4) Intoxications. Dializable intoxicants in man include:
    - (a) Some barbiturates.
    - (b) Diphenylhydantoin.
    - (c) Primidone.
    - (d) Digoxin.
    - (e) Potassium, sodium.
    - (f) Arsenic.
    - (g) Ethanol, methanol.
    - (h) Ethylene glycol.
    - (i) Sulfonamides.
    - (j) Nitrofurantoin.
    - (k) Kanamycin.
    - (l) Streptomycin.
    - (m) Neomycin.
    - (n) Chloramphenicol.
    - (o) Tetracycline.
  - (5) Do not wait until the prognosis is hopeless before considering this method of therapy.
- h. Contraindications for peritoneal dialysis include:
  - (1) Ruptured diaphragm.
  - (2) Extensive intra-abdominal adhesions.
  - (3) Although peritonitis was at one time considered to be a contraindication for peritoneal dialysis, clinical and experimental studies have disproved this generality.
    - (a) Peritoneal dialysis may be performed without any loss of efficacy in dogs with peritonitis.
    - (b) Peritoneal dialysis may be beneficial in the treatment of peritonitis because it removes exudate from the peritoneal cavity and facilitates contact of antibiotics with the peritoneum.
  - (4) Recent abdominal surgery is not an absolute contraindication to peritoneal dialysis as long as the abdominal wound is properly sutured and does not leak dialysate fluid.
7. Hemodialysis.
   a. There is a massive volume of literature pertaining to technical aspects and clinical value of hemodialysis in human medicine.
   b. Currently, economics, technical complications, and time have restricted the use of hemodialysis units in veterinary medicine.
   c. Development of simplified, reliable equipment which is technically easy to use may permit hemodialysis to be used on a larger scale in clinical veterinary medicine in the future.

d. The following discussion is presented with the objective of providing a conceptual understanding of hemodialysis.
e. Artificial kidneys have 3 primary components.
    (1) A dialyzer in which solute and water are removed from arterial blood by dialysis and ultrafiltration.
    (2) A dialysate delivery system which supplies and controls the flow and temperature of the dialysate solution.
    (3) Blood administration sets, cannulae, tubing, and other equipment to carry blood from the patient to the dialyzer and back to the patient.
f. Although there are a variety of dialyzers, construction principles are basically similar for all.
    (1) A tube carries blood from the patient into the dialyzer where it flows against one side of a thin (approximately 0.015 mm.) membrane with a surface area of approximately one square meter.
    (2) Dialysate solution (water and electrolytes) flows against the opposite side of the membrane, usually in a different direction. There is no direct contact between blood and dialysate solution.
    (3) Undesirable waste solutes dissolved in blood pass through the membrane into the dialysate solution by diffusion. Blood substances of large size or high molecular weight cannot pass through the small pores of the membrane. If desirable to remove fluid from the body, ultrafiltration can be utilized.
g. Recent development of a hollow-fiber membrane dialyzer* has allowed miniaturization of equipment and substantial reduction in cost. Additional advantages of this equipment include a small priming volume (approximately 100 ml.) and simplicity of operation. Although the units are disposable, they have been successfully re-used in human beings at least 3 times.
h. A major limiting factor in the use of hemodialysis in veterinary medicine is establishment of blood flow adequate for performing hemodialysis on anything but a short-term basis.

8. Renal transplantation.
    a. The surgical technique of kidney transplantation is not technically difficult, and can be satisfactorily performed with the equipment and personnel in most veterinary hospitals.
        (1) The transplanted kidney is usually placed in the iliac fossa.
        (2) The renal artery is anastomosed to the internal iliac, external iliac or hypogastric artery while the renal vein is anastomosed to the iliac vein.
        (3) The ureter of the transplanted kidney is transplanted directly into the urinary bladder.
    b. Host versus graft rejection phenomena is responsible for the economical and technical unfeasibility of this technique in clinical veterinary medicine.
        (1) Randomly selected canine renal homotransplants are usually rejected in less than one to two weeks.
        (2) Canine renal homotransplants obtained from littermates may

---
*Cordis-Dow Artificial Kidney, Cordis Corporation, Miami, Florida 33137.

survive for a longer period, but usually are rejected in four to six weeks.
- (3) Immunosuppression must be utilized to prevent host destruction of the renal graft.

c. All immunosuppressive techniques used clinically are designed to remove or destroy immunologically competent cells or their activity. Immunosuppressive techniques are broad spectrum in effect and as a result depress the host's body defense mechanisms. Fortunately, the body's immune response to the renal graft is often more readily suppressed by immunosuppressive agents than is the body's immune response to infectious agents.
- (1) Immunosuppressive agents available for use include:
  - (a) Cytotoxic drugs (corticosteroids, azothioprine).
  - (b) Extracorporeal irradiation.
  - (c) Graft irradiation.
  - (d) Thoracic duct drainage.
  - (e) Antilymphocyte globulin.
- (2) Cytotoxic drugs exert their effects by disturbing immune-cell function, especially that of short-lived lymphocytes. These drugs alter sensitization at the time when antigenic stimulation converts small lymphocytes to active sensitized cells. Once lymphocytes become sensitized, the cytotoxic agents commonly used often are ineffective at therapeutic dosages.
- (3) Radiation. Small lymphocytes are very sensitive to the effects of irradiation, but once sensitized become more radio-resistant.
- (4) The objective of thoracic duct drainage is to decrease the number of circulating lymphocytes by drainage of the thoracic duct.
- (5) Antilymphocyte serum and antilymphocyte globulin are effective agents in prolonging homograft survival, but their exact mode of action has not been established.

d. Experimental studies indicate that the host-graft reaction in the dog is more profound than in human beings. Use of homotransplantation in the dog probably will not achieve the degree of success that it has in man until more effective methods of establishing tissue compatibility and of controlling the rejection phenomenon are discovered.

9. Treatment of complications of chronic renal failure.
   a. Anemia.
      (1) Anemia caused by chronic generalized renal disease is unresponsive to therapy with hematinics such as vitamin B_{12}, iron, and folic acid.
      (2) Anabolic agents may be of value in treatment of the anemia of chronic uremia (see Conservative medical management of renal failure, in this chapter).
      (3) Blood transfusions are usually unnecessary, even in severely anemic patients. In the event signs caused by anemia develop, whole blood or packed red cell transfusions may be administered. Transfusions are of no therapeutic value other than to transiently correct inadequate numbers of RBC.
   b. Osteodystrophy.
      (1) Patients with renal failure have impaired ability to metabolize

vitamin D to its active form, and thus have impaired ability to absorb calcium from the intestines.
- (2) The severity of osteodystrophy may be minimized by reducing the oral intake of phosphorus and enhancing gastrointestinal loss of phosphorus.
- (3) Phosphorus intake may be reduced by feeding a low protein diet.
- (4) Intestinal excretion of phosphorus may be enhanced by administering oral nonabsorbable phosphate binding compounds such as aluminum hydroxide gels or basic aluminum carbonate gels.*
- (5) It is advisable to withhold specific calcium therapy in patients with chronic uremia. Although administration of calcium and vitamin D in large doses may overcome the intestinal block in calcium absorption, there is a danger that increased calcium absorption will produce metastatic calcification of soft tissues including the kidneys. This is undesirable since calcium is nephrotoxic.
 c. Hypocalcemic tetany.
   (1) Long-term therapy should be directed toward limiting the rise of the plasma concentration of phosphorus (see Osteodystrophy, in this chapter).
   (2) Hypocalcemic tetany must be treated symptomatically. The following methods may provide an immediate but short-lived response.
      (a) Intravenous administration of calcium solutions.
      (b) Avoid rapid alkalinizing therapy since an increase in plasma pH may decrease the concentration of ionized calcium (see Chapter 13, Extrarenal Manifestations of Uremia).
      (c) Oral administration of calcium salts is ineffective in producing a rapid and sustained elevation of the plasma concentration of calcium, especially in the presence of marked hyperphosphatemia.

IV. Summary of recommended therapy for renal failure of different degrees of severity.

A. *For specific details regarding rationale and dosages, refer to the preceding discussion of conservative medical management, diuresis, and peritoneal dialysis.*

B. *Polyuria, polydipsia, nonazotemia.*
  1. Avoid stress.
  2. Administer anabolic agents.
  3. Provide a balanced diet.
  4. Provide unlimited access to water.
  5. Administer B-complex vitamins orally.

C. *Polyuria, polydipsia, azotemia.*
  1. Avoid stress.
  2. Administer anabolic agents.
  3. Provide a low quantity, high quality protein diet.
  4. Provide unlimited access to water.

---

*Basaljel, Wyeth Laboratories, Philadelphia, Pa. 19101.

5. Orally administer B-complex vitamins.
6. Orally administer sodium chloride and sodium bicarbonate.

D. *Uremic crisis (polyuria, vomition, dehydration).*
1. Restrict oral intake of water until vomiting subsides.
2. Correct deficits or excesses of fluids and electrolytes (see Chapter 32, Fluid Therapy in Renal Failure).
3. Use osmotic diuresis, furosemide or ethacrynic acid.
4. Use peritoneal dialysis if diuretic therapy is ineffective.
5. Give vitamins parenterally.
6. Supply adequate nonprotein calories to minimize endogenous protein catabolism (see Chapter 32, Fluid Therapy in Renal Failure).
7. Administer anabolic agents.
8. Return to oral therapy as described for polyuria, polydipsia, azotemia as soon as possible.

E. *Uremic crisis (oliguria or anuria, vomition, dehydration).*
1. Restrict oral intake of water.
2. Correct deficits or excesses of fluids and electrolytes (see Chapter 32, Fluid Therapy in Renal Failure).
   a. Avoid overhydration.
   b. Avoid administration of potassium.
3. Try to initiate urine production with osmotic diuretics, furosemide or ethacrynic acid. *Do not overhydrate the patient while attempting to induce diuresis.*
4. Consider peritoneal dialysis if diuretic therapy is ineffective.
5. Give vitamins parenterally.
6. Supply adequate nonprotein calories to minimize endogenous protein catabolism (see Chapter 32, Fluid Therapy in Renal Failure).
7. Administer anabolic agents.
8. Return to oral therapy as described for polyuria, polydipsia, azotemia as soon as the patient can sustain adequate urine output.

F. *Nephrotic syndrome and polyuria.*
1. Proteinuria, nonedematous, nonazotemic.
   a. Avoid stress.
   b. Administer anabolic agents.
   c. Provide a diet with a sufficient quantity of high quality protein to balance protein loss in urine.
   d. Provide unlimited access to water.
   e. Orally administer B-complex vitamins.
2. Proteinuria, nonedematous, azotemic.
   a. Avoid stress.
   b. Administer anabolic agents.
   c. Cautiously supply additional high quality protein in the diet to balance protein loss in urine. Do not provide excessive protein since some may be deaminated and metabolized for energy. Monitor BUN and albumin concentration of serum.
   d. Provide unlimited access to water.
   e. Orally administer B-complex vitamins.
   f. Administer sodium chloride and sodium bicarbonate with caution.

Discontinue use of these drugs if edema develops. Oral calcium lactate may be provided to combat metabolic acidosis.
3. Proteinuria, edematous, nonazotemic.
   a. Avoid stress.
   b. Administer anabolic agents.
   c. Provide a diet with a sufficient quantity of high quality protein to balance protein loss in urine.
   d. Provide unlimited access to water unless the edema is of sufficient severity to threaten the life of the patient.
   e. Orally administer B-complex vitamins.
   f. Administer furosemide or ethacrynic acid to reduce or eliminate edema.
      (1) Depending on the underlying cause, it may be necessary to continue diuretic therapy for the life of the patient.
      (2) Prevent diuretic induced fluid and electrolyte deficits.
4. Proteinuria, edematous, azotemic.
   a. Avoid stress.
   b. Administer anabolic agents.
   c. Cautiously supply additional high quality protein in the diet to balance protein loss in urine. Do not provide excessive protein since some may be deaminated and metabolized for energy. Monitor BUN and albumin concentration of serum.
   d. Provide unlimited access to water.
   e. Orally administer B-complex vitamins.
   f. Administer sodium chloride and sodium bicarbonate with caution. Discontinue use of these drugs if the edema increases in severity. Oral calcium lactate may be provided to combat metabolic acidosis.
   g. Parenteral administration of plasma protein solutions may provide very transient benefit in relief of the severity of edema, but may aggravate the severity of uremic signs.
   h. Consider the use of aldosterone antagonists such as spironolactone.

G. *Polyuria, polydipsia, azotemia, congestive heart failure.*
   1. Management of patients with this combination of diseases provides a paradox in selection of treatment. Following careful evaluation of the patient's physical status, emphasis should be placed on eliminating signs which are the greatest threat to life.
   2. Avoid stress; provide rest.
   3. Digitalize the patient with caution.
   4. Administer anabolic agents.
   5. Provide a sodium free diet if pulmonary edema is of sufficient severity to cause respiratory distress.
   6. Provide unlimited access to water.
   7. Orally administer B-complex vitamins.
   8. If the patient does not have marked pulmonary edema, administer low dosages of sodium chloride and sodium bicarbonate with caution. Discontinue use of these drugs if respiratory stress develops. Oral calcium lactate may be provided to combat acidosis.
   9. Consider the use of diuretics to relieve edema caused by congestive heart failure and to augment water turnover.

REFERENCES

Ben-Ishay, Z., Wiener, J., Sweeting, J., Bradley, S. E., and Spiro, D.: Fine structural alterations in the canine kidney during hemorrhagic hypotension. Effects of osmotic diuresis. Lab. Invest., 17:190–210, 1967.

Berman, L. B.: Modification of protein catabolic rate and survival time in the anuric dog. Clin. Res., 7:282, 1959.

Blom Van Assendelft, P. M., and Dorhout Mees, E. J.: Urea metabolism in patients with chronic renal failure: Influence of sodium bicarbonate and sodium chloride administration. Metabolism, 19:1053–1063, 1970.

Bricker, N. S.: Chronic progressive renal disease: Pathologic physiology and relation to treatment. Progr. Cardiov. Dis., 4:170–199, 1961.

Butler, H. C.: Technique of kidney transplantation and its future in veterinary medicine. J.A.V.M.A., 147:1436–1443, 1965.

Butler, H. C.: Renal support systems and transplantations. In Scientific Presentations and Seminar Synopses of the 38th Annual Meeting of the American Animal Hospital Association. Elkhart, Ind., American Animal Hosp. Assoc., 1971.

Drobeck, H. P., Coulston, F., Beyler, A. L., and Potts, G. O.: Evaluation of anabolic, hormonal, hematopoietic and pathologic properties of stanozolal. Exp. Molecular Path., Suppl., 2:115–135, 1963.

Edney, A. T.: Observations on the effects of feeding a low protein diet to dogs with nephritis. J. Sm. Anim. Pract., 11:281–291, May, 1970.

Eng, K., and Stahl, W. M.: Correction of the renal hemodynamic changes produced by surgical trauma. Ann. Surg., 174:19–23, 1971.

Gault, M. H., Ferguson, E. L., Sidha, J. S., and Corbin, R. P.: Fluid and electrolyte complications of peritoneal dialysis. Ann. Int. Med., 75:253–262, 1971.

Gourley, I. M. G.: Prevention and treatment of acute renal failure in the canine surgical patient. J.A.V.M.A., 157:1722–1728, Dec. 1, 1970.

Grollman, A., Turner, L. B., and McLean, J. A.: Intermittent peritoneal lavage in nephrectomized dogs and its application to the human being. Arch. Int. Med., 87:379–390, 1951.

Houck, C. R.: Problems in maintenance of chronic bilaterally nephrectomized dogs. Amer. J. Physiol., 176:175–182, 1954.

Humphreys, C. F.: Effects of diet and cation exchange upon survival of nephrectomized dogs. J. Urol., 82:208–211, 1959.

Jackson, R. F.: The use of periteoneal dialysis in the treatment of uremia in dogs. Vet. Rec., 76:1481–1486, 1487–1490, 1964.

Ladd, M., and Raisz, L. G.: Response of normal dog to dietary sodium chloride. Amer. J. Physiol., 159:149–152, 1949.

Levin, N. W.: Furosemide and ethacrynic acid in renal insufficiency. Med. Clin. N. Amer., 55:107–119, Jan., 1971.

Low, D. G.: Conservative medical management of chronic renal disease. In Current Veterinary Therapy. Vol. 4. Edited by R. W. Kirk. Philadelphia, Pa., W. B. Saunders Co., 1971.

Lumb, G. A., Mawer, E. B., and Stanbury, S. W.: The apparent vitamin D resistance of chronic renal failure. A study of the physiology of vitamin D in man. Amer. J. Med., 50:421–441, 1971.

Meengs, W., Greene, J. A., and Weller, J. M.: Peritoneal clearance of urea and potassium and protein removal during acute peritonitis in dogs. J. Lab. Clin. Med., 76:903–906, 1970.

Montoreano, R., Mouzet, M. T., Cunarro, J., and Ruiz-Guinazu, A.: Prevention of initial oliguria of acute renal failure (in dogs) by the administration of furosemide. Postgrad. Med. J. Suppl.:7–10, April, 1971.

Mylon, E., and Goldstein, P.: Influence of protein reserves on nephrectomized and renal artery ligated dogs. Proc. Soc. Exp. Biol. Med., 69:198–200, 1948.

Naets, J. P., and Wittek, M.: Mechanism of action of androgens on erythropoiesis. Amer. J. Physiol., 210:315–320, 1966.

Padula, R. T., Camishion, R. C., Magee, J. H., Noble, P. H., and Cowen, G. S. M.: Evaluation of protective effects of osmotic diuretics. Curr. Top. Surg. Res., 1:177–187, 1969.

Perper, R. J., and Najarian, J. S.: A technique for transplantation of the canine kidney. M. V. P., 45:31–37, 1964.

Pierce, J. C., and Varco, R. L.: Technical considerations in the transplantation of the kidney to the dog's neck. J. Surg., Res., 4:275–280, 1964.

Stone, A. M., and Stahl, W. M.: Effect of ethacrynic acid and furosemide on renal function in hypovolemia. Ann. Surg., 174:1–11, July, 1971.

Weston, R. E., and Roberts, M.: Clinical use of stylet catheter for peritoneal dialysis. Arch. Int. Med., 115:659–662, 1965.

White, H. J. O.: Renal transplantation. J. Sm. Anim. Pract., 8:485–492, 1967.

Chapter 32
FLUID THERAPY IN RENAL FAILURE

I. **The type of parenteral fluid therapy employed in treatment of patients with renal failure is variable, depending on:**

   A. *The clinical status of the patient.*

   B. *The primary cause (prerenal, primary renal or postrenal) of the renal failure.*

   C. *The specific objectives of treatment.*

   As a generality, parenteral fluids may be administered to uremic patients for either or both of two purposes:
   1. To correct imbalances (deficits and excesses) in water, electrolyte, caloric, and acid-base metabolism, and to maintain a state of balance.
   2. To promote loss of metabolic end-products that accumulate in abnormal quantities as a result of renal failure. The latter may be accomplished by:
      a. Diuresis (see Intensive diuresis, in Chapter 31).
      b. Peritoneal dialysis (see Peritoneal dialysis, in Chapter 31).
      c. Hemodialysis (see Hemodialysis, in Chapter 31).

II. **Although it is true that fluid and electrolyte therapy is ultimately of little value without adequate renal function, adequate renal function is not synonymous with total renal function.**

   The more precisely parenteral fluids and electrolytes match body requirements at the time of administration, the less is the quantity of renal function that is required to be adequate.

III. **Principles of fluid therapy in renal failure**

   A. *Normal body composition*
      1. Water.
         a. Normally 55 to 75 per cent of body weight is water.
         b. About 25 to 35 per cent of body weight is extracellular water; the remainder is intracellular water.
      2. Electrolytes.
         a. Intracellular water contains high concentrations of potassium, phosphorus, and magnesium, but a low concentration of sodium.
         b. Extracellular water contains high concentrations of sodium and chloride, but low concentrations of potassium, magnesium and phosphorus.

c. Normally, extracellular electrolyte composition is maintained within narrow limits.
3. Acid-base balance.
   a. The kidney and the lungs are of great importance in maintaining acid-base balance.
   b. Normally, plasma bicarbonate concentration is maintained at about 25 mEq. per liter, and blood carbonic acid content is maintained at about 1.2 mEq. per liter.
   c. Blood pH is normally maintained between 7.31 and 7.42.

B. *Deviations of water, electrolyte, acid-base, and caloric balance associated with primary uremia.*
   1. Abnormalities of water, electrolyte, acid-base, and caloric balance are not invariably present in patients with generalized renal disease. Generally, compensatory mechanisms of the body are able to maintain a state of biochemical homeostasis which is compatible with normal activity unless oral intake is diminished or until a severe state of renal failure develops.
   2. Uremia associated with polyuria.
      a. Water. Because of obligatory osmotic diuresis associated with generalized nephron disease, a tendency toward dehydration develops.
      b. Electrolytes.
         (1) Varying degrees of body deficits of sodium, chloride, and calcium may be present.
            (a) The kidneys lose the ability to efficiently conserve these ions.
            (b) The development of hypocalcemia is related to a negative calcium balance and a decreased renal clearance of phosphorus.
         (2) A body deficit of potassium may exist, but serum potassium concentration is usually normal.
         (3) A body excess of phosphates and sulfates exists as a result of decreased renal clearance of these substances.
      c. Acid-base balance.
         (1) Acid-base balance may range from normal to a severe metabolic acidosis depending on the duration, severity, and type of renal disease.
         (2) Metabolic acidosis associated with renal failure develops as a result of:
            (a) Impaired tubular secretion of hydrogen ions.
            (b) Decreased renal clearance of dietary nonvolatile acids.
            (c) Impaired tubular secretion of ammonia.
            (d) Decreased ability of the kidneys to conserve bicarbonate ions.
      d. Caloric balance.
         (1) Usually a negative caloric balance exists, and the body is forced to catabolize its own tissues for energy.
   3. Uremia associated with oliguria or anuria.
      a. Water. Depending on the degree of oliguria and the magnitude of water loss by other routes (vomiting, diarrhea), water balance may be:
         (1) Normal
         (2) Positive (overhydration).

(3) Negative (dehydration).
   b. Electrolytes.
      (1) Body excesses of phosphates and sulfates exist.
      (2) Depending on the degree of oliguria and the severity of electrolyte losses by other routes, there may be a body excess of sodium, potassium, and chloride. Serum concentration of these ions may be increased.
   c. Acidosis may be present or absent. When present it is usually more severe in patients with oliguria or anuria than in patients with polyuria.
   d. Caloric balance. Usually a negative caloric balance exists.

IV. Detecting deviations from normal

A. Detecting dehydration
   1. Clinical signs. The following guidelines relate the percentage of body water deficit to total body weight. By relating the percentage of fluid deficit to body weight, an approximation of the quantity of fluid necessary to replace the deficits may be determined. Multiplication of body weight times the estimated percentage of dehydration will provide the amount of fluid required to replace the deficit.
      a. 5 per cent dehydration. The skin has a doughy consistency. This is the minimum amount of dehydration that can be detected by physical examination.
      b. 7 to 8 per cent dehydration.
         (1) The loss of skin pliability is sufficient to allow the skin to retain the abnormal position to which it is displaced.
         (2) The mucosa of the mouth may be dry.
         (3) If renal function is adequate, oliguria associated with urine of high S. G. will be present. If renal function is inadequate, the S. G. of the urine will be low, despite the body's need to conserve water.
         (4) The eyes are slightly depressed into the skull as a result of dehydration of the surrounding tissues. A decreased intraocular pressure may also be present.
      c. 10 to 12 per cent dehydration. The preceding signs are more severe; shock may be present in debilitated patients. Involuntary muscle twitching may be present (Fig. 32–1).
      d. 12 to 15 per cent dehydration. Shock is marked and death is imminent.
   2. Weight data.
      a. Knowledge of the animal's weight prior to illness may facilitate estimation of water loss.
      b. In addition to fluid deficit, weight loss may occur as a result of tissue wasting associated with chronic diseases. Rapid changes in body weight which occur over a short period of time are most useful as indices of alterations of body fluid balance.
   3. Laboratory data. In addition to the physical examination, laboratory data may be used to estimate the quantity of fluid deficit.
      a. Packed cell volume.
         (1) An increase in PCV may be caused by:
            (a) Dehydration and hemoconcentration.
            (b) Splenic contraction.

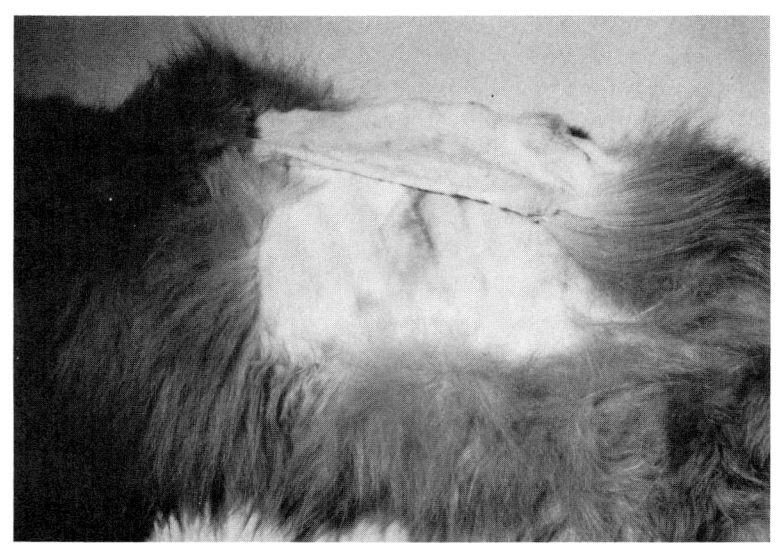

Figure 32-1. Severe dehydration in a 2-year-old male domestic shorthaired cat with chronic generalized renal disease. The skin retained for several minutes the abnormal position to which it was displaced.

- (c) Physiologic polycythemia (high altitudes, prolonged vigorous exercise).
- (d) Pathologic polycythemia (erythropoietin producing renal tumors or polycythemia vera — Rare).
- (2) An increase of PCV due to dehydration in an anemic patient may be erroneously interpreted as a normal value if not considered with the findings of the physical examination and the total protein concentration of serum.
- b. Total protein.
  - (1) An increase in total protein may be caused by:
    - (a) Dehydration and hemoconcentration.
    - (b) Disease states associated with hyperglobulinemia.
  - (2) An increase in total protein concentration due to dehydration in a hypoproteinemic patient may be erroneously interpreted as a normal value if not considered in association with the findings of the physical examination and PCV.
- c. By considering physical examination findings, PCV, and total protein concentration when evaluating patients for dehydration, the chance of erroneous conclusions is decreased.
  - (1) The likelihood of a patient having anemia and hypoproteinemia is not great, although it may occur in patients with the nephrotic syndrome or advanced chronic uremia.
  - (2) Once the presence of dehydration has been established, periodic reevaluation of PCV and total protein concentration is a better index of daily changes in hydration than is physical examination since the latter is more difficult to quantitate.

B. *Detecting electrolyte alterations*

1. History provides valuable information concerning the direction of alterations of some electrolytes.

a. Vomiting may result in significant loss of:
   (1) Sodium.
   (2) Potassium.
   (3) Chloride.
b. Diarrhea may result in significant loss of:
   (1) Sodium.
   (2) Potassium.
   (3) Bicarbonate.
c. Impaired renal function. See deviations of electrolytes associated with primary uremia, in this chapter.
2. Physical examination provides little information concerning electrolyte imbalances, except in instances of extremely severe imbalances. Signs that may be seen with severe abnormalities are:
   a. Hyperkalemia: cardiac conduction abnormalities, muscle weakness, mental confusion.
   b. Hypokalemia: muscle weakness.
   c. Hyponatremia: nausea, vomiting, muscle weakness, low specific gravity urine.
   d. Hypocalcemia: tetanic muscle spasms.
3. Laboratory aids.
   a. Serum electrolyte concentrations provide information concerning the quantity of electrolyte present compared to the quantity of water present. (i.e., the ratio of electrolyte to water).
   b. This data is valuable but should be interpreted considering:
      (1) The state of hydration of the patient.
      (2) The significance of concentration of the electrolyte vs. total body content.
   c. When serum concentration of the electrolyte is significant (hypocalcemia, hypercalcemia, hyperkalemia, or hypokalemia), appropriate action should be taken to correct the abnormality.
   d. When body content is significant (sodium balance), serum electrolyte concentration must be interpreted considering the state of hydration. For example:
      (1) A dog with edema may have a normal serum sodium concentration. However, since there is a body excess of extracellular fluid containing the normal sodium concentration, body content of sodium is increased. Administration of additional sodium to such a patient is contraindicated.
      (2) A dehydrated dog that has an increase in serum sodium concentration may still have a body deficit of sodium. More water than sodium may have been lost, causing an elevation of the serum sodium concentration.

C. *Detecting acid-base alterations.*
   1. History.
      a. History gives valuable information concerning the probable direction of alterations in acid-base balance.
         (1) Uremic patients frequently have metabolic acidosis.
         (2) Vomiting may cause metabolic alkalosis.
         (3) Diarrhea may cause metabolic acidosis.
         (4) Anorexia may result in mild metabolic acidosis.

b. The magnitude of the deviation is dependent on many factors, including:
   (1) Severity of the abnormality.
   (2) Duration of the abnormality.
   (3) Ability of the body to make compensatory alterations.
      (a) Compensatory alterations are made by the lungs and kidney.
      (b) Renal disease may affect the ability of the patient to compensate.
c. History may aid in determining the probable direction of an acid-base deviation, but it does not give quantitative information regarding the magnitude of change.
2. Physical examination.
   a. Physical examination is unreliable for detection of acid-base deviations.
      (1) Signs indicative of disturbances of acid-base balance are not specific.
      (2) Signs are frequently absent unless changes are severe.
      (3) Severe imbalances may be present without physical signs.
   b. Physical signs that may be observed include:
      (1) Increased rate and depth of respiration associated with metabolic acidosis. The body is eliminating carbon dioxide (and thus carbonic acid) in an attempt to restore the normal ratio (20 to 1) of bicarbonate to carbonic acid.
      (2) Decreased rate and depth of respiration associated with metabolic alkalosis. The body is retaining carbon dioxide (and thus carbonic acid) in an attempt to restore the normal ratio of bicarbonate to carbonic acid.
3. Laboratory aids.
   a. Urine pH.
      (1) A low urine pH is indicative of a large quantity of acid being excreted by the kidneys, This can be caused by many circumstances, including ingestion of proteins of animal origin, any cause of respiratory acidosis, or any cause of metabolic acidosis (see urinalysis, in Chapter 6).
      (2) Interpretation of urine pH with respect to acid-base balance.
         (a) Low urine pH (5.5 or below) indicates that the kidneys have some ability to excrete acid and that they are in fact excreting acid.
         (b) Low urine pH does not mean that the patient is invariably acidotic; blood pH and plasma bicarbonate values may be normal.
         (c) High urine pH (above 7) is indicative of any of the following:
            [1] The kidneys are unable to excrete acid.
            [2] Factors in the urinary tract, such as infection with urea splitting bacteria or diet, are altering urine pH.
            [3] The acid load presented to the kidney is relatively small, and there is no need to excrete additional acid in order to maintain acid-base balance.
            [4] The patient may be receiving alkalinizing drugs.
   b. Measurement of blood pH, plasma bicarbonate, and pCO_2.
      (1) The acid-base status of the patient can be precisely assessed by measuring any two of the following:

(a) Blood pH.
(b) Plasma bicarbonate concentration.
(c) Carbonic acid content of blood (essentially synonymous with pCO_2, although the units are different).
(2) Measurement of bicarbonate concentration alone gives valuable information in uremia since it is known that there is a tendency for metabolic acidosis with uremia.
(3) Determination of blood pH and plasma bicarbonate or pCO_2 is beyond the laboratory capability of most veterinary hospitals. Most human hospitals can make the determinations, but it is necessary to collect the sample anaerobically, and to inhibit metabolic processes in the sample. This can be accomplished as follows:
(a) Prepare an ice bath for the sample (a tray of ice cubes in a quart of water suffices).
(b) Completely fill the dead space of a 10 ml. syringe, fitted with a needle, with sodium heparin. Remove all air bubbles from the syringe and needle.
(c) Obtain a venous blood sample, preferably from the jugular vein. In order to obtain accurate values, blood samples must not be collected under a condition of venous stasis. In order to collect a sample without venous stasis:
[1] Occlude the vein.
[2] Make a venipuncture.
[3] Remove pressure from the vein.
[4] Allow blood to flow through the vein for several seconds.
[5] Gently aspirate blood into the syringe. Do not create excessive negative pressure by forceful movements with the syringe plunger as this may result in leakage of room air into the syringe barrel.
(d) Withdraw the needle and place a rubber stopper on the needle tip. Leave the syringe attached.
(e) Immerse the syringe with attached needle and rubber stopper in the ice bath immediately.
(f) The sample will provide satisfactory values provided determinations are made within two hours.

V. A plan for fluid therapy

A. As a generality, formulation of therapy for correction of abnormalities in fluid, electrolyte, acid-base, and caloric balance should be based on evaluation of three distinct categories.

1. Repair of deficits or excesses.
2. Maintenance therapy.
3. Correction of contemporary (continuous) abnormalities (deficits or excesses).

B. Repair of deficits

1. This therapy is designed to correct abnormalities that are detected at the time the patient is first examined.
2. See section IV (Detecting deviations from normal) in this chapter for estimation of these deficits.

298 DISEASES OF THE UPPER URINARY SYSTEM

    3. Rate of correction of deficits.
        a. Except in instances of hypovolemic shock or therapeutic use of osmotic diuretics, it is usually unnecessary and inadvisable to rapidly correct the entire deficit.
        b. Severe depletions should be treated aggressively, but as normalcy is approached, the compensatory mechanisms of the body should be allowed to maintain homeostasis. If shock is not present:
           (1) Administer about ½ of the total deficit during the first nine hours of therapy.
           (2) Administer approximately ¾ of the total deficit during the first 24 hours.
           (3) Complete deficit repair in 48 hours.
  C. *Maintenance therapy. Maintenance therapy consists of daily provision of water and electrolytes required by the body for physiological processes.*
    1. In normal dogs and cats, a certain quantity of fluids and electrolytes is lost daily via:
        a. Obligatory urine volume.
        b. Respiratory system.
        c. Skin (minor effect).
        d. Gastrointestinal tract (minor effect normally).

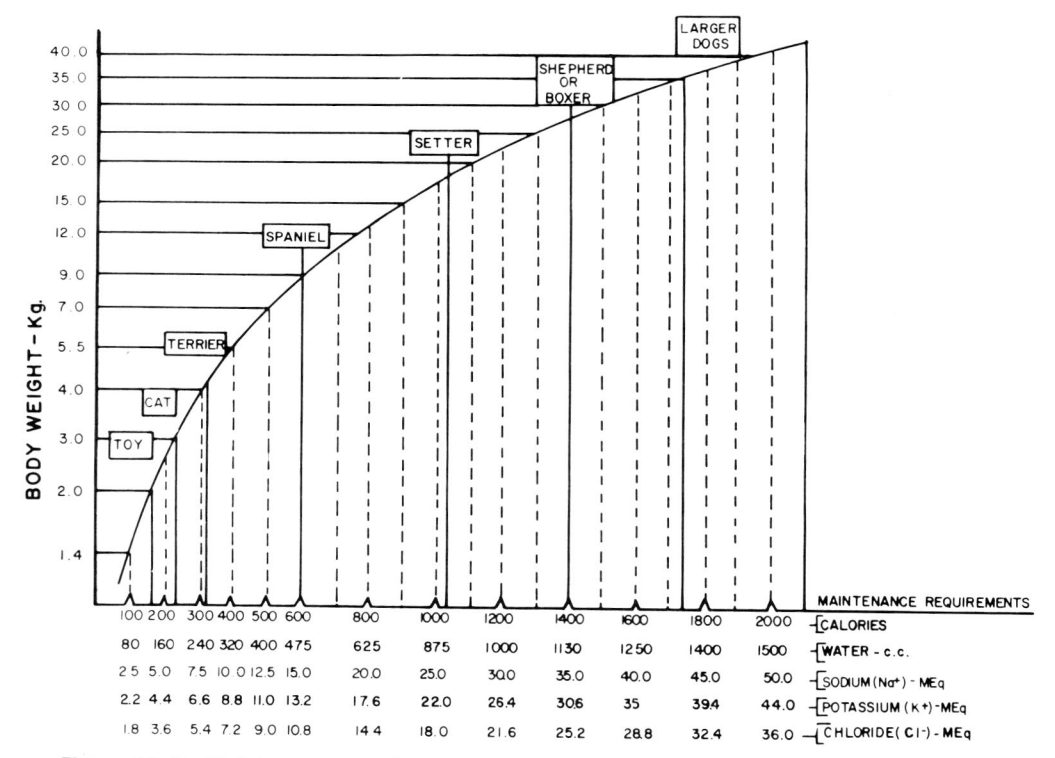

Figure 32-2. Maintenance requirements for calories, water and electrolytes of dogs and cats restricted to hospital confinement. (Modified from Harrison, J. B., Sussman, H. H., and Pickering, D. E.: Fluid and Electrolyte Therapy in Small Animals. J.A.V.M.A., *137*:637–645, 1960.)

2. If anorexia and lack of water intake occur, the daily requirement of exogenous metabolites must be replaced by other means.
3. Maintenance water and electrolyte requirements parallel caloric expenditure. See Figure 32-2 for data related to water, electrolyte and caloric requirements of caged dogs and cats.
4. If the patient eats and drinks normally, maintenance therapy is unnecessary.
5. Note from Fig. 32-2 that maintenance requirements for the patient should be supplied by solutions which are hypotonic as compared to plasma, and which contain concentrations of electrolytes dissimilar to that of plasma. The reason for these differences is that normal loss of water from the body exceeds normal loss of electrolytes, and that daily maintenance requirements are not related to plasma concentrations of electrolytes.
6. For short-term maintenance therapy where potassium losses are ignored, two volumes of 5% dextrose and one volume of lactated Ringer's solution provide adequate water and electrolyte therapy. Commercially prepared maintenance solutions are also available.*
7. See Nutritional replacement therapy and Oral fluid Administration, in this chaper, for methods of fulfilling maintenance requirements for calories.

D. *Therapy of contemporary gains or losses*
1. Contemporary therapy consists of:
   a. Replacement of continuing fluid and electrolyte losses due to polyuria, vomiting, diarrhea, etc.
   b. Correction of continuing fluid and electrolyte excesses such as edema, hyperkalemia, etc.
2. Since the patient is frequently hospitalized during the period of contemporary losses, the type and quantity of loss can be estimated to serve as a guide for therapy.

E. *Evaluation of patient response to fluid therapy*
1. Since many of the parameters used to determine the type and quantity of fluid for fluid therapy represent estimates rather than precise measurements, the patient should be reexamined at least once daily to evaluate the efficacy of therapy.
2. The quantity and type of fluid subsequently administered should be based on the knowledge of maintenance requirements and estimates of contemporary losses, and on the patient's physical status and body weight changes. Laboratory analyses (PVC and TP, serum electrolytes, blood pH, and plasma bicarbonate) and determination of urine volume may also be utilized. The total quantity of fluid administered should ultimately be determined by the patient's response to therapy, rather than by rigid adherence to an arbitrarily established dosage schedule.

VI. Oliguric versus polyuric renal failure

A. *Because there are significant differences in the type and magnitude of excesses and deficits of fluids and electrolytes that develop in patients with oliguric and nonoliguric*

---

*Normosol-M, Abbott Laboratories, North Chicago, Illinois 60064; Plasma-Lyte 56, Baxter Laboratories, Morton Grove, Illinois 60053.

primary renal failure, it is imperative to divide candidates for therapy of renal failure into those with oliguria and those with polyuria.

This division is based on the quantity of urine that the patient produces as a result of primary renal disease. Frequently patients with renal disease may be producing small quantities of urine of low specific gravity because dehydration has superimposed prerenal uremia on primary renal disease. Once rehydrated, polyuria ensues. Oliguria in this discussion refers to instances in which urine volume is scanty, despite correction of prerenal or postrenal factors.

B. *Oliguria*
   1. For patients with oliguria, a regimen of therapy characterized by fluid, electrolyte, and protein restriction should be adopted.
   2. Severe persistent oliguria is typically associated with fluid retention, hyperkalemia, and marked metabolic acidosis.
       a. Initial therapy should be formulated to correct existing deficits, without accentuating existing excesses.
       b. Once fluid, electrolyte, and acid-base alterations have been corrected, additional fluid therapy should be designed to provide for daily losses of fluids and electrolytes via the gastrointestinal, respiratory, integumentary, and urinary systems (maintenance therapy). Provisions should also be made for continuing fluid and electrolyte losses due to vomiting and diarrhea (contemporary therapy).
       c. Generally, parenteral fluids given to oliguric patients should contain minimal quantities of potassium, but should contain sufficient quantities of other electrolytes to replace daily body requirements. (2 parts 5% dextrose in water to 1 part lactated Ringer's solution).
       d. The quantity of fluid given should be adjusted so that body weight remains stable, or, in instances where the patient is not consuming calories, a slight but continuous loss of body weight occurs due to body catabolism. Significant increases in body weight indicate overhydration.
       e. If the patient will tolerate oral therapy, oral consumption of water should be restricted to that volume required for basal needs.
       f. In order to minimize the risk of accumulation of body fluid, administration of large quantities of sodium chloride should be avoided.
       g. Alterations in the serum concentration of potassium are especially important since relatively small changes in serum concentration can produce hazardous clinical changes.
           (1) Since the kidneys are the primary route of excretion of potassium, patients with oliguria are predisposed to hyperkalemia. It is emphasized, however, that, provided urine volume is adequate, severely damaged kidneys are capable of excreting a sufficient quantity of potassium to prevent clinically significant hyperkalemia.
           (2) Clinical signs of hyperkalemia usually appear when the serum concentration is between 7 to 10 mEq. per liter.
           (3) The urgency and regimen of treatment for hyperkalemia is dependent on the degree of cardiotoxicity.
           (4) In instances where clinical signs of cardiotoxicity are present

(bradycardia, arrhythmias, heart block) treatment should be directed toward promoting the transfer of potassium into cells. This may be accomplished by:
    (a) Intravenous administration of regular insulin (1/4 to 1/2 units per lb.) in 5% dextrose solution.
    (b) Administration of sodium bicarbonate. This promotes a shift of potassium into cells and hydrogen out of cells.
    (c) Intravenous administraion of calcium gluconate or calcium lactate. The pharmacologic action of calcium is antagonistic to that of potassium.

(5) Parenteral and oral administration of substances containing potassium must be avoided.

(6) Peritoneal dialysis using dialysate solutions that do not contain potassium may be of benefit (see Peritoneal dialysis, in Chapter 31).

(7) Clinical response to therapy should be monitored with electrocardiograms and serum concentration of potassium.

(8) In situations where hyperkalemia is less severe (serum concentrations of 6 to 7 mEq. per liter) treatment should be directed toward preventing excessive accumulation of potassium in the blood.
    (a) Oral administration of cation exchange resins* (50 Gm. per day in divided doses) have been effective in controlling hyperkalemia in nephrectomized dogs by inducing potassium loss in feces.
    (b) Dietary management and attempts to maintain nitrogen balance will reduce the quantity of potassium released from catabolism of exogenous and endogenous proteins.
    (c) The duration of therapy should be correlated with serum concentration of potassium in order to prevent hypokalemia. Therapy usually can be discontinued when the body can maintain the serum concentration of potassium below 6 mEq. per liter.

h. Energy should be supplied in the form of nonprotein high calorie diets** in order to minimize exogenous and endogenous metabolism of protein for energy.

i. Anabolic agents should be administered since they tend to stimulate appetite and promote positive nitrogen balance. Anabolic agents do not produce positive nitrogen balance unless caloric intake is adequate.

j. Drugs which are dependent on the kidneys for excretion in active or metabolized form should be given with caution in order to prevent development of toxic side reactions (see Chapter 33, Drug Therapy in Renal failure).

k. If the patient does not tolerate or respond to the oral and parenteral therapy outlined above, intermittent peritoneal dialysis or hemodialysis should be considered. If overhydration is a clinical problem,

---

*Kayexalate, Winthrop Laboratories, New York, N. Y. 10016
**Lipomul, The Upjohn Company, Kalamazoo, Michigan 49001; Controlyte Powder, Doyle Pharmaceutical Co., Minneapolis, Minnesota 55410.

302   DISEASES OF THE UPPER URINARY SYSTEM

peritoneal dialysis with solutions containing 4.25 or 7% dextrose should be used. By increasing the glucose content of the dialysate fluid, a substantial volume of fluid may be removed from the body (see Peritoneal dialysis, in Chapter 31).

C. *Polyuria*
1. Unlike oliguria and anuria, potential complications of polyuria include excessive loss of fluids and electrolytes, especially sodium.
2. While hyperkalemia is a common finding in oliguric renal failure, it is usually not a feature of polyuric renal failure since viable nephrons undergo compensatory adaptation and are capable of maintaining potassium balance (see Chapter 12, Pathophysiology of Renal Failure).
3. Patients with polyuric renal failure should receive conservative medical therapy characterized by (see Chapter 31, Treatment of Renal Failure):
    a. Unlimited access to water, unless they are vomiting. Maintenance of fluid and electrolyte balance may also require parenteral administration of isotonic, polyionic fluids such as lactated Ringer's solution.
    b. Dietary restriction.
    c. Oral administration of sodium chloride and sodium bicarbonate.
    d. Oral administration of multiple vitamins.
    e. Oral or parenteral administration of anabolic steroids.
    f. Avoidance of stress.

VII. Products for therapy

A. *Adequate correction of electrolyte and acid-base alterations of the uremic patient can be accomplished utilizing one or more of the following products.*
1. Lactated Ringer's solution.
    a. This solution closely approximates extracellular electrolyte composition, except lactate is present rather than bicarbonate.
    b. Its electrolyte composition makes it a fluid of choice for rehydrating a dehydrated uremic patient.
    c. For correction of severe acidosis, this solution should be supplemented with sodium lactate or sodium bicarbonate.
2. Sodium lactate* or sodium bicarbonate.**
    a. These solutions are designed specifically for treatment of acidosis.
    b. If plasma bicarbonate concentration is known, the required dosage of these solutions can be calculated.
        (1) One half of the total body bicarbonate is extracellular.
        (2) Extracellular fluid constitutes about 30 per cent of body weight.
        (3) Bicarbonate deficit (mEq./L.) is 25 minus the bicarbonate concentration (mEq./L) in the patient.
        (4) From the preceding, the total bicarbonate deficit can be calculated as:
        body wt. (kg.) $\times$ 0.3 $\times$ 2.0 $\times$ bicarbonate deficit = body wt. (kg.) $\times$ 0.6 $\times$ bicarbonate deficit (mEq./L) = mEq. of lactate or bicarbonate that should be administered to correct the deficit.

---
*1/6 M sodium lactate U.S.P. (contains 167 mEq. per liter of sodium and 167 mEq. per liter of lactate).
**Sodium bicarbonate, Abbott Laboratories (contains 44.6 mEq. of bicarbonate per 50 ml.).

c. If plasma bicarbonate is unknown, the severity of the uremia may serve as a rough guide for the quantity of bicarbonate or lactate to administer.

Severity of uremia	Probable bicarbonate deficit (mEq/L.)	HCO_3 needed (mEq/Kg. body wt.)
mild	5	3
moderate	10	6
severe	15	9

d. Oral replacement may be used provided the patient is not vomiting (1 grain of $NaHCO_3$ = approximately ¾ mEq.).
e. Acidosis should be corrected over a 48 hour period.
3. Potassium chloride.
   a. Solutions containing high concentrations of potassium are rarely indicated in uremic animals because potential exists for retention of potassium by the kidney.
   b. Occasionally a patient with profound polyuria, either of spontaneous or iatrogenic origin, will have hypokalemia. Therapy with potassium is indicated in such a patient. The kidneys are unable to conserve all of the potassium filtered, even in deficit states.
      (1) Replacement by the oral route is preferred because the slow rate of absorption of potassium from the gastrointestinal tract minimizes the possibility of iatrogenic hyperkalemia.
         (a) Potassium gluconate or potassium carbonate may be used.
         (b) Enteric coated potassium chloride USP may be used.[†]
         (c) Potassium bicarbonate may be used.[††]
      (2) Solutions containing up to 35 mEq. of potassium per liter can be administered subcutaneously without signs of local or systemic toxicity.
      (3) Caution must be used if potassium is administered by the intravenous route.
         (a) Potassium should not be administered at a rate greater than 0.5 mEq. per kg. per hr. to avoid hyperkalemia.
         (b) The patient should be frequently evaluated for evidence of hyperkalemia.
            1 — Auscultation for cardiac arrhythmias.
            2 — Electrocardiography.
            3 — Determination of serum concentration of potassium.
         (c) Potassium for parenteral administration may be obtained in vials containing 20 to 40 mEq. of potassium.[†††] Solutions containing high concentrations of potassium should be added to other parenteral solutions prior to administration.
      (4) The potassium deficit should be replaced over a period of 48 to 72 hours.
      (5) The rate of potassium replacement is less critical if renal function is adequate.

[†]Wolins Mfg. Corp., Farmingdale, New York.
[††]Mead-Johnson Laboratories, Evansville, Indiana.
[†††]Potassium Chloride Injection USP, Travenol Labs, Inc., Morton Grove, Illinois 60053.

DISEASES OF THE UPPER URINARY SYSTEM

B. *Nutritional replacement therapy*
1. Carbohydrate preparations.
   a. Glucose.
      (1) Metabolism of glucose nets the body less than four Calories per gram.
      (2) Glucose is readily available as a source of calories, but attempts to replace total daily caloric requirements with parenteral solutions are impractical.
      (3) Example:
         (a) An 18 kg. dog requires about 1200 Calories per 24 hours (Fig. 32-2).
         (b) Five per cent dextrose contains 50 grams of glucose per liter.
         (c) $\dfrac{1200 \text{ Calories}}{4 \text{ Calories/gm.}}$ / 300 gm.
         (d) This represents a dosage of 6 liters of 5% dextrose.
         (e) Although more concentrated solutions of glucose can be administered by the intravenous route, the rate of administration must be slow if loss in the urine is to be avoided.
         (f) It has been recommended that, in order to avoid glucosuria, glucose must not be administered intravenously at a rate which exceeds 1 gm. per kg. per hr.
   b. Fructose:
      (1) Has the same caloric value as glucose.
      (2) May be assimilated more rapidly than glucose, resulting in less loss in the urine.
   c. 10% invert sugar (half glucose, half fructose).
      (1) This sugar was administered to two 10 kg. beagles, at a total dose of 470 ml. One half of the solution was given in the first 15 minutes of therapy; the remaining half was administered during the following 30 minutes. It was found that:
         (a) About 80 per cent of the invert sugar was retained.
         (b) A slight positive balance of fluid existed.
      (2) Relation of this data to 24 hour caloric requirements.
         (a) From Figure 32-2 it is estimated that a 10 kg. dog requires about 575 Calories per day.
         (b) $\dfrac{575 \text{ Cal.}}{4 \text{ Cal./gm.}} = 140$ gm. of sugar
         (c) 470 ml. × 10% sugar × 80% retention = 38 gm. of sugar retained.
         (d) $\dfrac{140}{38} = 3$ to 4 daily administrations of 470 ml. of 10% invert sugar, to totally fulfill caloric requirements for a 10 kg. dog.
         (e) Administrations should be spaced throughout the day to facilitate a higher per cent of utilization and retention of the solutions.
   d. Ethanol.
      (1) Metabolism nets 5.6 Calories per gm.
      (2) Ethanol must be given slowly to prevent excessive CNS depression.
      (3) It is contraindicated in hepatic disease since most of the ethanol must be metabolized by the liver.

(4) Giving a combination of 5% dextrose, 5% alcohol has the following caloric advantage:
   5% alcohol + dextrose contains 450 Cal/L.
   5% dextrose contains   170 Cal/L.
e. Caloric therapy in renal disease.
   (1) In general, fluid therapy conducted for short intervals should emphasize correction of deficits or excesses of water and electrolytes.
      (a) A short-term negative caloric balance is less important than water and electrolyte imbalances.
      (b) Providing total caloric needs by the parenteral route is usually not feasible.
   (2) In uremic animals, there is an advantage in preventing catabolism of body protein as a source of calories, since nitrogenous products of protein catabolism contribute to uremia, and increase obligatory urine volume.
   (3) If osmotic diuresis is performed with 10% or 20% dextrose, some calories will be provided. Use of 5% dextrose, invert sugar, and alcohol will aid in preventing protein catabolism.
   (4) If the patient can tolerate oral medication, calories should be administered by the oral route.
      (a) Gavage may be required.
      (b) Commercial preparations high in calories may be used (see Chapter 31, Treatment of Renal Failure).
2. Amino acid therapy (parenteral).
   a. Most commercial preparations of amino acids are made from fibrin or casein that has been subjected to enzymatic or acid hydrolysis.
   b. Individual amino acids and some polypeptides are present in most products marketed.
   c. Requirements.
      (1) It is estimated that 2.0 mg. of nitrogen per Calorie per day is the basal requirement; growing animals may require five to 10 times this amount.
      (2) 2.0 mg. N × 6.25 (conversion factor) = 12.5 mg. of protein/Cal./day.
   d. Assimilation.
      (1) The patient should not be in a caloric deficit if the amino acids are to be incorporated into body protein.
      (2) If the patient has a caloric deficit, the amino acid will be deaminated and metabolized for energy.
      (3) Consequently it is necessary to provide adequate calories when giving amino acid solutions.
   e. Rate of administration.
      (1) Rapid administration of amino acids may cause nausea and vomiting.
      (2) Renal thresholds are present for amino acids. Rapid administration results in loss in urine.
      (3) In dogs, infusion of a daily dose in one to two hours generally will result in efficient utilization without side reactions.
   f. Calculation of dosage.

(1) 5% supplemented amino acid hydrolysates.*
   (a) These products contain 50 gm. of hydrolysate per liter, and are supplemented with amino acids to provide a balanced amino acid solution.
   (b) From Figure 32–2, it is apparent that an 18 kg. dog requires about 1200 Calories per day.
   (c) Protein requirements, therefore, are 1200 × 12.5 = 15,000 mg. = 15 gm.
   (d) This quantity (15 gm.) is supplied by 300 ml. of the protein hydrolysate.
(2) Some commercial veterinary products contain only a small quantity of amino acids. One product contains 290 mg. of amino acids per liter. It would require 50 liters of this product to provide daily requirements for a 20 kg. dog.
(3) Examine the label on the bottle to establish the amino acid content of the product.
f. Protein (amino acid) therapy in uremia.
   (1) Parenteral therapy with amino acid solutions is indicated when negative nitrogen balance exists.
   (2) In uremia, the patient frequently suffers from anorexia, vomiting, and diarrhea. Consequently a negative caloric balance exists.
   (3) Unless the caloric balance is restored prior to administration of amino acids, the amino acids will be metabolized as a source of energy. Production of nitrogen waste products will accentuate the uremia.
   (4) Non-nitrogen sources of calories should receive a high priority, and amino acid solutions should receive a low priority, when formulating fluid therapy for uremic patients. Unless the amino acids are incorporated into protein, they may do more harm to the uremic patient than good.
3. Lipid preparations.
   a. The theoretical advantage of high caloric value per unit volume exists, since lipids net about 9 Calories per gram.
   b. Some benefit may be derived from essential unsaturated fatty acids.
   c. Technical problems exist in manufacturing a stable preparation for parenteral use; therefore, parenteral lipid preparations are not commercially available in the United States at present.
   d. Oral administration of lipid preparations** by force feeding or gavage is an efficient method of supplying calories.

VIII. Routes and rates of fluid administration

A. Oral fluid administration
1. This is the route of choice except in cases of instantaneous need. Forced feeding or gavage may be used.
2. Advantages.
   a. Fluids may be rapidly administered without regard to their composition.

---

*Available as Aminosol, Abbott Laboratories, North Chicago, Illinois 60064, and Amigen, Baxter Laboratories, Morton Grove, Illinois 60053.
**Lipomul, The Upjohn Company, Kalamazoo, Michigan.

b. There is little likelihood of potential complications common to other routes of administration.
c. Sterility of preparations is unnecessary.
d. It is economical. Tap water, dog food, or commercial concentrates are cheaper than parenteral fluids.
e. Tonicity of the fluid is not critical.
f. This is the only route by which the total caloric needs of the patient are likely to be supplied.
3. Disadvantages.
a. Gastrointestinal disease (vomiting, diarrhea) may hinder or prevent use of this route.
b. Time required for absorption makes utilization slower as compared to parenteral routes.
c. Selective administration and precise control of dosage are difficult.
d. Some drugs may not be absorbed by the gastrointestinal tract.

B. *Intravenous fluid administration*
1. Advantages.
a. This is the fastest route for dispersion of solutions throughout the body.
b. Precise control of dosage is possible.
c. Within physiologic and pharmacologic limits, solutions can be used that differ from extracellular fluid in composition and tonicity.
2. Disadvantages.
a. It is time consuming.
b. A limited number of sites are available for administration of fluids.
c. Solutions must be sterile and pyrogen free.
d. There is a greater chance of side effects due to the rate of administration or the composition of the fluid.
3. Rate of intravenous fluid administration.
a. Rate of administration will depend on:
(1) Convenience in administration of the fluids. If the patient is cooperative, fluids may be administered slowly without constant supervision.
(2) Composition of the fluid. Solutions with a composition similar to extracellular fluid can be administered rapidly. Solutions containing high concentrations of potassium or calcium must be given slowly.
b. When fluids of extracellular composition must be administered rapidly, the following guide may be used.
(1) Use body weight as the guide for rate of administration.
(2) Assume that a fluid volume equal to blood volume can be administered in one hour.
(3) Estimate blood volume at 90 ml. per kg. of body weight.
(4) For example:
(a) A 3 kg. cat would receive fluids at the following rate:
3 kg. × 90 ml./kg. = 290 ml./hr. = 4.5 ml./minute.
(b) A 40 kg. dog would receive fluids at the following rate:
40 kg. = 90 ml./kg. = 3600 ml./hr. = 60 ml./minute.
(5) Regardless of the calculated rate, stop or decrease the rate of fluid administration if the patient demonstrates:

(a) Anxiety.
(b) A marked increase in heart rate, or an irregular cardiac rhythm.
(c) Shivering, shaking.
(d) Abnormal lung sounds suggestive of edema.
    (6) Revise the initial estimate downward if the patient has disease which predisposes to cardiovascular overload.
  c. Five per cent dextrose can usually be administered quite rapidly, but loss of glucose in the urine is minimized if it is administered slowly.
  d. Potassium must be administered slowly because of cardiotoxicity, and because renal excretion of this ion may be impaired in some renal diseases.

C. *Subcutaneous fluid administration*
  1. Advantages.
    a. It is less time consuming than intravenous therapy.
    b. The rate of administration is not critical.
    c. Slower absorption allows a greater margin of therapeutic error.
    d. Multiple sites are available for administration.
  2. Disadvantages.
    a. Only isotonic, nonirritating sterilized solutions may be utilized.
    b. Utilization is slower as compared to intravenous therapy.
    c. Fluids may not be absorbed if peripheral vascular perfusion is poor.
  3. Rate of administration. Rate is limited only by patient comfort and ability to absorb the fluid. Hyaluronidase may promote absorption.
  4. Site of injection.
    a. It is preferable to place the fluids over the dorsum so that absorption occurs as the fluids gravitate to the dependent portions of the body.
    b. Place the fluids over the thorax if a ventral abdominal incision is present, to avoid gravitation of the fluids to the suture line.
  5. Precaution on the administration of 5% dextrose subcutaneously.
    a. Injection of 5% dextrose can lead to transient electrolyte and water depletion. In cases where electrolyte depletion and hypovolemia already exist this may aggravate the condition.
    b. Mechanism:
      (1) Glucose diffuses more slowly than do electrolytes.
      (2) After injecting glucose subcutaneously, there is a diffusion of electrolytes and water into the 5% glucose pool to a point of equilibrium with extracellular fluid concentrations of the electrolytes. During this time further water and electrolyte depletion occurs. As glucose is reabsorbed, equilibrium is reestablished.

D. *Intraperitoneal route*
  1. This route is useful for dialysis in uremia (see Chapter 31, Treatment of Renal Failure).
  2. In all other situations, this route is of value only when rapid absorption is desired and the intravenous route cannot be utilized.
  3. Potential complications include peritonitis and injury to abdominal organs.

E. *Rectal route*
  1. Advantages.
     a. Simple.
     b. Rapid.
  2. Disadvantages.
     a. This route cannot be used if diarrhea is present.
     b. Even in the patient without diarrhea:
        (1) Absorption of water is unreliable.
        (2) Certain ions may be lost.
           (a) Potassium.
           (b) Bicarbonate.

F. *Intramedullary route (bone marrow cavity)*
  1. Advantages.
     a. Rapid absorption of fluid is possible.
     b. This route may be useful in treatment of patients in which a venipuncture cannot be made.
  2. Disadvantages.
     a. Potential for osteomyelitis exists.
     b. Administration of fluids by this route has been reported to be associated with pain in some instances.

REFERENCES

Bland, J. H.: Clinical Metabolism of Body Water and Electrolytes. Philadelphia, Pa., W. B. Saunders, Co., 1963.

Danowski, T. S., Greenman, L., Mateer, F. M., Parsons, W. B., Weigland, F. A., Mermelstein, H., and Peters, J. H.: Carboxylic cation exchange resin effects in dogs. J. Clin. Invest., *30*:984–994, 1951.

Hammond, P. B.: Drugs altering the fluid balance. *In* Veterinary Pharmacology and Therapeutics. 3rd edition. Edited by L. M. Jones. Ames, Iowa, Iowa State University Press, 1965.

Harrison, J. B., Sussman, H. H., and Pickering, D. E.: Fluid and electrolyte therapy in small animals. J.A.V.M.A., *137*:637–645, 1960.

Johnson, G., and Lamber, J.: Responses to fluid and electrolyte overloads. Ann. Surg., *167*:561–567, 1968.

Katsikas, J. L., and Goldsmith, C.: Disorders of potassium metabolism. Med. Clin. N. Amer., *55*:503–512, March, 1971.

Kaufman, C. F., and Kirk, R. W.: The utilization, excretion and diuretic effects of intravenously administered glucose, invert sugar, and fructose in the dog. J. Amer. Anim. Hosp. Assoc., *6*:252–259, Nov., 1970.

Pickering, D. E., and Fisher, D. A.: Fluid and Electrolyte Therapy: A Unified Approach. Portland, Oregon, Medical Research Foundation of Oregon, 1959.

Smith, C. R.: Fluid therapy. *In* Canine Medicine. 3rd edition. Santa Barbara, Calif., American Veterinary Publications, Inc., 1968.

Smith, C. R., Hamlin, R. L., and Powers, T. E.: Subcutaneous fluid therapy. J.A.V.M.A., *146*:1045–1048, May 15, 1965.

Tasker, J. B.: Fluids, electrolytes, and acid-base balance. *In* Clinical Biochemistry of Domestic Animals. Vol. 2. 2nd edition. Edited by J. J. Kaneko and C. E. Cornelius. New York, Academic Press, 1971.

Welt, L. G., Hollander, W., and Blythe, W. B.: The consequences of potassium depletion. J. Chronic Dis., *11*:213–254, 1960.

Whang, R., Reyes, R., Rogers, D., and Bryant, M.: Response of serum magnesium and potassium to glucose and insulin infusion in uremic dogs. Metabolism., *18*:439–443, 1969.

Wynn, V.: A metabolic study of acute water intoxication in man and dogs. Clin. Sci., *14*:669–680, 1955.

Zontine, W. J., and Donovan, M. L.: Effect of hypodermoclysis with dextrose in dogs. Amer. J. Vet. Res., *30*:605–609, April, 1969.

Chapter 33

DRUG THERAPY IN RENAL FAILURE

I. **Drugs are often administered to uremic dogs and cats without knowledge of the animals' normal metabolic pathways, and without knowledge of whether or not the drugs' pharmacologic action will be affected by the uremic state.**

It is likely that clinical deterioration of patients with renal failure is often attributed to progression of the underlying renal disease without considering the possibility that deterioration may be related, at least in part, to toxicity induced by administration of drugs.

II. **Since there are significant species differences in pathways of drug metabolism, determination of drug toxicity and major pathways of elimination of drugs from the body must be evaluated in the species in question.**

   A. *In human patients with renal failure, toxicity caused by administration of a variety of drugs at recommended therapeutic dosages has been well documented.*

   B. *Evaluation of drug metabolism in uremic dogs and cats has been virtually nonexistent.*

   C. *Extrapolation of data obtained by evaluation of drugs in one species for use in other species must be done with great caution.*

   D. *Quantitative comparisons between dosage, plasma concentration, and response of various drugs must be evaluated in uremic and nonuremic patients before the degree of toxicity can be defined and placed in perspective.*

III. **Pathogenesis of drug toxicity in renal failure**

   A. *The kidneys are the major route of excretion of active and metabolized drugs from the body. The liver is the major extrarenal site.*

   B. *Toxic manifestations of drugs may be enhanced in uremic patients by any one or a combination of the following:*
   1. Delayed renal excretion.
      a. Delayed clearance may be caused by:
         (1) Altered glomerular filtration.
         (2) Altered tubular reabsorption.
         (3) Altered tubular secretion.
      b. As a result of decreased renal clearance, substances normally eliminated from the body increase in concentration.

(1) Increase in plasma concentration of drug metabolites with no pharmacologic or biologic activity is of no significant clinical importance.
(2) The pharmacologic or biologic action of active metabolites may be intensified or prolonged.
 2. Reduced rate of metabolism.
 3. Altered sensitivity to pharmacologic activity.
   a. Increased sensitivity. In some species (man, rabbits, rats), renal failure enhances individual susceptibility to the effects of barbiturates. Metabolism of barbiturates is normal. It has been hypothesized that the increased sensitivity of uremic individuals to barbiturates is related to alteration in the "blood-brain" barrier or alteration in plasma protein binding capacity.
   b. Decreased sensitivity. Larger than normal doses of insulin are required in uremic human patients in order to achieve a therapeutic response. The decrease in sensitivity of uremic human beings to insulin is thought to be related to altered cellular sensitivity to insulin.

IV. Recommendations for drug therapy in patients with renal failure

A. *Modification of drug dosage may be accomplished in any of three ways.*
 1. Constant dose, varying interval method.
   a. Administer the normal recommended dose of the drug.
   b. Lengthen the interval between maintenance therapy.
   c. Because the plasma concentration of the drug may significantly vary during the period between maintenance dosage administration, this method of dosage should be used only when satisfactory response can be achieved in the presence of intermittent therapeutic concentrations of the drug (e.g., steroids).
 2. Varying dose, constant interval method.
   a. The drug should be administered at a dosage below that recommended for patients with normal renal function.
   b. The recommended interval between maintenance therapy should not be altered.
   c. Since this method reduces the variation in plasma concentration of the drug between maintenance therapy, it may be used with drugs that require a relatively constant plasma concentration to be effective.
 3. Varying dose, varying interval method.
   a. Administer the drug at a dosage below that recommended for normal renal function, but above that administered in the varying dose, constant interval method.
   b. Lengthen the interval between maintenance therapy.
   c. By using appropriate modifications of the constant dose, varying interval and varying dose, constant interval methods, the limitations inherent to each technique may be minimized.

B. *In man, dosage principles for administration of drugs to patients with renal failure have been formulated on the basis of knowledge of the serum half-life of drugs, and the degree of renal functional impairment of the patient.*

Clinical trials have revealed that, provided drug dosage is properly modified, many drugs can be given with relative safety.

C. *The following generalities recommended for dogs and cats with renal failure have*

TABLE 33-1. Major Route of Drug Excretion in Dogs and Cats

Drug	Route of Excretion
Chloramphenicol	Renal and hepatic
Erythromycin	Renal
Gentamicin	Renal
Kanamycin	Renal
Lincomycin	Renal
Neomycin	Renal
Nitrofurans	Renal
Penicillin	Renal
Polymyxin B	Renal
Streptomycin	Renal
Tetracycline	Renal
Tylosin	Renal and hepatic

Adapted from:
1. Jones, L. M.: Veterinary Pharmacology and Therapeutics. 3rd ed. Ames, Iowa, Iowa State University Press, 1965.
2. Manufacturers' description of drugs.
3. Wyman, J. B., Karlson, A., Wakim, K. G., and Cain, J. C.: Pancreatic, hepatic and renal excretion of antibiotics in dogs. Observations on erythromycin, lincomycin, kanamycin, and colistimethate excretion. Arch. Surg., 97:46–50, July, 1968.

been established on the basis of published reports of concepts related to drug toxicity associated with renal failure.

Because of the paucity of such information in the veterinary literature, some generalities have not been substantiated by experimental and clinical investigations in dogs and cats. The generalities are intended as guidelines only, and should not be interpreted as rigid facts.

1. The best cure is prevention.
   a. Avoid "shotgun therapy."
   b. Do not administer drugs to uremic patients unless there is a specific indication for their use.
2. In the absence of quantitative data about serum half-life and renal functional capacity, establish the main route of excretion of the drug (Table 33-1). Use the working hypothesis that drugs which are primarily excreted by the kidneys will accumulate to a variable degree in patients with renal failure. Therapeutic dosage levels may therefore be achieved by less frequent administrations or administration of smaller doses.
3. If the use of drugs that are primarily excreted by the kidneys is essential, carefully evaluate the patient for signs of toxicity known to be associated with the drugs. If the drug is potentially nephrotoxic, use serial evaluations of urinalyses and serum concentration of BUN or creatinine as indices of toxicity.
4. Selection of drugs for treatment of patients with renal failure should always be based on:
   a. The manufacturer's recommendations.
   b. Knowledge of reported toxic reactions which may be caused by the drug.
5. Avoid use of drugs which increase protein catabolism, including:
   a. Thyroid preparations.
   b. Corticosteroids.
   c. Tetracyclines.

(1) Tetracyclines have been found to induce uremia in normal human patients, and to potentiate uremia in patients with renal disease. Provided the drug is withdrawn, changes in patients without renal disease are usually reversible.

(2) The significance of tetracycline toxicity in dogs and cats has not been well documented.
   (a) Tetracycline has been incriminated in the production of renal disease in two dogs.
   (b) Experimental studies have revealed that tetracycline degradation products can produce azotemia in dogs.
   (c) Experimental studies have revealed that tetracycline can produce renal lesions in dogs.

(3) The pathogenesis of azotemia associated with administration of tetracyclines has not been well defined.
   (a) The significance of renal lesions associated with tetracycline administration has not been determined.
   (b) It has been hypothesized that, in high concentrations, tetracyclines exert an inhibiting effect on hepatic enzyme systems. Inability of the liver to synthesize amino acids into proteins results in metabolism of amino acids for energy. As a result, the concentration of nitrogenous waste products which must be excreted by the kidneys is increased.
   (c) Experimental studies in dogs and rats have revealed that osmotic diuretic agents have a protective effect on azotemia induced by tetracycline.

6. Avoid use of potentially nephrotoxic drugs if toxicity is related to the blood concentration of the drug. Some examples of these drugs are:
   a. Kanamycin.
   b. Neomycin.
   c. Vancomycin.
   d. Amphotericin B.
   e. Polymyxin B.
   f. Gentamicin.
   g. Bacitracin.

7. If use of drugs is absolutely imperative in terms of life of the patient, do not allow potential toxicity to interfere with choice of the most effective agent. If the alternative to using the drug is death, the risk is justified.

8. Selection of drugs for use in urinary tract infections because they are excreted in significant concentrations by the kidney should be carefully evaluated in patients with renal failure. Reduction in renal function may prevent effective concentrations of the drug in the urinary tract. For example, the concentrations of sulfas and nitrofurans in the urine of human patients with renal failure have been found to be too low to be of therapeutic value.

9. In man, normal therapeutic dosages of chloramphenicol may be given to patients with severe renal failure because extrarenal sites of excretion and inactivation exist.

10. Although the excretion of penicillin G is prolonged in human patients with renal failure, its slight toxicity allows normal therapeutic dosages to be administered to patients with severe uremia. Similar conclusions have been established in dogs and cats on the basis of empirical clinical observation.

11. Cardiac glycosides.
    a. Digoxin and other cardiac glycosides are excreted primarily by the kidneys in active and degraded form.
    b. Cardiac glycosides have a prolonged action in renal failure, and therefore maintenance dosages may have to be reduced accordingly.
12. Anesthetics and analgesics.
    a. Inhalant anesthetics are preferred in patients with renal failure because variables associated with drug metabolism and renal excretion are eliminated. They also have the advantage of permitting rapid change in depth of anesthesia and allowing rapid recovery following withdrawal.
    b. Halothane has been effectively used at the University of Minnesota to anesthetize uremic dogs and cats prior to renal biopsy. Although halothane causes a variable reduction in renal blood flow, it is apparently not nephrotoxic.
    c. Several reports have incriminated methoxyflurane anesthesia in the production of polyuric renal failure in man.
        (1) Polyuric renal failure following methoxyflurane anesthesia of obese human beings has been correlated with elevated levels of inorganic and organic fluoride-containing metabolites of methoxyflurane.
        (2) Precipitation of oxalate crystals in renal tubules and excretion of oxalate in urine have also been reported in patients who develop renal failure following methoxyflurane anesthesia.
        (3) Anesthesia of human patients with methoxyflurane is not consistently associated with detectable nephrotoxicity.
        (4) It has been hypothesized that rapid metabolism of a large quantity of this fat-soluble agent in obese patients for prolonged periods of time provides optimum circumstances for development of renal dysfunction.
        (5) The presence of a dose-response relationship, or factors in addition to methoxyflurane, in the development of tubular dysfunction has not been established.
        (6) The combined use of tetracycline and methoxyflurane in man has been reported to cause severe renal failure.
        (7) There have been no reports incriminating methoxyflurane as a cause of renal dysfunction in dogs and cats, nor have there been any reports which conclusively establish that it cannot be nephrotoxic.
    d. Medium- and short-acting barbiturates are primarily inactivated by the liver and can be given to uremic dogs and cats as a method of induction for inhalant anesthesia.
    e. If the patient is severely depressed, local or regional techniques of anesthesia should be considered.
    f. Ketamine should be used with caution in cats with renal failure since this drug is excreted in urine in active form. The use of this drug in uremic patients must be investigated before any definite statements can be made.

REFERENCES

Adriani, J.: The Pharmacology of Anesthetic Drugs. Springfield, Ill., Charles C Thomas, 1970.
Benitz, K. F., and Diermeier, H. F.: Renal toxicity of tetracycline degradation products. Proc. Soc. Exp. Biol. Med., *115*:930–935, 1964.

Blackmore, W. P., Erwin, K. W., Wiegand, O. F., and Lipsey, R.: Renal and cardiovascular effects of halothane. Anesthesiology, 21:489–495, 1960.
Byles, P. H., and Dukin, A. B.: The pharmacodynamics of methoxyflurane. In Textbook of Veterinary Anesthesia. Edited by L. R. Soma. Baltimore, Md., The Williams and Wilkins Co., 1971.
Cale, J. O., Parks, C. R., and Jenkins, M. T.: Hepatic and renal effects of methoxyflurane in dogs. Anesthesiology, 23:248–250, 1962.
Deutsch, S.: Anesthetic effects on the kidney. The Kidney, 4:1–6, 1971.
Domer, F. R.: Animal Experiments in Pharmacological Analysis. Chapter 19: Techniques for evaluation of drugs acting on the kidneys. Springfield, Ill., Charles C Thomas, 1971.
Frascino, J. A., Vanamee, P., and Rosen, P. P.: Renal oxalosis and azotemia after methoxyflurane anesthesia. New Eng. J. Med., 283:676–679, 1970.
Handley, C. A.: Changes in renal function produced by morphine in normal dogs with diabetes insipidus. J. Pharmacol. Exp. Ther., 99:33–37, 1950.
Klide, A. M., and Soma, L. R.: Epidural anesthesia in the dog and cat. J.A.V.M.A., 153:165–173, 1968.
Kunin, C. M.: Problems of drug therapy in renal failure. A guide to the use of antibiotics in patients with renal disease. Ann. Int. Med., 67:151–158, 1967.
Kuzucu, E. Y.: Methoxyflurane, tetracycline and renal failure. J.A.M.A., 211:1162–1164, 1970.
MacDonald, A. G.: The effect of halothane on renal cortical blood flow in normotensive and hypotensive dogs. Brit. J. Anesth., 41:644, 1969.
Marcus, F. I., Peterson, A., Salel, A., Scully, J., and Kapada, G. G.: The metabolism of tritiated digoxin in renal insufficiency in dogs and man. J. Pharmacol. Exper. Therap., 152:372–382, 1966.
Mathog, R. H., Thomas, W. G., Hudson, W. R., and Durhan, N. C.: Ototoxicity of new and potent diuretics. Acta Otolaryngal., 92:7–13, 1970.
Mazze, R. I., Shue, G. L., and Jackson, S. H.: Renal dysfunction with methoxyflurane. J.A.M.A., 216:278, 1971.
Merkle, R. B., McDonald, F. D., Waldman, J., Maynard, G. D., Fleming, P. J., and Murray, W. J.: Renal function after methoxyflurane anesthesia. J.A.M.A., 218:841–844, 1971.
Pan, S. Y., Scadute, L., and Callen, M.: Pharmacology of terramycin in experimental animals. Ann. N. Y. Acad. Sci., 53:238, 1950.
Panner, B. J.: Toxicity following methoxyflurane anesthesia. I. Clinical and pathological observations in two fatal cases. J.A.M.A., 214:86–90, 1970.
Papper, S., and Papper, E. M.: The effect of preanesthetic, anesthetic and post operative drugs on renal function. Clin. Pharmacol. Ther., 5:205–215, 1964.
Polec, R. B., Yeh, S. D. J., and Shils, M. E.: Protective effect of ascorbic acid, iso-ascorbic acid and mannitol against tetracycline induced nephrotoxicity (in dogs). J. Pharmacol. Exp. Ther., 178:152–158, 1971.
Reidenberg, M. M.: Renal Function and Drug Action. Philadelphia, Pa., W. B. Saunders Co., 1971.
Sedwitz, J., Bateman, J. C., and Klopp, C. T.: Oxytetracycline studies in dogs. Antibiotics & Chemotherapy. 3:1015–1019, 1953.
Soma, L. R.: Textbook of Veterinary Anesthesia. Baltimore, Md., The Williams and Wilkins Co., 1971.
Taves, D. R., Freeman, R. B., and Gillies, A. J.: Fluoride concentrations in nephrotoxicity. J.A.M.A., 214:91–95, 1970.
Theye, R. A., and Maher, F. T.: The effects of halothane on canine renal function and oxygen consumption. Anesthesiology., 35:54–60, 1971.
Westermark, L., and Wahlin, A.: Blood circulation in the kidney of the cat under halothane anesthesia. Acta Anaesth. Scand., 13:185–208, 1969.
Wyman, J. B., Karlson, A., Wakim, K. G., and Cain, J. C.: Pancreatic, hepatic and renal excretion of antibiotics in dogs. Observations on erythromycin, lincomycin, kanamycin, and colistimethate excretion. Arch. Surg., 97:46–50, 1968.

DISEASES OF THE UPPER AND LOWER URINARY SYSTEM

Chapter 34
UROLITHIASIS

I. **Composition of uroliths**
   A. *Knowledge of the composition of uroliths is of clinical significance because prognosis and choice of prophylactic procedures are dependent upon composition.*
   B. *On the basis of mineral content, uroliths may be divided into four general categories.*
   1. Phosphate uroliths.
      a. Sixty to 90 per cent of all uroliths in dogs are composed of phosphates.
      b. Usually these uroliths are yellow to white, fairly hard, and yield a chalklike powder when crushed.
      c. Usually they are radiopaque.
      d. The uroliths are composed of varying amounts of Mg^{++}, NH_4^+, and Ca^{++} together with phosphate. Because of composition, such phosphates are commonly referred to as "triple phosphates."
   2. Urate uroliths.
      a. Prevalence varies with different surveys, but they comprise about 10 per cent of all uroliths in dogs.
      b. Usually these uroliths are yellow in color, brittle, and have concentric eggshell-like laminations.
      c. Often they are radiotranslucent.
      d. The uroliths are composed of NH_4 urate.
   3. Cystine uroliths.
      a. Prevalence varies with different surveys, but they comprise about five per cent of all uroliths in dogs.
      b. These uroliths are creamy yellow and smooth, and can be easily crushed.
      c. Often they are radiotranslucent.
      d. Cystine uroliths are composed of the amino acid cystine.
   4. Oxalate uroliths.
      a. Prevalence varies with different surveys, but they probably comprise about 10 per cent of all uroliths in dogs.
      b. These uroliths are very hard and brittle. The edges of sharp crystals often protrude from the surface.
      c. Usually they are radiopaque.
      d. The uroliths are composed of calcium oxalate.
   C. *Urolithiasis also occurs in the cat but is far less common than in the dog.*
   Debris obstructing the urethra of male cats is not organized as are uroliths. Thus the term urolithiasis does not accurately describe this condition (see cystitis—urethral obstruction complex in the cat). Most uroliths in cats occur in females, and are composed of phosphates.
   D. *Many uroliths that are predominantly of one type of mineral will have traces of another type of mineral.*
   For example, urate calculi frequently have traces of phosphates.

E. *Most uroliths contain an organic matrix which is located between layers of inorganic material.*

This matrix is mucoprotein.

F. *Commercial kits* are available for analysis of uroliths.*

II. Etiology

A. *Numerous theories concerning urolith formation have been proposed, but none has been completely accepted.*

The etiology is probably not the same for different types of uroliths.

B. *Predisposing factors may be important in urolith formation.*

However, definition of predisposing factors has not adequately explained the etiology since such factors do not always cause urolithiasis. For example:
1. Cystine uroliths probably occur only in dogs with cystinuria, but not all dogs with cystinuria develop cystine uroliths.
2. Ammonium urate uroliths occur predominantly in the dalmatian, and are probably related to this breed's high rate of excretion of uric acid. Many dalmatians, however, excrete large amounts of uric acid and do not develop urate uroliths.

C. *The following generalizations regarding etiology may be modified when more precise information is obtained.*
1. Phosphate uroliths are often associated with alkaline urine. Since infection frequently causes urine to become alkaline, infection has been assumed to play a significant role in the etiology, or the growth, of phosphate uroliths.
2. Urate uroliths have been associated with the hereditary trait of dalmatian dogs to excrete large quantities of uric acid in urine. They are occasionally found in other breeds that excrete large amounts of uric acid.
3. Cystine uroliths occur in dogs with cystinuria. Uroliths composed of cystine have been found in many breeds including the dachshund, Welsh corgi, Irish terrier, chihuahua, Scottish terrier, Labrador retriever, bulldog, German shepherd, boxer, poodle, cairn terrier, cocker spaniel, bassett, Shetland collie, and mongrel breed.
4. Urine stasis is a predisposing factor to urolith formation regardless of mineral type.
5. Vitamin A deficiency plays no established role in urolith formation in the dog.

III. Breed, sex, and site predilection of urolithiasis

A. *Breed predilection*
1. Uroliths are more common in chondrodystrophied breeds (e.g., cocker spaniel, dachshund, Pekingese).
2. Cystine uroliths have frequently been reported in male Welsh corgis and dachshunds.
3. Dalmatians are predisposed to urate uroliths.
4. Boxers, German shepherds, and Labrador retrievers may be more resistant to the formation of uroliths than other breeds.

---

*Oxford Stone Analysis Set for Urinary Calculi, Oxford Laboratories, 1149 Chess Drive, Foster City, California 94404.

B. *Sex predilection.*

Except for the following, each sex appears to be affected equally.
1. Cystine uroliths have been reported exclusively in male dogs.
2. Urate uroliths have been reported more frequently in male dogs.
3. Phosphate uroliths are reported more frequently in female dogs.

C. *Site predilection*
1. Uroliths are predominantly located in the bladder and urethra in dogs. In man, however, uroliths are primarily located in the kidneys and ureters.
2. Cystine, urate, and oxalate uroliths are most frequently found in the urethra of male dogs.
3. Phosphate uroliths are more frequently found in the urinary bladder of female dogs.

IV. Clinical history

A. *As a generality, urolithiasis is observed in dogs with a mean age of about 6 years.*

Dogs from a few weeks to 16 years of age, however, have been affected with urolithiasis.

B. *The history is dependent upon the location of the urolith.*
1. Urethral uroliths in male dogs may be associated with:
   a. Dysuria or anuria.
   b. A distended or turgid abdomen.
   c. Signs of uremia, which occur if urine flow has been obstructed for a sufficient period of time (approximately 48 hours).
2. Bladder uroliths.
   a. Bladder uroliths may be detected on routine physical examination of patients with no signs having been observed by the owner.
   b. They are usually associated with clinical signs similar to those of cystitis.

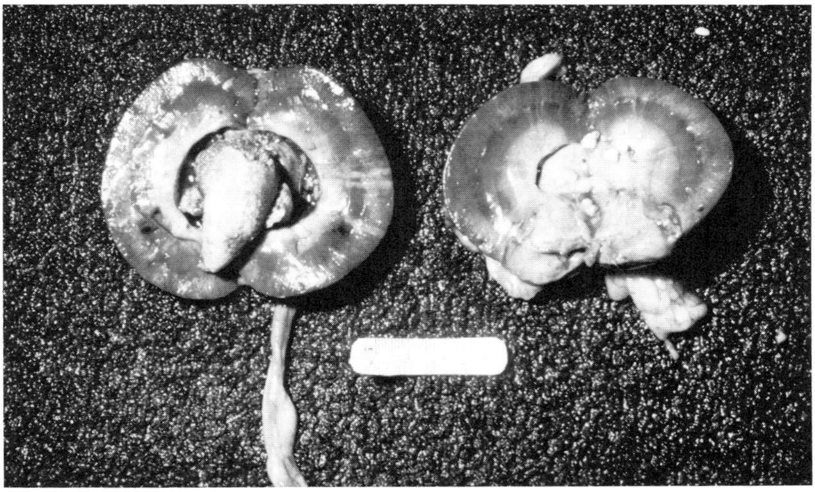

Figure 34-1. Multiple phosphate renoliths in the renal pelves of a 7-year-old female dachshund dog. Microscopic examination of sections of kidney revealed the presence of chronic generalized pyelonephritis. (Courtesy of Dr. Kenneth H. Johnson, College of Veterinary Medicine, University of Minnesota.)

322 DISEASES OF THE UPPER AND LOWER URINARY SYSTEM

(1) Hematuria is common and frequently is more severe at the end of micturition.
(2) Micturition is usually characterized by frequent passage of small amounts of urine (dysuria).
3. Renal uroliths.
   a. During the early stages of formation of renoliths, clinical signs may be absent.
   b. Extensive pyelitis or pyelonephritis associated with renoliths may cause depression, anorexia, hematuria, and reluctance of the patient to move (Fig. 34–1).
   c. Signs of uremia may be present in cases of bilateral renolithiasis associated with loss of the functional capacity of at least three fourths of the nephrons.

V. **Findings detected during physical examination are dependent on the location of calculi.**

   A. *Urethral uroliths (male)*
   1. Signs of uremia may be present.
   2. A tense, distended abdomen may occur as a result of distention of the urinary bladder.
   3. Uroliths may be palpable in that portion of the urethra posterior to the penis.
   4. Persistent dribbling of urine may occur.

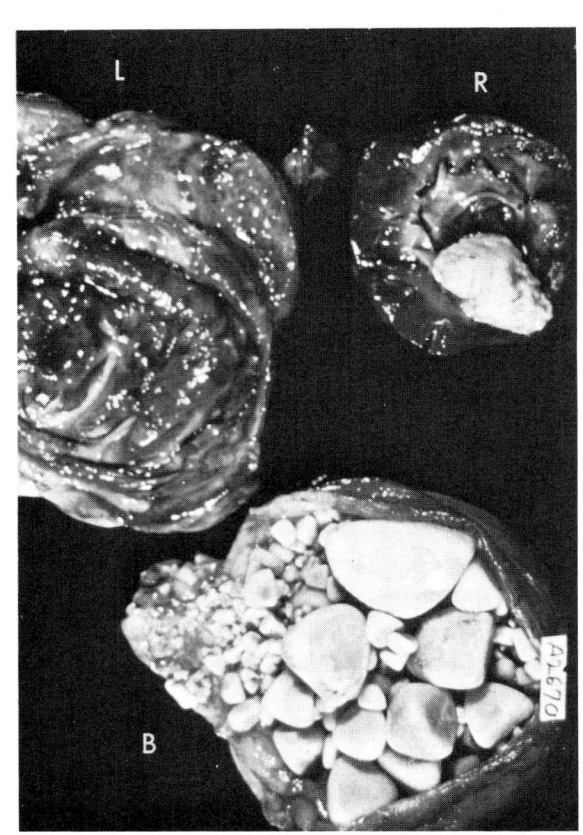

Figure 34–2. Advanced pyonephrosis of the left kidney (*L*), less advanced pyonephrosis and nephrolithiasis of the right kidney (*R*), and cystic calculi in an 11-year-old female mixed breed dog. The urinary bladder (*B*) contained more than 500 calculi, and calculi obstructed the left and right ureters. Numerous calculi were passed during micturition. The dog died as a result of chronic renal failure.

B. *Bladder uroliths*
1. Uroliths may be palpable. Abdominal palpation may reveal:
   a. A firm nonyielding mass in the bladder if a solitary urolith is present.
   b. A grating feeling confined to the bladder if multiple uroliths are present.
2. Usually no other findings detected by physical examination are specifically related to cystoliths.

C. *Renal uroliths*
1. In the absence of infection, abnormalities are usually not detectable unless bilateral renoliths are associated with sufficient renal damage to cause uremia.
2. If infection is present, there may be:
   a. Pain in the area of the kidneys.
   b. Palpable enlargement of the affected kidney(s).

D. *When uroliths are present in multiple sites, combinations of the above signs may occur* (Fig. 34-2).

VI. A diagnosis of urolithiasis may be based on typical findings of the:

A. *History*

B. *Physical examination*
1. One should suspect the presence of urethral uroliths in male dogs when urethral catheters cannot be passed into the bladder. The latter may also be associated with urethral strictures or space occupying lesions which partially or totally occlude the urethral lumen.
2. One should suspect the presence of cystic uroliths if during catheterization with a metal catheter, grating of the catheter against calculi is detected. Extreme caution must be used to prevent damage to the urethra or bladder with metal catheters.
3. The diagnosis may frequently be established on the basis of palpation alone. Palpation per rectum should be performed to detect uroliths in the bladder neck or proximal urethra.

C. *Urinalysis.*

Findings detected by urinalysis are often consistent with bacterial cystitis (see Urinalysis, in Chapter 6).

D. *Radiography (see Chapter 8, Radiographic Evaluation of the Urinary System)*

Radiographic evaluation of the urinary tract is indicated when cystitis fails to respond to antibiotic therapy, or recurs following discontinuation of therapy, in order to eliminate the presence of cystic uroliths (Figs. 34-3 and 34-4).

VII. Treatment

A. *Urethral obstruction*
1. If obstruction of the urethra has been present for a sufficient period of time, the patient may be in poor physical condition due to postrenal

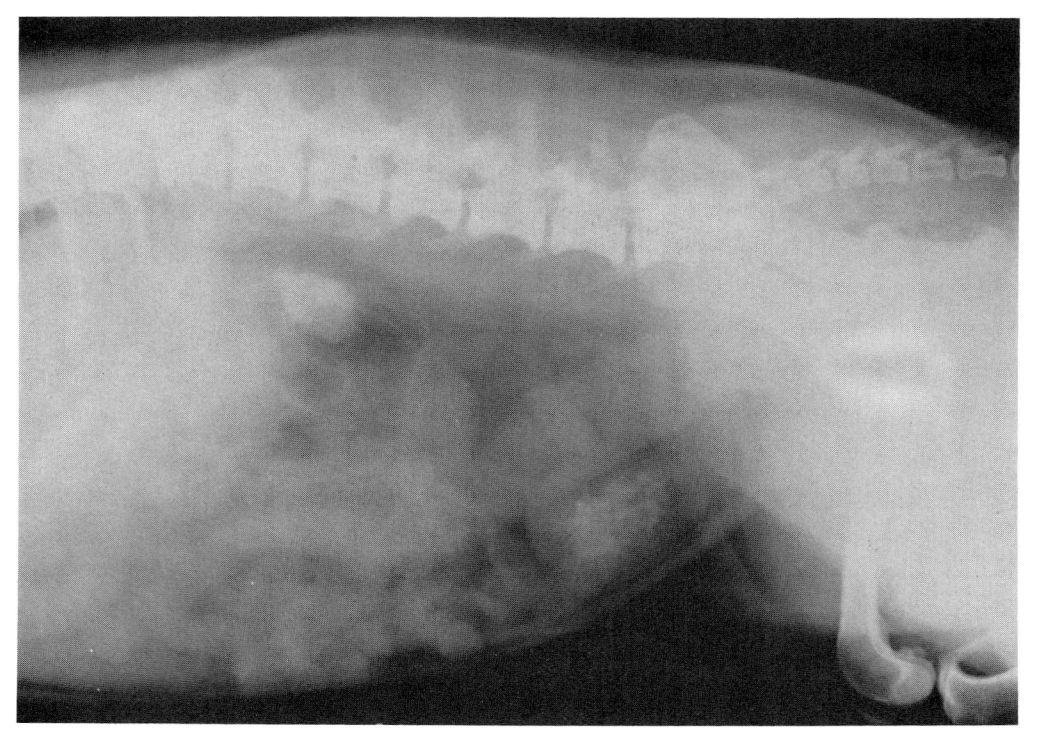

Figure 34–3. Survey radiograph of the abdomen of a 3-year-old female Pekingese dog. A solitary urolith is present in the left kidney and multiple uroliths are present in the urinary bladder.

uremia. Under these circumstances, treatment must be aimed at reestablishing urine flow.
2. Urethral uroliths may be removed by any one of several nonsurgical techniques.
   a. If obstruction is encountered when attempting to catheterize a patient, a catheter of smaller diameter may be used in attempt to bypass the urolith. The catheter may be allowed to remain in the bladder until the patient's physical condition improves sufficiently to permit removal of the urolith.
   b. Urethral uroliths may be pushed back into the bladder with the aid of a catheter.
      (1) The diameter of the catheter selected for use should be as large as is consistent with atraumatic technique.
      (2) The catheter should be liberally coated with sterilized water soluble lubricant.
      (3) A mixture composed of 1 part sterilized water soluble lubricant and 1 part sterilized water should be injected through the catheter as the urolith is being advanced toward the urinary bladder. This mixture will lubricate the urethral mucosa, which is often inflamed and swollen, and will tend to flush uroliths ahead of the catheter.
      (4) Care must be used not to traumatize the urethra while performing this procedure. Excessive force must not be used.

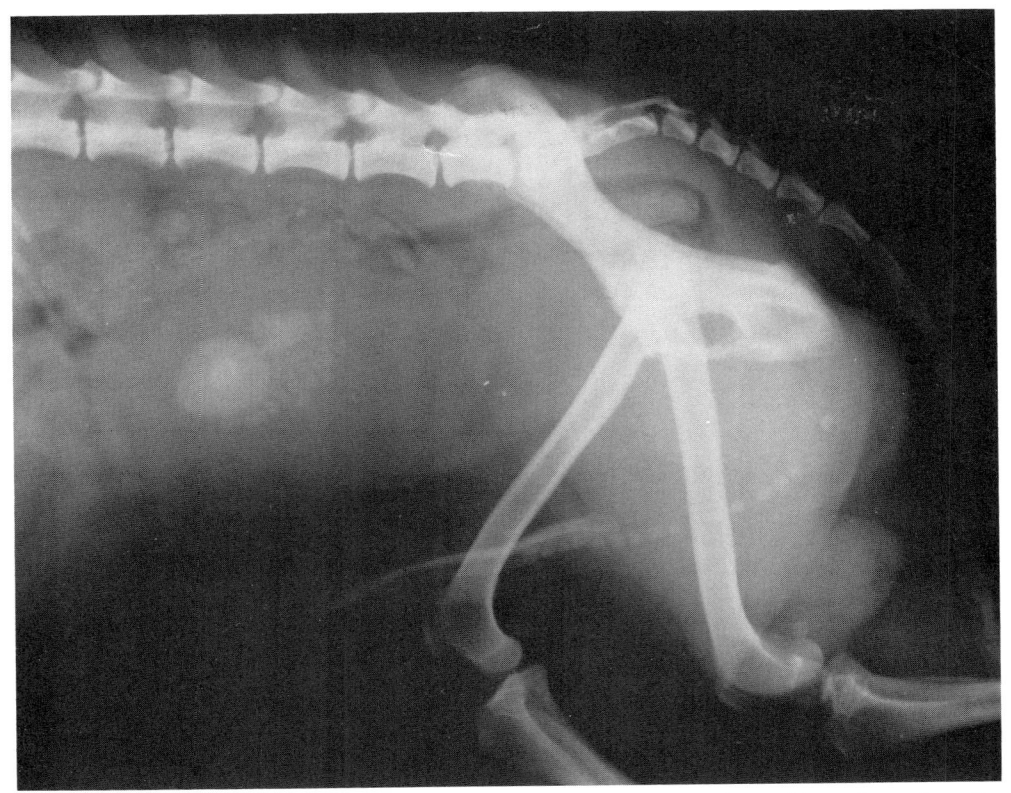

Figure 34–4. Abdominal radiograph of a 7-year-old male chihuahua with cystic and urethral calculi. The wall of the urinary bladder is markedly thickened. (J.A.V.M.A., *159*:1755–1757, 1971.)

    c. Uroliths lodged in the urethra of male dogs can frequently be removed by dilating a portion of the urethra with fluid under pressure. Sudden release of the pressure will be followed by forceful movement of the fluid, and often urethral uroliths, in the direction of decreased pressure (hydropropulsion).
      (1) To perform this technique, a large volume syringe (20 to 35 ml.), a sterilized bovine teat cannula, and sterilized water or physiologic saline solution are required.
      (2) Depending on the condition of the patient, sedation or general anesthesia may be required. If the patient is uremic, topical application of 2% lidocaine gel* to the urethral mucosa in combination with parenteral administration of tranquilizers may be adequate.
      (3) First, a liberal quantity of dilute, sterilized lubricant should be injected through a catheter into the urethral lumen adjacent to the urolith.
      (4) An assistant should then occlude the lumen of the pelvic urethra by applying digital pressure against the ischium through the ventral wall of the rectum (Fig. 34–4).
      (5) Next a bovine teat cannula, with attached syringe loaded with

---

*Anestacon, Conal Pharmaceuticals, Chicago, Illinois 60640

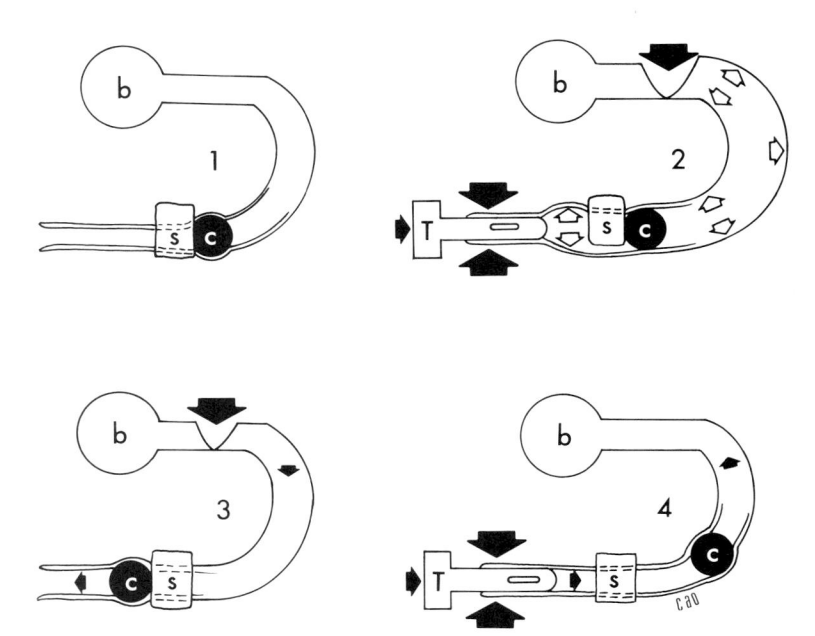

Figure 34-5. Schematic drawings illustrating removal of urethral calculi with the aid of fluid under pressure: **1,** Diagram of urethral calculus lodged behind os penis; **2,** diagram illustrating dilatation of urethral lumen by injecting fluid under pressure. Pressure applied to the external urethral orifice and the pelvic urethra (large black arrows) has created a closed system. **3,** diagram illustrating sudden release of digital pressure at the external urethral orifice and subsequent movement of fluid and calculus toward the external urethral orifice; **4,** diagram illustrating sudden release of digital pressure at the pelvic urethra and subsequent movement of fluid and calculus toward the bladder. *b,* Urinary bladder; *s,* os penis; *c,* calculus; *T,* teat cannula (J.A.V.M.A., *159*:1755–1757, 1971.)

saline, should be placed into the penile urethra via the external orifice.

(6) The external urethral orifice should then be compressed around the teat cannula by digital pressure. In this fashion, a portion of the urethra from the external urethral orifice to the bony pelvis becomes a closed system.

(7) Saline should then be injected into the urethra until a definite rebound is perceived through the syringe plunger. This should cause a palpable increase in the diameter of the pelvic urethra (Fig. 34–5).

(8) Next, the teat cannula should be removed and pressure applied to the external urethral orifice should be rapidly released to permit rapid and forceful expulsion of saline out of the urethra. If the uroliths are small enough to pass through the distended portion of the cavernous urethra which is located in the ventral groove of the penis, they will be moved toward the external urethral orifice (Fig. 34–5).

(9) It is often necessary to repeat the procedure more than once in order to expel all uroliths from the urethra.

(10) If the urethral uroliths are too large to pass through the ventral groove of the os penis, the procedure should be modified. Instead of releasing pressure applied to the external urethral orifice, pressure applied to the pelvic urethra should be rapidly released.

In this fashion the saline will be forcibly advanced into the urinary bladder, and will often carry uroliths with it (Fig. 34–5).
- (11) If it is necessary to repeat the procedure more than once to remove all the uroliths from the urethra, it may be advantageous to alternate with both variations of the technique.
3. Urethral uroliths may be removed by surgical techniques.
   a. Urethrotomy should be considered to provide temporary relief of urethral obstruction when nonsurgical treatment is unsuccessful.
   b. Urethrostomy should be considered when prophylactic therapy of urolithiasis is not feasible or is unsuccessful. This technique will prevent normal ejaculation, and therefore may be contraindicated in dogs to be used for natural breeding.
   c. Consult veterinary surgical textbooks for specific details about the techniques of urethrostomy and urethrotomy.
4. If patients with obstructive uropathy are poor surgical risks due to severe postrenal uremia, decompression of the bladder should be accomplished by periodic cystocentesis (see cystocentesis in Chapter 5). Cystocentesis should be repeated until the condition of the patient will permit surgical intervention.

B. *Cystolithiasis, nephrolithiasis and ureterolithiasis*
1. In dogs and cats, surgical removal remains the treatment of choice for uroliths in the urinary bladder, ureters and kidneys. Consult veterinary surgical textbooks for specific details about the techniques of cystotomy, nephrotomy and ureterotomy.
2. Clinical trials have revealed that certain drugs may be of value in dissolving uroliths in man, but the efficacy of these drugs in dogs and cats has not been established.
   a. Allopurinol* has been used to dissolve uric acid uroliths in man.
   b. Although Methylene blue has been used to dissolve uroliths in man, clinical trials must be conducted prior to its use in nonhuman species. Methylene blue may cause hemolytic anemia in the cat.

VIII. Prophylaxis.

A. *Surgical removal of uroliths is followed by recurrence in 10 to 20 per cent of the cases.*

For this reason, prophylactic procedures should be initiated in all patients that have had uroliths.

B. *The type of prophylactic treatment used is dictated by the mineral composition of the urolith.*
1. Phosphate uroliths.
   a. Phosphate uroliths are usually associated with infection and alkaline urine.
   b. Surgical removal of phosphate uroliths is a necessary prerequisite to elimination of urinary tract infection. Effective eradication of infection is essential for prophylaxis of phosphate uroliths. (see Treatment of bacterial cystitis, in Chapter 38).
   c. Polydipsia and polyuria induced by oral administration of NaCl may be of value.

---

*Zyloprim, Burroughs Wellcome and Co., Research Park Triangle, North Carolina.

(1) The dosage for the dog is 1 to 10 Gm. of salt per day, given in divided doses.

(2) Polyuria dilutes minerals and decreases the opportunity for crystallization.

2. Urate uroliths.
   a. Induce polydipsia and polyuria, and if necessary, alkalinize the urine by administration of $NaHCO_3$ and NaCl. Strive to double the urine volume, and keep the urine pH above 6.5.
   b. Eliminate urinary tract infection if present (see treatment of bacterial cystitis, in Chapter 38).
   c. In instances of recurrence, the use of allopurinol may be considered. This drug has been found to have prophylactic value in some human patients who have a history of recurrent uric acid urolith formation. Clinical studies concerning the use of this drug in dogs are underway. Pertinent points concerning allopurinol are:
      (1) It inhibits conversion of hypoxanthine to xanthine, and xanthine to uric acid. A decrease in urinary excretion of uric acid, but an increase in excretion of hypoxanthine and xanthine may occur.
      (2) It is used in man at a dosage of 200 to 400 mg. daily. Although a precise dose for dogs has not been established, 30 mg. per kg. per day in divided doses has resulted in a decrease in uric acid excretion in the urine of the dog.
      (3) Several side-effects of drug use have been noted in humans. Consult the manufacturer's recommendations for details.
      (4) Indefinite use is necessary if a prophylactic effect is to be maintained.
      (5) Xanthine urolith formation is a potential complication in dogs treated with the drug.
   d. Do not administer urinary acidifiers, since urates are less soluble at a low pH and in the presence of NH_4^+.
   e. The efficacy of a low purine diet in the prevention of urate uroliths in the dog is debatable. Theoretically, a low purine diet (milk, cheese, and muscle, instead of glandular organs) should decrease urate excretion. The value of such diets in reducing the recurrence of urate uroliths has not been documented, but neither has it been proved to be without value.

3. Cystine uroliths.
   a. Induce polydipsia and polyuria, and if necessary alkalinize the urine by administration of $NaHCO_3$ and NaCl. Strive to double the urine volume and keep the urine pH above 7.5.
   b. Eliminate urinary tract infection, if present (see Chapter 38, Bacterial Cystitis).
   c. Consider the use of D-penicillamine* for recurrent cystine urolith formation. This drug:
      (1) Combines with one-half the cystine molecule (cysteine) and decreases urinary excretion of the less soluble cystine.
      (2) Has been reported to be of prophylactic value following use in two dachshunds.
      (3) Must be used indefinitely to maintain its prophylactic effect.

---
*Cuprimine, Merck, Sharp and Dohme, West Point, Pa.

(4) May cause vomiting in the dog. It causes many side-effects in man, including skin rash, fever, and arthralgia.
    d. Do not administer urinary acidifiers, especially methionine, since low urine pH enhances cystine precipitation and methionine administered orally may increase cystine excretion.
4. Oxalate calculi.
    a. Induce polydipsia and polyuria by administering NaCl.
    b. Eliminate urinary tract infection if present (see Chapter 38, Bacterial Cystitis).

REFERENCES

Appleman, R. M., Hallenbeck, G. A., and Shorter, R. G.: Effect of reciprocal allogenic renal transplantation between dalmatian and non-dalmatian dogs on urinary excretion of uric acid. Proc. Soc. Exp. Biol. Med., *121*:1084–1097, 1966.

Bovee, K. C.: Cystinuria and cystine calculi. *In* Current Veterinary Therapy. Vol. 4. Edited by R. W. Kirk. Philadelphia, Pa., W. B. Saunders Co., 1971.

Beeler, M. F., Veith, D. A., Morriss, R. H., and Biskind, G. R.: Analysis of urinary calculi: Comparison of methods. Am. J. Clin. Path., *41*:553–560, 1964.

Brodey, R. S.: Canine urolithiasis. A survey and discussion of 52 clinical cases. J.A.V.M.A., *126*:1–9, 1955.

Chernesky, S. J. K., and Cawley, A. J.: Successful surgical treatment of bilateral renal calculi in a dog. Canad. Vet. J., 7:18–22, 1966.

Clark, W. T.: A study of the amino acids in urine from dogs with cystine urolithiasis. Vet. Rec., *88*:414–417, 1971.

Cornelius, C. E., Bishop, J. A., and Schaffer, M. H.: A quantitative study of amino aciduria in dachshunds with a history of cystine urolithiasis. Cornell Vet., *57*:177–183, 1967.

Duncan, H., and Curtiss, A. S.: Observations on uric acid transport in man, the dalmatian and the non-dalmatian dog. Henry Ford Hosp. Med. J., *19*:105–114, 1971.

Finco, D. R.: Current status of canine urolithiasis. J.A.V.M.A., *158*:327–335, 1971.

Finco, D. R., Kurtz, H. J., and Porter, T. E.: Renal and ureteral urolithiasis in a dog. J.A.V.M.A., *157*:837–840, 1970.

Finco, D. R., Rosin, E., and Johnson, K. H.: Canine urolithiasis: A review of 133 clinical and 23 necropsy cases. J.A.V.M.A., *157*:1225–1228, 1970.

Frimpter, G. W., Thouin, P., and Ewalds, B. H.: Penicillamine in canine cystinuria. J.A.V.M.A., *151*:1084–1086, 1967.

Gordon, N.: Surgical anatomy of the prostate gland, bladder, and urethra in the male dog. J.A.V.M.A., *136*:215–221, 1960.

Gourley, I. M. G., Leighton, R. L., and Swanwick, P. M.: Surgical procedures for nephrotomy and ureterotomy in the dog. Pract. Vet., *43*:11–22, 1971.

Haugh, I., Lonsdale, K., and Mason, P.: Crystallography and calculi. J. Sm. Anim. Pract., *7*:565–570, 1966.

Jackson, O. F., and Sutor, D. J.: Ammonium acid urate calculus in a cat with a high uric acid excretion possibly due to renal tubular reabsorption defect. Vet. Rec., *151*:335–337, 1970.

Kidder, D. E., and Chivers, P. R.: Xanthine calculi in a dog. Vet. Rec., *83*:228–229, 1968.

Medway, W., Archibald, J., and Bishop, E. J.: Canine renal disorders. IV. Nephrolithiasis. No. Amer. Vet., *36*:125–128, 1955.

Osbaldiston, G. W., and Lowrey, J. L.: Allopurinol in the prevention of hyperuricemia in dalmatian dogs. Vet. Med/S.A.C., *66*:711–715, 1971.

Piermattei, D. L., and Osborne, C. A.: Nonsurgical removal of urethral calculi from male dogs. J.A.V.M.A., *159*:1755–1757, 1971.

Weaver, A. D.: Canine urolithiasis: Incidence, chemical composition and outcome of 100 cases. J. Sm. Anim. Pract., *11*:83–92, 1970.

Weaver, A. D.: Surgical treatment of bilateral renal calculi in a bitch. J. Sm. Anim. Pract., *12*:319–325, 1971.

White, E. G., and Porter, P.: Urinary calculi. *In* A Textbook of Veterinary Clinical Pathology. Edited by W. Medway, J. E. Prier, and J. S. Wilkinson. Baltimore, Md., The Williams and Wilkins Co., 1969.

White, E. G., Treacher, R. J., Jolly, D. W., Worden, A. N., Clark, W. T., Goulden, B. E., Haugh, I., Lonsdale, K., and Mason, P.: Symposium on urolithiasis in the dog. J. Sm. Anim. Pract., *7*:529–570, 1966.

Chapter 35
DISEASES OF THE URETER

I. As a generality, the ureters are not commonly affected by primary diseases.

When the ureters are affected by disease processes, the primary abnormality usually is present in the urinary bladder or kidneys. Signs of ureteral disease usually cannot be distinguished from, or are overshadowed by, signs related to the underlying abnormality.

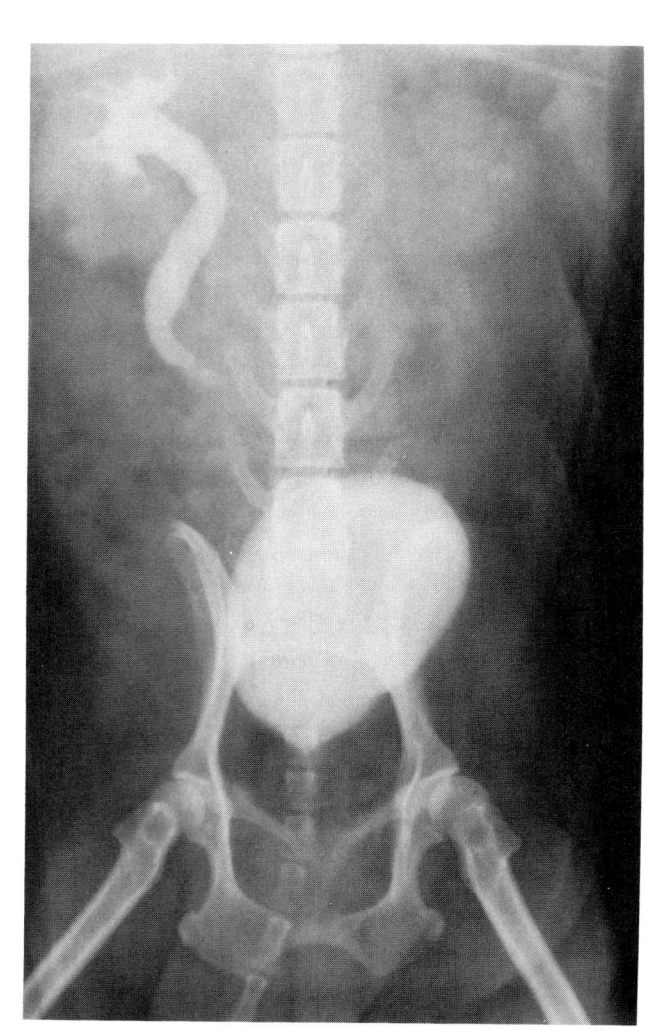

Figure 35-1. Intravenous urogram of a 6.5-year-old female English pug dog. Obstruction of the right ureter with a urolith has resulted in dilatation of the renal pelvis and ureter proximal to the site of obstruction. (J.A.V.M.A., *157*:837–840, 1970.)

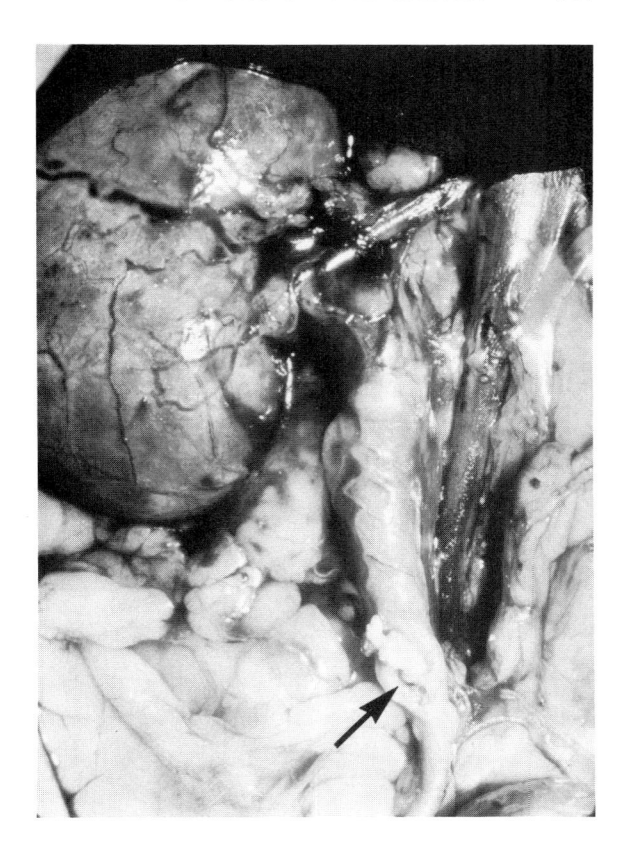

Figure 35-2. Urolith in the right ureter of a 6½-year-old female English pug dog. The ureter has been incised to demonstrate the urolith (arrow). (J.A.V.M.A., *157*:837–840, 1970.)

II. Obstructive ureteropathy

A. *The ureters may be occluded by:*
1. Intrinsic disease processes.
   a. Calculi (Figs. 35-1 and 35-2).
   b. Neoplasms.
   c. Blood clots.
2. Extrinsic disease processes.
   a. Abdominal neoplasms that impinge upon one or both ureters.
   b. Ligation of a ureter during abdominal surgery.
   c. Displacement of the urinary bladder.

B. *The significance of obstructive ureteropathy is the effect that it has upon the kidney(s) (see Chapter 22, Hydronephrosis).*

C. *Although obstruction of the ureters is usually unilateral, it may be bilateral.*
1. Bilateral obstruction usually occurs as a result of lesions at the trigone of the urinary bladder.
2. Bilateral ureteral obstruction may precipitate a uremic crisis.
3. Unilateral ureteral obstruction is usually not an immediate threat to life since uremia does not occur. Severe hydronephrosis may develop.

D. *Clinical Findings*
1. Bilateral obstruction of the ureter will be associated with signs of renal failure.

2. Abdominal palpation may reveal enlargement of one or both kidneys if the patient has survived for a sufficient period of time.
3. Increase in renal size may be noted on survey radiographs, while dilated renal pelves and ureters are typical findings on intravenous urograms.

E. *Treatment must be directed toward elimination of the cause of obstruction and restoration of renal function.*

This may be difficult or impossible, depending on the nature of the underlying cause and the degree of nephron obstruction that has occurred (see Chapter 22, Hydronephrosis).

F. *Prognosis is dependent on the likelihood of successful treatment of the primary cause and on the potential for recovery of sufficient renal function to maintain life.*
1. If the cause of obstruction is removed prior to the development of significant structural renal damage, a good prognosis is justified.
2. If the obstructive lesion has been present for a sufficient period of time to cause severe bilateral hydronephrosis, the prognosis will be guarded to poor in most instances.

III. Trauma

The ureters of dogs and cats are occasionally ruptured following severe abdominal trauma (see Chapter 36, Physical Injuries).

IV. Calculi

A. *Ureteral calculi are uncommonly encountered in the dog and cat, although they have been reported (Figs. 35–1 and 35–2).*

The infrequent occurrence of ureteral calculi in these species may be related, at least in part, to the relative infrequency with which renal calculi occur in dogs and cats. Ureteral calculi originate from the renal pelves (see Chapter 34, Urolithiasis).

B. *In man, calculi that migrate through a ureter stimulate severe abdominal pain.*
Severe abdominal pain was observed in two dogs with ureteral calculi.

V. Neoplasia

The paucity of reported cases of primary and secondary benign and malignant tumors in the ureters of dogs and cats indicates that they are rarely encountered. On occasion, neoplasms originating from abdominal organs or tissues will encroach upon a ureter and occlude its lumen.

VI. Vesico-ureteral reflux

A. *Definition*

Vesico-ureteral reflux is regurgitation of urine from the bladder into the ureter.

B. *Pathophysiology*
1. Well defined ureterovesical valves are not present; however, the oblique course of the ureters through the bladder wall prevents retrograde flow

of urine from the bladder. The ureterovesical valve protects the kidneys from contamination with infected bladder urine.
2. The length of the intravesical portion of the ureter plays an important role in vesico-ureteral reflux.
   a. The longer it is, the less likely it is to allow reflux.
   b. Ureters with relatively short intravesical portions are more likely to allow reflux.
   c. Any abnormality that shortens the intravesical portion of the ureter predisposes the patient to vesico-ureteral reflux. In man, abnormalities which have the potential to cause vesico-ureteral reflux include:
      (1) Weakness of the vesical trigone.
      (2) Obstruction of the lower urinary tract.
      (3) Disturbance of innervation to the vesical trigone due to any cause.
      (4) Ectopic or duplicated ureters.
      (5) Inflammation. Inflammation itself usually does not cause reflux if the ureterovesical valve is normal, but it may aggravate reflux if other causes are present.

C. *Significance of vesico-ureteral reflux in man*
   1. Mechanical emptying of the bladder is one important mechanism by which the bladder eliminates bacteria.
   2. If cystitis occurs in association with vesico-ureteral reflux, the latter may perpetuate the infection. Even if the bladder is capable of completely eliminating all urine from its lumen, it will be recontaminated with infected refluxed urine returning from the ureter.
   3. Vesico-ureteral reflux is a significant factor associated with pyelonephritis in man because it permits bacteria to reach the kidneys (see Chapter 19, Pyelonephritis).

D. *Significance of vesico-ureteral reflux in dogs*
   1. Investigations performed in experimental dogs have revealed the following:
      a. Vesico-ureteral reflux may occur in normal dogs.
         (1) The incidence of vesico-ureteral reflux in normal dogs has not been established.
         (2) Occurrence of vesico-ureteral reflux varies with age.
            (a) It is least common in newborn puppies and dogs over seven years of age.
            (b) It is most common in dogs seven to 12 weeks of age.
         (3) Presence or absence of radiographically demonstrable vesico-ureteral reflux may be affected by:
            (a) Depth of anesthesia.
            (b) Patient positioning. Dogs with reflux demonstrated in the lateral recumbent position may not have reflux when placed in the ventrodorsal position.
      b. Some investigators have concluded that vesico-ureteral reflux does not occur in normal dogs. If detected, they argue that it is caused by the technique of evaluation.
      c. Vesico-ureteral reflux has been observed in dogs with experimentally induced bladder infection.
   2. The clinical significance of vesico-ureteral reflux in dogs has not been

established. In one study, vesico-ureteral reflux was reported to occur in association with:
- a. Urolithiasis. Reflux was demonstrated in five of 21 dogs with urolithiasis.
- b. Prostatic enlargement.
- c. Infection of the urinary tract.
- d. Neoplasia of the urinary bladder.
- e. Diverticula of the bladder wall.

E. Diagnosis
1. In man, vesico-ureteral reflux may be demonstrated by:
   a. Contrast cystography.
   b. Delayed or voiding contrast cystography.
   c. Voiding cystourethrography.
   d. Voiding cinecystography.
2. In dogs, vesico-ureteral reflux has been demonstrated by:
   a. Contrast cystography.
   b. Voiding cystourethrography.
      (1) Anesthetize the patient.
      (2) Catheterize the patient with a sterilized, nylon, disposable catheter.
      (3) Remove all residual urine from the bladder with the patient in lateral recumbency.
      (4) Instill radiopaque contrast media into the bladder via the catheter. The radiopaque material should be allowed to enter the bladder by gravity flow. It was recommended that the receptacle containing the radiopaque media be held approximately three feet above the patient's body.
      (5) Expose films as soon as spontaneous voiding around the catheter occurs.
   c. Voiding cinecystography. In one study, this technique increased the accuracy of detection of vesico-ureteral reflux by only four per cent when compared to the technique of micturating cystourethrography.

F. Treatment
1. Treatment of vesico-ureteral reflux in man consists of a variety of medical and surgical methods.
2. If vesico-ureteral reflux is associated with bacterial infection of the urinary system, long-term antibacterial therapy is instituted.
3. Consult medical textbooks of urology for specific details.
4. Lack of information precludes a discussion of treatment of vesico-ureteral reflux in dogs and cats.

VII. Ectopic ureters

A. *Normally the ureters terminate in the urinary bladder at the trigone.*

B. *Termination of one or both ureters outside the urinary bladder may occur as a result of faulty differentiation of mesonephric and metanephric ducts.*

C. *With one exception, urinary incontinence associated with ectopic ureters has only been encountered in female dogs.*

1. Affected dogs have a history of persistent urinary incontinence since birth or weaning.
2. Either or both ureters may be involved.
3. The ectopic ureters may terminate in the uterus, vagina, or urethra.

D. *Ectopic ureters are often associated with additional acquired and congenital anomalies of the urinary system.*
   1. Megaureter and hydronephrosis without evidence of obstruction to urine flow often involve the affected ureter(s) and kidney(s).
   2. Hypoplasia of the kidney, urinary bladder, and urethra has been observed.
   3. Pyelonephritis of the kidney associated with the ectopic ureter has been observed. Since there is no functional sphincter of the ectopic ureter, reflux predisposes the associated kidney to ascending bacterial infection.
   4. An ectopic urethra was reported in one patient with an ectopic ureter.
   5. Abnormalities in the urethral sphincter which also contribute to the urinary incontinence have been observed in several dogs in which the ectopic ureter terminated in the urethra.
   6. A progressive decrease in the severity of the urinary incontinence has been observed in some female dogs which also had an acquired generalized progressive disease of the associated kidney. The latter may have been caused by pyelonephritis. As a result of progressive destruction of functioning nephrons, a stage was ultimately reached in which urine formation by the affected kidney progressively decreased.

E. *With one exception, ectopic ureters in male dogs have not been associated with urinary incontinence.*

   An ectopic ureter associated with urinary incontinence has been observed in a male wire haired fox terrier (Fig. 22–6).

   Ectopic ureters in male human beings rarely result in urinary incontinence because the site of the ectopic termination of the ureter is usually in the prostatic urethra. As a result, urine dribbles back into the urinary bladder.

F. *Diagnosis*
   1. A history of persistent urinary incontinence in a female dog since birth should provide a high index of suspicion of ectopic ureter(s).
   2. Observation, with the aid of a vaginal endoscope, of an abnormal orifice which communicates with the vagina provides significant evidence.
   3. Failure to observe ureteral orifices at the trigone of the bladder via cystoscopy provides supportive evidence of ectopic ureters.
   4. Radiology.
      a. When an abnormal orifice in the vagina is detected, catheterization of the orifice followed by retrograde ureteropyelography is the best method of establishing a definitive diagnosis (Fig. 35–3).
      b. Although intravenous urography may be of value, visualization of the exact termination of the ureter may be difficult or impossible because of:
         (1) Lack of sufficient contrast media in the distal segment of the ureter. The latter may be caused by ureteral peristalsis.
         (2) Poorly functioning renal tissue drained by the ectopic ureter (see Chapter 8, Radiographic Evaluation of the Urinary System).

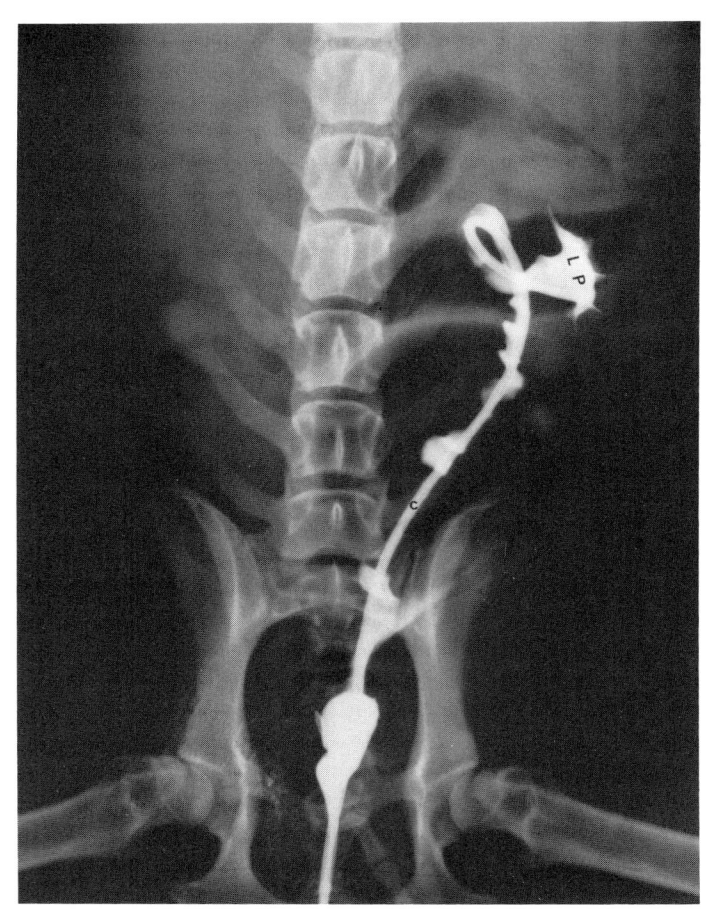

Figure 35-3. Retrograde ureteropyelogram of a 21-month-old nonspayed female English bulldog with an ectopic ureter. Because the ureter terminated in the urethra, the dog had urinary incontinence since birth. *LP* = left kidney pelvis. *c* = Radiopaque fiber catheter. (J. Amer. Animal Hosp. Assoc., *3*: 111–122, 1967.)

      (3) Accumulation of contrast media in the urinary bladder resulting in interference of visualization of the distal portion of the ureter.

      (4) Ureteral visualization may be improved with high dose urography.

  c. A vaginogram may be useful in puppies and small breeds of dogs.

      (1) To perform a vaginogram, tilt the animal with head down and distend the vagina with contrast material. In order to increase the viscosity of the contrast solution, combine it with sterile lubricant (see Urethrography, in Chapter 8).

      (2) Reflux of the radiopaque material into ectopic ureters may be observed.

5. The diagnosis may also be established by injecting sterile, colored dye into the urinary bladder. In patients with urinary incontinence due to an ectopic ureter, normal colored urine should appear at the vulva.

6. Exploratory laparotomy.

  a. Lack of termination of the ureter at the trigone of the urinary bladder confirms a diagnosis of ectopic ureter.

  b. Saline injected into an ectopic ureter should escape through the vulva.

G. *Treatment*
   1. There is no effective medical treatment for patients with urinary incontinence due to an ectopic ureter.
   2. Surgical repair is the treatment of choice.
       a. Try to control infection of the urinary tract prior to surgery.
       b. Any one or more of the following are indications for transplantation of the ureter into the urinary bladder:
           (1) Normal function and normal gross anatomical appearance of the kidney drained by the ectopic ureter.
           (2) Extravesicular termination of both ureters.
           (3) Hypofunction of both kidneys. Nephrectomy is not the treatment of choice in this instance since it may precipitate a uremic crisis.
       c. Indications for nephrectomy and ureterectomy include:
           (1) An abnormal kidney drained by the ectopic ureter. This method of correction should only be considered if the contralateral kidney is functioning normally.
           (2) Intractable infection of the urinary bladder, ureter, or kidney.

H. *Prognosis*
   1. If surgical correction of an ectopic ureter is feasible, a guarded to good prognosis is justified.
   2. If the ectopic ureter terminates in the urethra, the dog may continue to exhibit urinary incontinence following surgery as a result of an abnormal urethra.

REFERENCES

Boyarsky, S., Gottshalk, C. W., Tanagho, E. A., and Zimskind, P. D.: Urodynamics. Hydrodynamics of the Ureter and Renal Pelvis. New York, N. Y., Academic Press, 1971.
Christie, B. A.: Incidence and etiology of vesicourethral reflux in apparently normal dogs. Invest. Urol., 9:184–194, 1971.
Goulden, B. E.: Diagnosis of vesico-ureteral reflux. New Zealand Vet. J., 16:167–175, 1969.
Grana, L., Kidd, J., Idriss, F., and Swensen, O.: Effect of chronic urinary tract infection on ureteral peristalsis. J. Urol., 94:652–657, 1965.
Kim, H. L., Labay, P. C., Boyarsky, S., and Glenn, J. F.: An experimental model of ureteral colic. J. Urol., 104:390, 1970.
King, L. R., and Idriss, F. S.: The effect of vesicoureteral reflux on renal function in dogs. Invest. Urol., 4:419–427, 1967.
Lenaghan, D., and Cussen, L. J.: Vesicoureteral reflux in pups. Invest. Urol., 5:449–461, 1968.
Orr, W. A., and Gillenwater, J. Y.: Creation of vesicoureteral reflux in the canine experimental model. Invest. Urol., 8:604–609, 1971.
Osborne, C. A., and Perman, V.: Ectopic ureter in a male dog. J.A.V.M.A., 154:273–278, 1969.
Osborne, C. A., and Hanlon, G. F.: Canine congenital ureteral ectopia: Case report and review of literature. Anim. Hosp., 3:111–122, 1967.
Pollock, S., and Schoen, S. S.: Urinary incontinence associated with congenital ureteral valves in a bitch. J.A.V.M.A., 159:332–335, 1971.
Seidenberg, L., and Knecht, C. D.: Ectopic ureter in the dog. J.A.V.M.A., 159:876–877, 1971.
Sellards, H. G.: The effect of vesicoureteral reflux on renal growth and development in puppies. Invest. Urol., 9:95–97, 1971.
Sommer, J. L., and Roberts, J. A.: Ureteral reflux resulting from chronic urinary infection in dogs. Long term studies. J. Urol., 95:502–510, 1966.
Theran, P., Henry, W. B., and Thornton, G. W.: Ureteral calculi–ruptured ureter. J.A.V.M.A., 147:260–267, 1965.
Theran, P., and Thornton, G. W.: Abscessed right ureter. J.A.V.M.A., 149:1195–1201, 1966.

Chapter 36
PHYSICAL INJURIES

I. Renal trauma

   A. *Etiology*
   1. The kidneys of dogs and cats are sometimes injured by blunt abdominal trauma, and, less commonly, by penetrating wounds.
   2. Serious traumatic injuries to the kidneys are not a common clinical entity. The reasons may be that:
      a. The kidneys are not rigidly fixed in position.
      b. The kidneys are protected by vertebrae, ribs, and the lumbar muscles.
      c. The kidneys are surrounded by a tough, inelastic fibrous capsule.

   B. *Pathophysiology*
   1. Provided the renal capsule remains intact, renal injury associated with abdominal trauma is usually characterized by contusions and the formation of subcapsular hematomas. Such injuries are rarely associated with clinical signs, and result in little, if any, permanent loss of renal parenchyma.
   2. Trauma of sufficient severity to cause rupture of the renal capsule and parenchyma may be associated with an immediate threat to life due to exsanguination.
      a. Rupture of large arteries or veins, or avulsion of the renal artery and vein from the renal hilus may result in hemorrhage and death from shock in a very short period of time.
      b. If the rent does not communicate with the peritoneal cavity, large retroperitoneal hematomas may develop.
      c. If the rent communicates with the peritoneal cavity, hemoperitoneum may develop.
      d. If the rent in the renal parenchyma extends into the collecting system, blood clots may form which obstruct urine flow.
      e. Rents in the kidney which permit communication of the collecting system with the abdominal cavity or retroperitoneal tissues may be associated with formation of an inflammatory mass as a result of perirenal extravasation of urine.
   3. Following vascular damage, thrombi may form. Since the renal vasculature consists of a system of end-arteries without significant collateral blood supply, the portion of the renal parenchyma supplied by thrombotic vessels will undergo infarction.

   C. *Clinical findings*
   1. History. Significant observations may include:
      a. Recent trauma.
      b. Gross hematuria.

c. Oliguria or anuria if the patient is in a state of shock, or if the lesion is bilateral.
2. The physical findings associated with renal trauma are variable, being dependent on the primary cause, the location and extent of injury, and the duration of the disease process.
   a. In cases associated with severe hemorrhage, the clinical findings will be characteristic of hemorrhagic shock.
   b. If the patient survives, a progressively enlarging mass may be palpated in the area of the kidney.
      (1) The mass may be a retroperitoneal or subcapsular hematoma.
      (2) The mass may be composed of inflammatory tissue caused by perirenal extravasation of urine.
   c. Pain may be detected at the site of injury.
   d. Signs associated with renal failure will not develop if only one kidney is affected.
   e. Lesions caused by trauma to other organs and systems of the body may be detected.
3. Laboratory findings.
   a. Evaluation of laboratory tests of renal function will not reveal any abnormalities unless:
      (1) The patient has poor renal perfusion and prerenal uremia. In the latter instance, abnormal elevation of BUN or creatinine will be associated with a high urine specific gravity (above 1.025).
      (2) Both kidneys have generalized lesions.
   b. Urinalysis typically reveals gross or microscopic hematuria and proteinuria. There is no good correlation between the severity of hematuria and the extent or severity of renal injury.
   c. If hemorrhage remains unchecked, serial evaluation of hemograms will reveal a progressive decline in PCV.
   d. Abdominal paracentesis may also be of value in establishing the presence of significant renal trauma.
      (1) Slow withdrawal of the needle from the peritoneal cavity is imperative since in many instances only a thin layer of free peritoneal fluid is present between the parietal and visceral peritoneum.
         (a) If this layer is traversed too rapidly, the tip of the needle may not be in the correct position for a sufficient period of time to recover abnormal accumulations of fluid.
         (b) A negative tap does not exclude the presence of significant visceral damage.
      (2) If paracentesis yields blood-tinged fluid or nonclotted blood, major visceral damage should be suspected.
      (3) Aspiration of blood that clots indicates that the needle has entered a vessel in the abdominal wall, mesentery, or viscera, and is usually of little significance or consequence.
      (4) If in spite of negative paracentesis abdominal injury is still suspected, several hundred milliliters of a polyionic, isotonic solution, such as lactated Ringer's solution, should be injected into the peritoneal cavity and then immediately withdrawn. Following removal, the fluid should be evaluated for gross and microscopic abnormalities.

4. Radiographic findings. Suspicion of renal injury may be confirmed by various radiographic techniques.
   a. Survey radiography.
      (1) If extensive perirenal hemorrhage has occurred, survey radiographs may reveal irregularity, enlargement, or loss of the normal renal outline.
      (2) Injuries to other organs and tissues may be detected.
   b. Contrast radiography.
      (1) Excretory urography may be of value in determining the site and extent of renal damage, and may reveal perirenal extravasation of urine. Abnormalities of the renal pelvis caused by lesions in the adjacent parenchyma, or formation of blood clots in the pelvis, may be observed. Excretory urograms may also permit evaluation of the patency and configuration of the lower urinary tract.
      (2) Because the total quantity of radiopaque medium excreted during intravenous urography performed by conventional techniques may be reduced as a result of nephron damage and poor renal perfusion, a sufficient quantity of medium may not accumulate in the collecting system to provide diagnostic radiographs. For this reason high dose excretory urography should be performed (see High dose urography, in Chapter 8).
      (3) Although it is commonly implied that intravenous urograms are helpful in evaluating the functional capacity of the kidneys, this generally must be kept in proper perspective. Because of the numerous variables that affect the degree of visualization provided by contrast agents, intravenous urograms cannot be used as a quantitative index of renal function (see Chapter 8, Radiographic Evaluation of the Urinary System). Since the success of nephrectomies is ultimately related to the functional capacity of the contralateral kidney, renal function should be evaluated with more reliable renal function tests.
   c. Renal angiography.
      (1) In human medicine, renal angiography is considered to be the radiographic procedure of choice for evaluation of kidneys suspected of having traumatic injuries.
      (2) Angiography has been found to be superior to other contrast radiographic techniques in detection of traumatic lesions such as aneurysms, infarcts, and arteriovenous fistulas.

D. *Diagnosis*
   1. Traumatic damage to the kidneys that is sufficiently severe to be associated with clinical signs can usually be diagnosed on the basis of the history, physical examination, radiographic findings, and laboratory findings.
   2. In some instances, exploratory laparotomy must be used to confirm or eliminate a diagnosis of renal trauma.

E. *Treatment*
   1. The therapeutic objectives for management of renal trauma are the same as those for management of trauma of other organs and tissues of the body. In order of priority they should be to:

a. Control hemorrhage.
   b. Debride devitalized tissue.
   c. Repair injured structures.
2. The ultimate objective should be preservation of life and conservation of renal function.
3. Most renal lesions respond to nonsurgical therapy. If subcapsular or perirenal hemorrhage is self-limiting, cage rest and "tincture of time" may be the only treatment required. In such cases, hematomas will usually undergo spontaneous resolution in a period of seven to 10 days.
4. In instances of renal trauma associated with gross hematuria, a marked diuresis should be induced in order to minimize the chance of blood clots forming in the excretory pathway and obstructing the outflow of urine.
5. Exploratory laparotomy is indicated if:
   a. The patient is in a state of shock due to intra-abdominal hemorrhage.
   b. Palpable masses in the kidney continue to increase in size.
   c. Significant perirenal extravasation of contrast medium is detected.
6. Abdominal compression bandages will not effectively control severe hemorrhage from the kidney.
7. Management of renal injuries found at laparotomy is dependent on the type and severity of injury, and the condition of the patient. Conservation of viable renal tissue should receive a high priority.
   a. In instances in which the renal capsule is torn, closure with simple sutures is usually not possible because of swelling and loss of tensile strength of the injured capsule and parenchyma.
      (1) In experimental dogs, forceful attempts to approximate swollen renal lacerations with tension sutures placed through the capsule and parenchyma resulted in additional laceration of the kidneys.
      (2) When sutures were tied tight enough to control hemorrhage, the blood supply to the area was disrupted, and extensive necrosis and fibrosis of tissue resulted.
   b. Rents in the renal capsule and parenchyma are best repaired with the aid of hemostatic agents such as oxidized regenerated cellulose* and gelfoam.** Strips of fascia obtained from the sheath of the rectus abdominus muscle have also been successfully used to repair capsular lesions in canine kidneys.
   c. Extensive electrocautery should be avoided since it induces a significant degree of destruction of adjacent renal parenchyma and delays healing.
   d. In instances in which severe injury is confined to one pole of the kidney, partial nephrectomy using the transverse technique of amputation should be employed.
   e. Nephrectomy should be reserved for extensive injuries characterized by pulpefaction of most of the parenchyma, avulsion of the renal pedicle, or uncontrollable hemorrhage. The ultimate success of nephrectomy is dependent on the presence of adequate function in the opposite kidney.

F. *Prognosis*

If severe renal trauma is treated early and vigorously, the prognosis for life is usually guarded to good.

---
*Surgicel, Johnson and Johnson, New Brunswick, N.J. 10903.
**Gelfoam, The Upjohn Co., Kalamazoo, Michigan 49001.

342   DISEASES OF THE UPPER AND LOWER URINARY SYSTEM

II. Traumatic rupture of the ureter and renal pelvis

A. Rupture of a ureter or renal pelvis is not commonly encountered in dogs and cats, but may occur as a result of trauma or poor surgical technique.

B. Unless both ureters or renal pelves are affected, signs associated with renal failure will not develop.

C. Following rupture of a ureter or renal pelvis, leakage of urine outside the urinary tract will stimulate the formation of inflammatory tissue.

If urine outflow to the associated kidney is obstructed, varying degrees of hydronephrosis will develop (Fig. 36-1).

D. Clinical findings

1. Significant facts in the history may be:
   a. Recent trauma.
   b. Evidence of pain in the sublumbar area when the owner handles the patient.
2. Physical examination may reveal:
   a. Pain in the sublumbar area.
   b. A palpable mass in the sublumbar area.
   c. Enlargement of the associated kidney.

E. Radiographic findings

1. A sublumbar soft tissue mass may be detected on survey radiographs.
2. Leakage of contrast media into the peritoneal cavity or retroperitoneal tissue may be detected by intravenous urography.

F. Diagnosis

A history of recent trauma or surgery combined with the presence of a sublumbar mass and typical radiographic findings are sufficient to establish a diagnosis. The diagnosis may be confirmed by exploratory laparotomy if necessary.

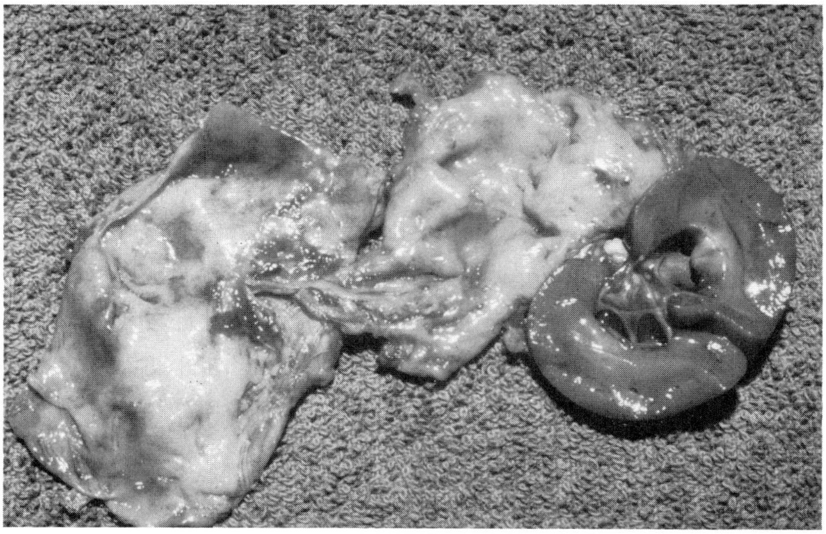

Figure 36-1. Chronic inflammatory reaction surrounding the ureter, and hydronephrosis which occurred as sequelae to traumatic rupture of the ureter in a 6-month-old female domestic short-haired cat.

PHYSICAL INJURIES

G. *Treatment*
1. Treatment is limited to surgical intervention.
2. If the ureter is damaged, resection of the lesion and ureteral anastomosis should be considered.
3. If unilateral nephrectomy is contemplated, it is imperative to confirm the presence of adequate function in the contralateral kidney.

H. *Prognosis*

If the lesion is unilateral and the opposite kidney has adequate function, a guarded to good prognosis is usually justified.

III. Trauma to the urinary bladder

A. *Contusions and abrasions of the urinary bladder are often caused by external abdominal trauma, vigorous abdominal palpation, and catheterization.*
1. Clinical findings usually consist of hematuria and proteinuria.
2. Treatment is usually unnecessary unless bacterial infection develops as a complication. If this happens, treatment should consist of measures to eliminate cystitis (see Chapter 38, Bacterial Cystitis).

B. *Rupture of the urinary bladder*
1. Etiology
   a. In small animal practice, rupture of the urinary bladder is most commonly encountered in:
      (1) Male dogs.
         (a) The more frequent occurrence of bladder rupture in male than in female dogs is associated with the limited potential of the long, narrow male urethra to rapidly dilate.
         (b) The urethra of female dogs is relatively short and wide and is not surrounded by any structure which prevents rapid dilatation of the urethral lumen.
      (2) Male tomcats with obstructed urethras. Rupture of the urinary bladder in obstructed tomcats is usually associated with overzealous attempts to dislodge a urethral plug by digital compression of an inflamed and distended bladder.
   b. Uncommonly, perforation of the bladder may be caused by instrumentation, bone fragments from a fractured pelvis, or penetrating abdominal wounds.
2. Pathophysiology.
   a. Rupture of the urinary bladder is a medical emergency since it may result in death within 24 to 48 hours from onset. In some instances, however, patients may survive several days following traumatic rupture of the bladder without therapy.
   b. Anuric dogs with rupture of the urinary bladder may die more rapidly than dogs which have been bilaterally nephrectomized.
      (1) Although unproven by experimental study, it is hypothesized that this difference is related, at least in part, to more severe changes in fluid and electrolyte balance in bladder rents which communicate with the peritoneal cavity.
         (a) Following accumulation of hyperosmolal urine in the peritoneal cavity, iso-osmolal fluid from the extravascular spaces is absorbed into the peritoneal cavity in order to establish osmotic

equilibrium. At the same time, high concentrations of solutes excreted in urine diffuse back into the body in order to establish solute equilibrium.
  (b) Obviously the magnitude of these changes is dependent on urine osmolality and the rate of urine formation.
 (2) If patients with ruptured urinary bladders are oliguric because of renal hypoperfusion associated with shock, the onset of significant shifts in fluid and electrolyte balance may require more time to develop than would be the situation in patients with good renal function.
 (3) A more rapid demise of a patient with a ruptured urinary bladder may be related to augmentation of hyperkalemia as a result of peritonitis and cellular necrosis.
 c. Rupture of the urinary bladder is typically associated with a sudden increase in intravesical pressure in a bladder distended with urine.
 (1) Rapid increase in intravesical pressure may be caused by external trauma or vigorous abdominal palpation.
 (2) When intravesical pressure reaches a critical limit, the wall of the bladder splits, usually at the vertex.
 (3) Because of the anatomical location of the urinary bladder in dogs and cats, rents in the bladder wall usually communicate with the peritoneal cavity.
 (4) Although uncommon, extraperitoneal rupture of the urinary bladder may occur.
  (a) Extraperitoneal extravasation of urine may not be associated with uremia, but rather tissue necrosis and cellulitis.
  (b) In one case reported in a dog, extraperitoneal extravasation of urine resulted in formation of a urine fistula which communicated with the exterior of the body through an opening in the medial aspect of the thigh.
3. Clinical findings.
 a. Clinical findings associated with rupture of the urinary bladder are variable, depending on the precipitating cause and the duration of rupture.
 b. Significant findings in the history may include one or more of the following:
 (1) Recent trauma.
 (2) Attempts to manually express a bladder distended with urine.
 (3) Sudden onset of signs.
 c. In cases associated with trauma, signs characteristic of shock or disorders caused by trauma to other organs and tissues may obscure signs related to the urinary system. Signs caused by bladder rupture usually develop in a matter of hours, but in exceptional instances may not become obvious for longer periods of time.
 d. Significant findings obtained from the physical examination may include:
 (1) Progressive depression.
 (2) Vomiting.
 (3) Normal to subnormal temperature. If a septic peritonitis develops, the temperature may become abnormally elevated.

(4) Ascites. After a variable period of time, variable quantities of fluid accumulate in the peritoneal cavity.
  (a) Because concentrated urine is irritating to tissues, signs associated with peritonitis (i.e., abdominal pain, spasm of abdominal musculature, stiff gait) may become evident.
  (b) The intensity of these signs progressively increases with time.
(5) Abnormal micturition.
  (a) The patient may be anuric.
  (b) Some patients may void a small quantity of bloody urine.
(6) Inability to palpate the urinary bladder.
e. Significant laboratory findings may include the following:
  (1) Evaluation of a hemogram may reveal abnormal elevation in PCV provided significant hemorrhage has not occurred.
    (a) Accumulation of hypertonic urine in the peritoneal cavity will be associated with a shift of fluid into the peritoneal cavity.
    (b) Depending on the magnitude of fluid shift, varying degrees of hemoconcentration will result.
  (2) The total WBC count may be elevated in response to stress (mature neutrophilia) or peritonitis (immature neutrophilia).
  (3) Abnormal elevations in serum BUN or creatinine concentrations. The magnitude of abnormal increase will be dependent on:

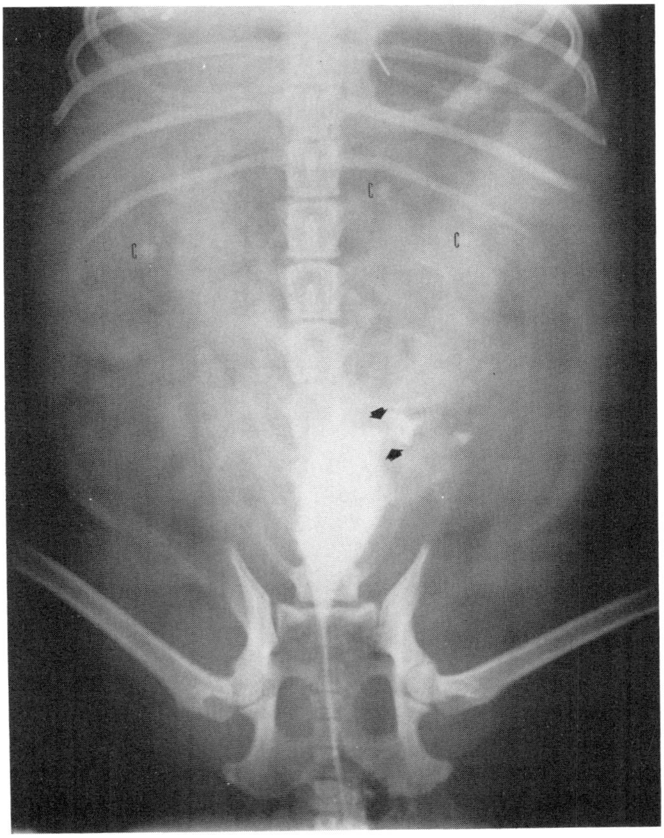

Figure 36-2. Positive contrast cystogram of a 4.5-year-old female wire-haired fox terrier with rupture of the urinary bladder. Radiopaque dye has entered the peritoneal cavity through a rent in the left cranial aspect of the bladder (arrows). The presence of fluid in the abdominal cavity has obscured visualization of abdominal viscera. Several uroliths have escaped from the bladder into the peritoneal cavity. The bladder ruptured following obstruction of the urethra with a urolith. *c*, Calculi.

(a) The length of time elapsed between rupture of the bladder and evaluation of BUN or creatinine.

(b) The magnitude of hemoconcentration.

(4) Comparison of the concentration of BUN of serum or plasma to that of aspirated peritoneal fluid will typically reveal a significantly higher concentration of BUN in peritoneal fluid.

(5) Depending on the presence or absence of bacteria in urine at the time of rupture, cytologic evaluation of peritoneal fluid will reveal that it is an exudate (septic) or a modified transudate (nonseptic).

(6) In uncomplicated cases, urinalysis will usually reveal hematuria and proteinuria. If the patient has concomitant cystitis, changes characteristic of inflammation will be present (see Urinalysis, in Chapter 6).

4. Radiographic findings.
   a. Radiographic techniques are the most reliable methods with which to confirm a diagnosis of a ruptured urinary bladder.
   b. Survey radiographs of the abdomen of patients with ruptured urinary bladders are usually characterized by:
      (1) Absence of the outline of the urinary bladder.
      (2) Typical "ground glass" appearance characteristic of accumulation of abdominal fluid.
   c. Survey films may also reveal:
      (1) Calculi in the abdominal cavity if they were present in the bladder prior to rupture (Fig. 36–2).
      (2) Traumatic lesions in other organs and tissues.
   d. Following survey radiography, pneumocystography or retrograde positive contrast cystography should be employed (Figs. 36–2 and 36–3).
      (1) Regardless of technique, it is essential to distend the bladder to full capacity with the contrast agent in order to avoid missing the presence of relatively small tears in the bladder wall. Failure to perceive back pressure while injecting contrast agents with a catheter and syringe provides supportive evidence of a ruptured bladder.
      (2) If pneumocystography is chosen:
         (a) Lateral abdominal views should be exposed with the patient in a standing position in order to demonstrate accumulation of air in the portion of the peritoneal cavity just ventral to the vertebral column (Fig. 36–3).
         (b) If the patient is unable to stand, the x-ray beam and cassette should be positioned so that the movement of free air toward the uppermost portion of the peritoneal cavity can be demonstrated.
      (3) Positive contrast cystography may also be used to confirm a diagnosis of rupture of the urinary bladder.
         (a) To perform this technique, a dilute solution (2.5 to 5.0 per cent) of organic iodinated radiopaque material should be instilled into the urinary bladder. Conventional ventrodorsal, lateral, and oblique views of the abdomen should then be exposed. The exact site of rupture is pinpointed by escape of contrast medium from the bladder lumen into the peritoneal cavity (Fig. 36–2).

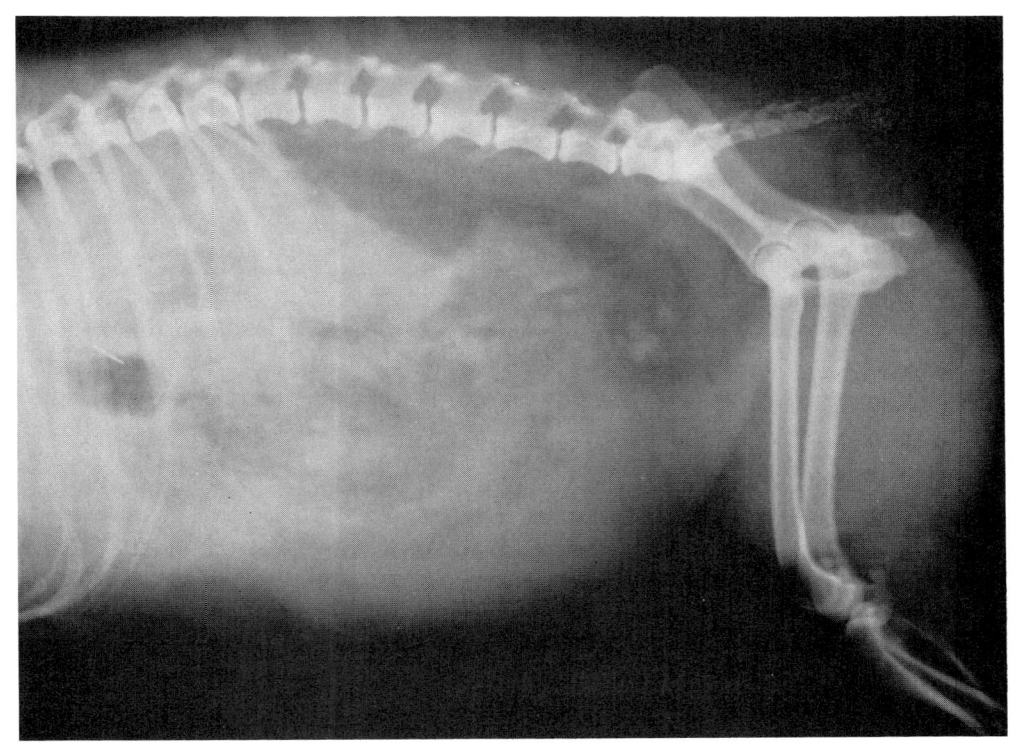

Figure 36-3. Pneumocystogram of the dog with the ruptured urinary bladder described in Figure 36-2. A large quantity of air has escaped from the lumen of the urinary bladder and accumulated under the lumbar vertebrae. Multiple uroliths are present in the urinary bladder. Several uroliths are present in the abdominal cavity. Abdominal fluid obscures visualization of abdominal viscera.

Films should be exposed as soon as the contrast medium has been injected into the bladder because contrast medium that has escaped from the bladder lumen will rapidly diffuse into the peritoneal cavity.
- (b) Positive contrast cystography is superior to pneumocystography in the diagnosis of bladder rupture because it permits determination of the exact point of rupture and does not require special positioning of the patient or x-ray unit.
- (c) Although some investigators object to the use of positive contrast cystography for diagnosis of ruptured urinary bladders on the grounds that the radiopaque medium is irritating to the peritoneal cavity, the objection must be kept in perspective. It is doubtful that diluted radiopaque media is significantly more irritating than urine. Since treatment of rupture of the urinary bladder is associated with a laparotomy and lavage of the peritoneal cavity, and because of rapid absorption of radiopaque media from the peritoneal cavity, the objection to the presence of irritating contrast medium in the peritoneal cavity is eliminated.
5. Catheterization.
   a. Catheterization of the urinary bladder should be performed with strict aseptic technique in order to prevent contamination of the peritoneal cavity with bacteria.

b. Since a small quantity of urine may remain in a ruptured bladder, and since the catheter may pass through a rent in the bladder wall into the urine-filled peritoneal cavity, collection of urine by catheterization does not exclude the presence of a ruptured urinary bladder.

c. The use of radiopaque catheters in conjunction with radiographic techniques has some advantages.
    (1) Visualization of a radiopaque catheter that has passed through the bladder lumen into the peritoneal cavity will confirm the presence of a ruptured bladder.
    (2) Since all bladders do not rupture at the vertex, however, failure to insert the catheter into the peritoneal cavity does not eliminate the possibility of a ruptured bladder.

d. Introduction of a known volume (25 to 50 ml.) of air or sterile fluid into an empty bladder with the aid of a catheter and syringe, followed by attempts to recover the air or fluid may be of diagnostic value. Inability to recover most of the air or fluid from the bladder suggests its escape into the peritoneal cavity. This suspicion should be confirmed by other techniques since recovery of fluid or air from an intact bladder may be impaired by faulty placement of the catheter.

6. Diagnosis.
    a. The most important aspect in diagnosis of rupture of the urinary bladder is recognizing that it can occur, especially in association with violent external trauma. The urinary bladder of any patient subjected to severe abdominal trauma should be carefully evaluated to be sure that it is intact.
    b. Physical examination, pertinent laboratory data, and evaluation of the history will usually allow a tentative diagnosis of ruptured urinary bladder to be established.
    c. Contrast cystography should be used to confirm the diagnosis.

7. Treatment.
    a. Tears in the wall of the urinary bladder of sufficient size to cause clinical signs rarely, if ever, heal spontaneously. For this reason surgical repair must be employed.
    b. If the patient is uremic, fluid therapy and diuresis should be instituted at the time of surgery, and should be continued until the patient can tolerate oral therapy.
    c. If the patient is in extremely poor physical condition, peritoneal dialysis may be utilized to ameliorate signs of uremia prior to surgery.
    d. Depending on the status of the patient, inhalant or epidural anesthesia should be employed.
    e. In addition to examination of the urinary bladder, all of the tissues and organs of the abdominal cavity should be inspected for the presence of lesions at the time of laparotomy.
    f. The edges of the rent in the bladder wall should be debrided, and approximated with a simple continuous suture line in the mucosa and an inverting Cushing suture line in the serosa.
    g. Following repair of the bladder wall, the peritoneal cavity should be thoroughly lavaged with physiologic saline solution.
    h. Antibiotics should be administered if sepsis has complicated the syndrome.

8. Prognosis.
   a. The prognosis for recovery from a ruptured urinary bladder is related to the precipitating cause.
      (1) Rapid surgical correction of a traumatic rent in the urinary bladder, combined with a good pre- and postoperative care, will usually be associated with complete recovery.
      (2) The prognosis for patients with rupture of the urinary bladder caused by nontraumatic diseases (inflammation, neoplasia) may be less favorable.

IV. Rupture of the urethra

   A. *Rupture of the urethra is not a common occurrence in small domestic animals, but may be caused by pelvic fractures, bite wounds, urethral obstruction, or improper catheterization.*

   B. *Periurethral extravasation of urine will result in severe cellulitis.*

   If the inflammatory process occludes the urethral lumen, obstructive uropathy will result.

REFERENCES

Archibald, J., Putnam, R. W., and Summer-Smith, G.: Partial nephrectomy—a technique. J. Sm. Anim. Pract., *10*:415–417, 1969.

Battershell, D. J.: Traumatic diverticulum of urinary bladder. J.A.V.M.A., *155*:67–68, 1969.

Gerlaugh, R., Demuth, W. E., Rattner, W. H., and Murphy, J. J.: The healing of renal wounds. II. Surgical repair of contusions or lacerations. J. Urol., *83*:529–534, 1960.

Lang, E. K., Trichel, B. E., and Turner, R. W.: Renal arteriography in the assessment of renal trauma. Radiology, *98*:103, 1971.

Meynard, J.: Traumatic rupture of the bladder in the dog. A clinical study of nine cases. J. Sm. Anim. Pract., *2*:131–134, 1961.

Murphy, J. J., Glantz, W., and Schoenberg, H. W.: The healing of renal wounds. III. A comparison of electrocoagulation and suture ligation for hemostasis in partial nephrectomy. J. Urol., *85*:882–883, 1961.

Putnam, R. W., Pennock, P. W., and Archibald, J.: Emergency surgery following urogenital trauma. Mod. Vet. Pract., *50*:34–41, 1969.

Rawlings, C. A.: Urinary bladder rupture and fistula. J.A.V.M.A., *155*:123–128, 1969.

Stirling, C. W., and Lands, A. M.: Experimental study of injuries of the kidney. J. Urol., *37*:466–479, 1937.

Chapter 37
OBSTRUCTIVE UROPATHY

I. Definition

Obstructive uropathy refers to any cause of obstruction to urine outflow from the body.

II. Etiology

A. Abnormalities causing obstruction may be located in the urethra, urinary bladder, ureters, or renal pelves.

B. Urethra
   1. The most common cause of urethral obstruction in male dogs is urinary calculi (see Chapter 34, Urolithiasis).
   2. The most common cause of urethral obstruction in male cats is material composed of mucus, triple phosphate crystals, and cellular debris (see Chapter 39, Cystitis—Urethral Obstruction Complex in the Cat).
   3. Urethral obstruction may also occur as a result of:
      a. Acquired strictures caused by trauma and inflammation.
      b. Congenital strictures.
      c. Neoplasia of the urethra or periurethral structures.
   4. See Chapter 45, Diseases of the Urethra, for information about specific diseases.

C. Urinary bladder
   1. Diseases of the bladder that cause obstructive uropathy include any abnormality which prevents urine outflow through the urethra or urine inflow from the ureters.
      a. Bladder neoplasms (see Chapter 41, Neoplasms of the Urinary Bladder).
      b. Granulomas of the uterine stump (spay granulomas).
      c. Herniation, torsion, or prolapse of the bladder (see Chapter 43, Abnormal Locations of the Urinary Bladder).
      d. Calculi.

D. Ureters and renal pelves
   1. Obstructive uropathy due to primary diseases of the ureters or renal pelves occurs much less commonly than obstructive uropathy due to primary diseases of the lower urinary tract.
   2. Potential causes include:
      a. Calculi.
      b. Blood clots.
      c. Neoplasms.
      d. Lesions in adjacent structures that compress the excretory pathway.

3. Urine flow from both kidneys must be obstructed before the patient will become uremic.
4. See Chapter 35, Diseases of the Ureter, for information about specific diseases.

III. Pathophysiology

A. *Obstructive uropathy may cause uremia if the outflow of urine from both kidneys is blocked. Uremia may occur as a result of:*
   1. Retention of metabolic waste products caused by the obstructive lesion (postrenal uremia).
   2. Destruction of the renal parenchyma caused by urine back pressure.
   3. Both of the above.

B. *Postrenal uremia*
   1. Back pressure induced by obstruction to urine outflow impairs the mechanisms of tubular reabsorption and tubular secretion. Significant reduction in glomerular filtration and renal blood flow also occurs.
   2. If the patient has total obstruction of the ureters for a period of four to six days, death from uremia will result. Death caused by total urethral obstruction may not occur as rapidly since urine must distend the bladder prior to cessation of renal function.
   3. Death is caused by alteration of fluid and electrolyte balance and accumulation of metabolic waste products rather than by structural damage to nephrons (see Chapter 13, Extrarenal Manifestations of Uremia, and Chapter 12, Pathophysiology of Renal Failure).

C. *If the obstructive lesion is allowed to persist, and if the patient survives, varying degrees of hydronephrosis will cause primary uremia (see Chapter 22, Hydronephrosis).*

D. *Complete unilateral obstruction is compatible with life, provided the opposite kidney is capable of adequate function (see Chapter 22, Hydronephrosis).*

E. *The pathophysiology associated with partial obstruction of the urinary tract is highly variable, being dependent on cause, location, and degree of obstruction.*

IV. Clinical findings, diagnosis, treatment, and prognosis of obstructive uropathy. See specific diseases mentioned under etiology.

DISEASES OF THE LOWER URINARY SYSTEM

Chapter 38
BACTERIAL CYSTITIS

I. **Pathogenesis of bacterial cystitis**
  A. *Routes of infection*
    1. Ascending migration from the lower urinary and genital tract is the most frequent route of infection.
    2. Hematogenous dissemination.
    3. Descending migration from the kidneys and ureters.
  B. *Normal defense mechanisms of the urinary bladder*
    1. The mechanical flushing action of frequent micturition is an important mechanism which prevents bacterial infection of the urinary bladder.
      a. Urine is normally completely expelled from the urinary bladder several times daily.
      b. Any bacteria present in the bladder lumen are likewise expelled.
    2. The epithelial barrier that exists between the lumen of the urinary tract and the underlying tissues provides an intrinsic antibacterial defense mechanism.
    3. It has been hypothesized that urine has antibacterial action.
  C. *Factors predisposing to bacterial cystitis include:*
    1. Retention of urine in the bladder. This may be caused by:
      a. Urethral stricture or obstruction due to:
        (1) Periurethral masses.
        (2) Urethral calculi.
        (3) Trauma.
        (4) Primary urethral neoplasms.
      b. Neurologic derangement of micturition caused by:
        (1) Spinal cord disease including:
          (a) Intervertebral disc syndrome.
          (b) Vertebral column displacement.
          (c) Neoplasia of the spinal cord or surrounding structures.
          (d) Myelitis.
          (e) Ossifying pachymeningitis.
        (2) Pelvic nerve disease including:
          (a) Trauma.
          (b) Idiopathic causes.
        (3) Chronic distention of the bladder.
      c. Acquired or congenital defects of the bladder wall including:
        (1) Diverticula.
        (2) Mechanical abrasion by calculi.
        (3) Neoplasia.

DISEASES OF THE LOWER URINARY SYSTEM

   2. Glucosuria. Glucose provides a good media for bacterial growth. Persistent glucosuria is associated with:
      a. Diabetes mellitus.
      b. Primary renal glucosuria (see Primary renal glucosuria, in Chapter 15).
      c. Inherited renal disease (see Familial renal disease in Norwegian elkhound dogs and Renal cortical hypoplasia, both in Chapter 15).
   3. Trauma caused by:
      a. Catheterization.
      b. Physical injuries.

II. Etiologic agents

Numerous bacterial organisms have been isolated from the urine of dogs and cats with bacterial cystitis. Common isolates include:

A. *Gram negative organisms*

   1. *Escherichia coli.*
   2. *Pseudomonas* spp.
   3. *Proteus* spp.

B. *Gram positive organisms*

   1. *Streptococcus* spp.
   2. *Staphylococcus aureus.*

III. History

A. *Abnormalities referable to body systems other than the urinary tract are usually absent in patients with uncomplicated cystitis.*

   1. Body temperature is usually normal.
   2. The patient is usually alert.
   3. Appetite is usually not affected.

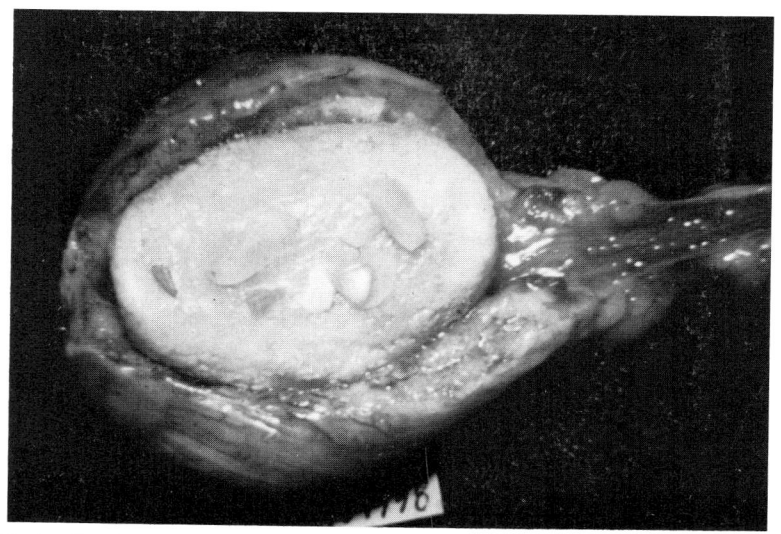

Figure 38–1. Cystic calculus and chronic cystitis in a 5-year-old female beagle dog. The dog had severe dysuria. (Courtesy of Dr. Kenneth H. Johnson, College of Veterinary Medicine, University of Minnesota.)

B. *Abnormalities referable to the urinary tract are often characterized by:*
   1. Dysuria (Fig. 38-1).
   2. Frequent attempts to micturate.
   3. Hematuria which is frequently most severe at the end of urination (see Chapter 3, Evaluation of the Clinical History in Diseases of the Urinary System).

IV. Physical examination

A. *Frequently no abnormalities are detected by physical examination.*

B. *Thickening of the bladder wall may be palpated, especially if the cystitis is chronic.*

C. *The genitourinary tract should be carefully examined to exclude or detect abnormalities other than cystitis that might cause hematuria or straining* (Fig. 38-1).

V. Clinical course

A. *Acute cystitis*
   1. If treated adequately, rapid remission of clinical signs usually occurs.
   2. Recurrence may occur if predisposing factors are not corrected.

B. *Chronic or recurrent cystitis may occur following:*
   1. No treatment or inadequate treatment of acute cystitis.
   2. Persistence or development of predisposing factors.
   3. Spontaneous reinfection.
   4. Infection with drug-resistant organisms.

VI. Diagnosis

A. *The history and clinical signs provide supportive evidence.*

B. *Abnormalities indicative of inflammation (proteinuria, hematuria, pyuria) detected by urinalysis provide supportive evidence (see Urinalysis, in Chapter 6).*

C. *Urine culture and* in vitro *sensitivity testing.*
   1. Culture a midstream urine sample, a sample obtained by catheterization, or a sample obtained by cystocentesis with a syringe and 22 gauge needle (see Chapter 5, Collection of Urine, and Bacterial culture of urine, in Chapter 6).
   2. Withdraw treatment at least five days prior to obtaining urine for culture to avoid inhibition of *in vitro* bacterial growth.

D. *Radiography*
   1. See Chapter 8, Radiographic Evaluation of the Urinary System for technique.
   2. Radiography is often indicated to detect diseases in which bacterial infection is not the only abnormality, such as:
      a. Urolithiasis.
      b. Neoplasms of the bladder.
      c. Diverticula of the bladder wall.
   3. Radiographic detection of diffuse thickening of the bladder wall is suggestive of chronic cystitis, but also may occur in association with diffuse neoplasia. Surgical biopsy may be necessary to differentiate the conditions (Fig. 38-2).

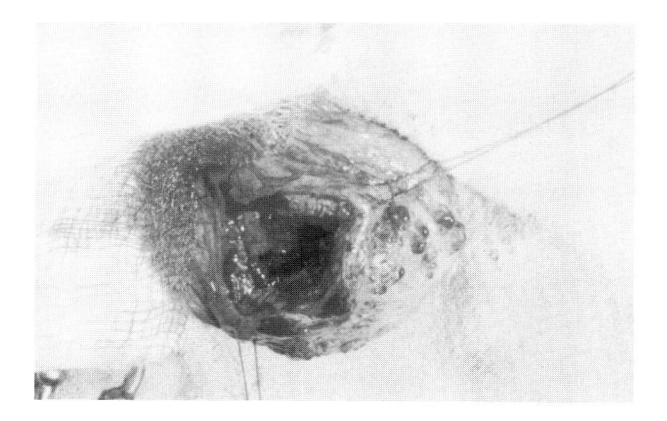

Figure 38-2. Generalized chronic cystitis of the urinary bladder of a 7.5-month-old male Irish setter. The musculature of the bladder wall was replaced with inflammatory cells and fibrous connective tissue. Differentiation of these changes from neoplasia was based on the microscopic appearance of the lesion.

VII. Treatment

    A. Correct predisposing causes if present.

    B. Antibacterial therapy

        1. Although routine culture and sensitivity testing of urine obtained from patients with acute cystitis is advisable, treatment without culture and sensitivity is often dictated by economic practicality.

            a. If bacteriologic information is not available, antibiotic choice should be based on known properties of antibiotics in combating urinary tract infection caused by commonly isolated organisms.

            b. Broad spectrum antibacterial agents commonly used for the treatment of cystitis include:

                (1) Chloramphenicol (10–25 mg./lb. repeated t.i.d. orally).
                (2) Gentamicin (2 mg./lb. repeated b.i.d. S.Q. or I.M.).
                (3) Sulfonamides.
                    (a) Sulfamethazine or sulfamerazine (25 mg./lb. orally or I.V., repeated b.i.d.).
                    (b) Sulfisoxazole (20 mg./lb. orally repeated q.i.d.).
                (4) Tetracycline hydrochloride (8 mg./lb. repeated t.i.d. orally; 3 mg./lb. repeated b.i.d., I.M.).
                (5) Ampicillin (5 mg./lb. repeated q.i.d. orally, I.M., or I.V.).

            c. Common antibacterial agents which are predominantly effective against Gram negative organisms include:

                (1) Streptomycin (5–7 mg./lb. repeated b.i.d., I.M.).
                (2) Nitrofurantoin (2 mg./lb. repeated b.i.d., orally).
                (3) Neomycin sulfate (5 mg./lb. repeated b.i.d., I.M. or I.V.).
                (4) Kanamycin sulfate (3 mg./lb. repeated b.i.d., I.M.).

            d. Common antibiotics predominantly effective against Gram positive organisms include:

                (1) Penicillin G., procaine (10,000 U/lb., o.d., I.M.).
                (2) Tylosin (5 mg./lb. repeated t.i.d., orally; 1 mg./lb., I.M. or I.V. repeated b.i.d.).

        2. In chronic cystitis, culture and antibiotic sensitivity testing are essential if response is to be obtained (see Bacterial culture of urine, in Chapter 6).

3. Schedule for antibiotic therapy.
   a. The dosage and the interval between doses should conform to recommendations of the manufacturer.
   b. Duration of therapy.
      (1) Duration of therapy should be based on elimination of urinary tract infection as detected by urinalysis in addition to the overall clinical response of the patient.
      (2) Some clinicians advocate the use of quantitative bacterial culture of urine as an index of response (see Bacterial culture of urine, in Chapter 6).
      (3) General plan.
         (a) Treat for a specified period.
            [1] Treat acute cystitis for at least one to two weeks.
            [2] Treat chronic cystitis for at least three to five weeks. Therapy for more prolonged periods may be required.
         (b) Perform a complete urinalysis three or four days prior to scheduled discontinuation of therapy.
         (c) If the urinalysis is normal, discontinue treatment. Repeat a urinalysis one week following discontinuation of therapy. Lack of abnormalities in the second specimen usually represents a satisfactory response.
         (d) If urinalysis findings are indicative of persistent or recurring infection, continued therapy is essential.
         (e) Persistent or recurring infection should be handled by changing antibiotic products, as suggested by sensitivity testing, until a satisfactory agent is found. Each product should be used for a sufficient period of time to evaluate its effectiveness.
         (f) In some patients with chronic cystitis, elimination of bacterial infection may prove to be impossible. In such cases it may be necessary to provide antibacterial therapy for the life of the patient.

C. *Urinary tract "antiseptics"*
   1. Methenamine:
      a. Acts by the formation of formaldehyde in the body.
      b. Requires an acid urine for effectiveness (pH 5.5 or lower).
      c. Is less effective than specific antibiotic therapy.
      d. Is indicated for long-term therapy in instances of some antibiotic resistant organisms or for prophylactic antibacterial therapy.
   2. Urinary acidifiers.
      a. Several products are available including ammonium chloride, methionine, mandelic acid, ethylenediamine dihydrochloride, and vitamin C.
      b. Urinary acidifiers should not be used as the primary treatment of bacterial cystitis, since more effective agents are available.
      c. Dosage of these drugs should be adjusted on the basis of response: urine pH should be monitored until it is established that acidification of urine is accomplished. Urine pH should be maintained at 6.5 or lower.
      d. Assuming that adequate acidification of urine is accomplished there is no therapeutic advantage of one acidifier over another.

3. Both antiseptics and acidifiers are used with the intention of:
    a. Creating an environment in the urinary tract which is unsuitable for bacterial growth.
    b. Enhancing the pharmacologic action of some antibiotics.

D. *Ancillary measures.*

1. Induce polydipsia and compensatory polyuria by increasing oral salt intake.
2. Provide the patient with the opportunity to void urine frequently.

REFERENCES

Aronson, A. L., and Kirk, R. W.: Rational use of antimicrobial drugs. *In* Current Veterinary Therapy. Vol. 4. Edited by R. W. Kirk. Philadelphia, Pa., W. B. Saunders Co., 1971.

Bohne, A. W., Osborne, R. W., and Hettle, P. J.: Regeneration of the urinary bladder in the dog following total cystectomy. Surg. Gynec. Obstet., *100*:259–264, 1955.

Darwish, M. E., Staubitz, W. J., Schueller, E. F., Rubin, M. I., and Neter, E.: Antibody response of dogs to experimental infection of bladder pouch. Invest. Urol., *6*:66, 1968.

Froe, D. L., and Williams, B. J.: An evaluation of anti-microbial sensitivity testing. M. V. P., *52*:45–49, 1971.

Gregory, J. G., Wern, A. J., Sansone, T. C., Murphy, J. J.: Bladder resistance to infection. J. Urol., *105*:220–222, 1971.

Hutch, J. A.: The role of urethral mucus in the bladder defense mechanism. J. Urol., *103*:165–167, 1970.

Kirk, R. W., and Jones, W. O.: Urinary tract infections. *In* Current Veterinary Therapy. Vol. 4. Edited by R. W. Kirk. Philadelphia, Pa., W. B. Saunders Co., 1971.

Malholland, S. G., Perez, J. R., and Gellinwater, J. Y.: The antibiotic propensities of urine. Invest. Urol., *6*:569–581, 1969.

Masih, B. K., Drouin, G., and Hinman, F.: Voiding and intrinsic defenses of the lower urinary tract of the female dog. I. Effects of episiotomy, colostomy, dilatation and urinary diversion. J. Urol., *104*:130–136, 1970.

Masih, B. K., and Hinman, F.: Voiding and intrinsic defenses of the lower urinary tract in the female dog. II. Effect of immunosuppressive drugs on canine urethral and vesical flora. Invest. Urol., *8*:494–498, 1971.

Mather, G. W.: Treatment of bacterial cystitis. J.A.V.M.A., *155*:2059–2061, 1969.

Mosier, J. E.: Treatment of cystitis. Anim. Hosp., *2*:11–14, 1966.

Piermattei, D. L.: A comparison of nitrofurantoin and dihydrostreptomycin in the treatment of experimental feline Escherichia coli urocystitis. Amer. J. Vet. Res., *23*:428–434, 1962.

Powers, T. E.: Antimicrobial therapy in small animal medicine. *In* Scientific Presentations and Seminar Synopses. 38th Annual Meeting, American Animal Hospital Association, Elkhart, Indiana, 1971.

Short, E. C., and Hammond, P. B.: Ammonium chloride as a urinary acidifier in the dog. J.A.V.M.A., *144*:864–867, 1964.

Chapter 39
CYSTITIS–URETHRAL OBSTRUCTION COMPLEX IN THE CAT

I. Introduction

A. *A clinical syndrome exists in both female and male cats that is characterized by dysuria and hematuria.*

Urethral obstruction frequently complicates the disease in the male, but rarely occurs in the female. Clinical signs indicate that the bladder and urethra are involved in this disease complex. Some evidence obtained at necropsy has been interpreted to suggest that primary renal disease exists with this complex. Whether the morphologic lesions noted were due to the primary disease, or secondary changes due to obstruction has not been resolved.

B. *The prevalence of this disease is reported to be between three and 10 per cent in the male cat; no statistics are available concerning its prevalence in the female.*

C. *Material that causes urethral obstruction of the male cat may be composed of mucoid material alone, mucoid material in combination with struvite (triple phosphate) crystals and cellular debris or crystals alone.*

Organization of crystals and mucus into a formed calculus is lacking; consequently, the term urolith or calculus is inappropriate for this material (Figs. 39–1 and 39–2).

II. Etiology

A. *Numerous factors have been incriminated including:*

1. Primary bacterial infection.
2. Diets high in mineral content.
3. Alkaline urine.
4. Vitamin A deficiency.
5. Pre-puberal castration.
6. Ingestion of dry cat foods (low water intake).
7. Viral infection.

362 DISEASES OF THE LOWER URINARY SYSTEM

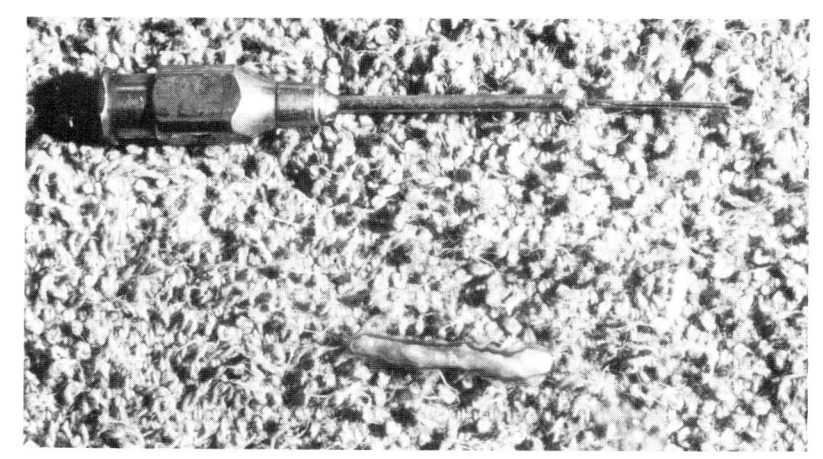

Figure 39–1. Urethral plug removed from the obstructed urethra of an 18-month-old male Siamese cat. The cat had severe cystitis (see Fig. 39–2.)

B. *Bacterial infection*
   1. Observations supporting the theory that bacterial infection is the primary cause of this disease include the following:
      a. Bacterial cystitis can cause dysuria and hematuria.
      b. Debris resulting from sloughing of cells and inflammatory exudate could result in urethral obstruction.
      c. Bacteria can sometimes be isolated from the urine of affected cats.
   2. Observations refuting the theory include the following:
      a. Bacteria cannot be consistently isolated from the urine of cats affected with cystitis or urethral obstruction or both.

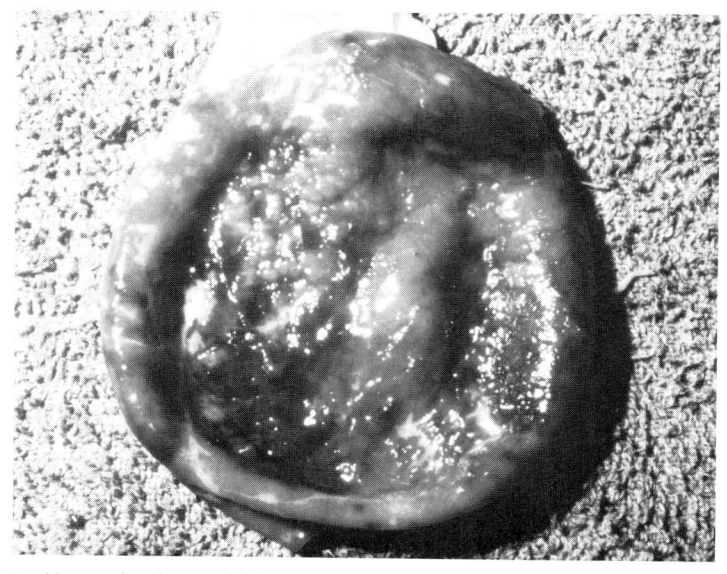

Figure 39–2. Hemorrhagic cystitis in an 18-month-old male Siamese cat. The cat had recurrent episodes of urethral obstruction.

b. When the bacterial isolates are obtained, it is not possible to establish whether their role is primary or secondary.
C. *Dietary intake of minerals (ash)*
   1. Observation supporting the theory:
      a. Increasing dietary mineral intake causes a slight increase in the quantity of struvite crystals in the urine.
   2. Observations refuting the theory:
      a. Efforts to induce urethral obstruction by feeding a high mineral diet to kittens have failed.
      b. There is no apparent relationship between crystal content of urine and urethral obstruction.
D. *Vitamin A deficiency*
   1. Observations supporting the theory:
      a. Vitamin A deficiency in rodents is associated with urolithiasis.
   2. Observations refuting the theory:
      a. Vitamin A deficiency has not been documented in affected cats.
      b. Vitamin A has not been demonstrated to be of prophylactic or therapeutic value in this disease.
E. *Alkaline urine*
   1. Alkaline pH of urine has been incriminated as a factor in the disease because of its relationship to crystal formation.
      a. Struvite crystals have less tendency to form below a urine pH of 6.8.
      b. As urine pH increases, the solubility of struvite decreases and crystallization increases.
   2. Alkaline urine may result from:
      a. Bacterial infection of the urinary tract.
      b. Urinary stasis.
      c. Diet (unlikely).
   3. It is probable that alkaline urine is caused by several factors, and cannot be incriminated as the primary cause of the disease.
F. *Pre-puberal castration*
   1. Castration prior to sexual maturity may affect the normal development of the genitalia.
   2. It has been hypothesized that the urethral diameter of the tomcat is decreased in size in the castrated male. Recent studies comparing the size of the urethra in cats neutered at five months and non-neutered males revealed that no difference in urethral diameter was present.
   3. Differences in the anatomy of the male and female urethra are undoubtedly related to the high incidence of urethral obstruction in males as compared to females.
G. *Ingestion of dry cat foods*
   1. It is reported that cats consuming dry foods ingest less water, resulting in the production of a more concentrated urine.
   2. Formation of crystals and aggregation of cellular debris is more likely to occur when the urine is concentrated.
   3. This disease complex does not occur exclusively in cats consuming dry food. It is probable that the role of dry foods in this disease is secondary rather than primary.

364 DISEASES OF THE LOWER URINARY SYSTEM

    H. *Viral infection*
        1. Urethral obstruction has been produced in normal male cats by injecting bacteria-free urine from obstructed cats into the bladder of normal cats.
        2. Three viruses, a picornavirus, a syncytial virus, and a Herpes-like virus, have been isolated from cats with urethral obstruction. Picornavirus was capable of inducing urethral obstruction when inoculated into the urinary bladder, or when cats were exposed by aerosol inoculation.
        3. Mineral crystals were observed in cell cultures infected with one or more feline viruses (syncytial virus and Herpes-like virus). It was implied that if viruses can induce mineral crystal formation in vitro, the possibility exists that the same phenomenon may occur in vivo.
        4. A mucoprotein, unique to cats with urethral obstruction, has been isolated from the urine. It has been hypothesized that this mucoprotein may serve as the matrix for the aggregation of debris that causes urethral obstruction.

    I. *Summary — etiology of feline cystitis–urethral obstruction complex*
        1. At present the viral theory of etiology is most attractive; primary bacterial infection is a likely cause in some cases also.
        2. Many factors that may influence the clinical course of the disease are probably of secondary etiologic significance.
            a. Alkaline urine.
            b. Crystalluria.
            c. Dry cat foods.
            d. Diets high in mineral content.
        3. Some factors are of no etiologic significance.
            a. Vitamin A deficiency.
            b. Castration.

III. History

    A. *Signs are usually limited to dysuria and hematuria in the female.*

    B. *In the male, dysuria and hematuria may be noted initially.*

    These actions are often misinterpreted by owners to indicate constipation. If obstruction occurs, the cat may lick its penis frequently. If obstruction persists, additional signs may be observed, including:
    1. Depression.
    2. Vomiting.
    3. Anorexia.
    4. Frequent, but unsuccessful attempts to urinate.

    C. *A seasonal incidence (highest in December through March) has been reported.*

    D. *Recurrent obstruction is a common complaint.*

IV. Clinical examination

    A. *In the absence of urethral obstruction:*
        1. Physical findings may be negative.
        2. The bladder is usually empty because of dysuria; occasionally pain is elicited by palpation of the bladder.
        3. Rectal temperature is normal.

B. *When urethral obstruction is present:*
  1. The bladder is firm and distended.
  2. Examination of the penis may reveal that it is inflamed and discolored. Occasionally the obstructing material may protrude from its tip.
  3. Affected cats may be alert or depressed, depending on the duration and degree of obstruction.
  4. Body temperature may be normal or subnormal.
  5. Dehydration may be severe.

V. Laboratory findings

A. *Urinalysis*
  1. Urine pH may be acid or alkaline.
  2. Tests for detecting the presence of protein and occult blood are frequently positive.
  3. Microscopic examination of urine sediment usually reveals a preponderance of red cells and a moderate number of leukocytes. Occasionally bacteria are observed. Struvite crystals are often present.

B. *BUN, creatinine*
  1. Early during the course of obstruction, values are elevated due to postrenal uremia.
  2. Primary renal uremia may develop if obstruction has been of sufficient duration.

C. *Both blood pH and plasma bicarbonate may be decreased; a metabolic acidosis may be present, depending on the duration of the obstruction.*

VI. Diagnosis

A. *Usually a diagnosis can be made on the basis of history and physical examination.*

B. *Inability to express urine from a moderately enlarged bladder by abdominal palpation is not diagnostic since male cats normally resist this technique.*

In instances of marked bladder distention, palpation should be performed with caution in order to avoid rupture of the bladder.

C. *Difficulty or inability to express urine from the cat while under anesthesia, or inability to inject a sterile solution into the bladder via a urethral catheter indicates the presence of urethral obstruction.*

VII. Treatment

A. *Provide relief of dysuria in the non-obstructed cat.*
  1. Urine culture should be performed to determine if bacterial infection is present. If bacteria are present, the patient should be treated for bacterial cystitis (see Chapter 38, Bacterial Cystitis).
  2. If urine culture is sterile, symptomatic treatment is indicated.
     a. Administration of smooth muscle relaxants may provide symptomatic relief of dysuria.
     b. Administration of sodium chloride will induce polydipsia and polyuria. This provides a "flushing action" in the urinary tract and decreases the concentration of the urine.
     c. An acid pH of the urine (6.5 or lower) will minimize crystalluria. It

may be necessary to administer urinary acidifiers to accomplish the objective. The dosage of acidifiers should be adjusted on the basis of urine pH. Administration of urinary acidifiers to uremic cats is contraindicated since they will aggravate the severity of metabolic acidosis.

B. *Urethral obstruction. Emergency treatment of the male cat with urethral obstruction should be directed toward re-establishing urine flow.*
  1. Manipulation of the penis. Occasionally the material obstructing the urethra may be dislodged by massaging the distal portion of the penis between the thumb and fingers.
  2. Reverse flushing of the urethra.
     a. Restraint of the patient.
        (1) If the cat is severely depressed, reverse flushing can usually be accomplished without pharmacologic restraint.
        (2) Generally, sedation or anesthesia is required.
           (a) Local anesthesia. Instillation of topical anesthetics such as 2% lidocaine may facilitate catheterization by relieving pain.
           (b) Regional anesthesia (epidural).
              [1] Two ml. of 2% procaine can be injected into the epidural space at the lumbosacral junction.
              [2] Maintain the cat in a horizontal position following the injection.
           (c) General anesthesia.
              [1] Thiamylal sodium*.
              [2] Induce anesthesia with thiamylal sodium and maintain it with methoxyflurane or halothane.
              [3] Ketamine hydrochloride**.
                 [a] The only route of excretion of this drug is by the kidney.
                 [b] Pending controlled studies in uremic cats, this drug should be used with caution in cats with impaired renal function.
     b. A sterilized straight lacrimal cannula, a sterilized 3½ French catheter† or sterilized synthetic tubing†† can be used as a catheter for reverse flushing. If synthetic tubing is used it should be prepared by cutting one end at a 45 degree angle and flaring the opposite end with the heat of a burning match.
     c. A sterilized water soluble lubricant should be applied to the catheter. The penis should be extruded from the sheath and pulled slightly posterior in order to provide a direct pathway for the catheter (see Chapter 5, Collection of Urine).
     d. The catheter should be inserted into the urethra 2 to 3 cm., or until the obstruction is encountered.
     e. Sterilized saline should be injected into the urethra. Saline and obstructing debris will often be forced around the catheter and out of the urethra.
     f. If the obstruction cannot be removed in this manner, the tip of the

---

*Surital, Parke-Davis and Co., Detroit, Michigan.
**Ketaset, Bristol Laboratories, Syracuse, New York 13201.
†Brunswick sterile disposable feeding tube and urethral catheter, Brunswick Laboratories, Inc. St. Louis, Missouri; Tomcat catheters, Sherwood Medical Industries, Inc., St. Louis, Missouri 63103.
††Intramedic Polyethylene Tubing, PE 60 to 90, Clay Adams Inc., New York, N. Y.

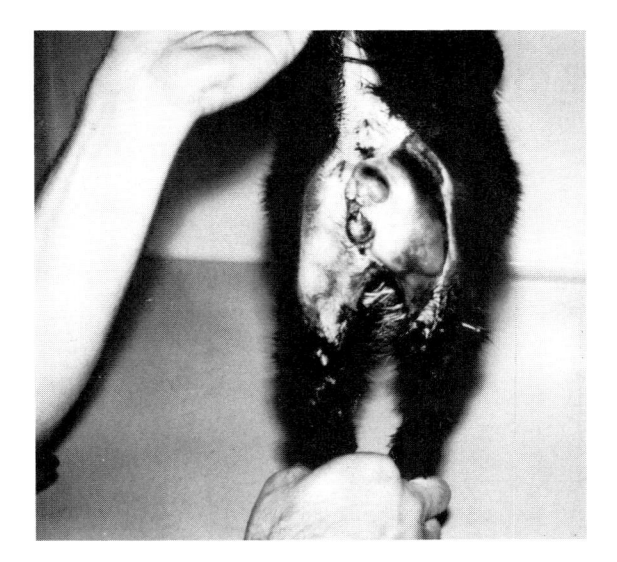

Figure 39–3. Cellulitis in an adult male domestic short-haired cat caused by periurethral extravasation of urine following rupture of the urethra. The urethra was ruptured with a metal catheter one week previously while attempts were being made to remove a urethral plug.

      penis should be firmly compressed around the catheter, and sterilized saline should be injected into the urethra. The obstructing material may be forced into the bladder. Care must be used not to damage the urethra during this procedure (Fig. 39–3). Gentle, steady digital pressure applied to the bladder at this time may help to dislodge urethral plugs. Compression of the bladder must be performed with care in order to avoid rupture.
   g. When the obstruction is relieved, most of the urine should be manually expressed from the bladder.
   h. In some cats, prolonged distention of the bladder may result in atony. Normal bladder function may return provided urine is manually expressed from the bladder several times per day. Alternatively, an indwelling catheter may be placed in the bladder. Digital manipulation must be gentle in order to prevent persistent hematuria.
   i. Although other solutions (1/12 N sulfuric acid, procaine, Renacidin*, tap water) have been advocated for use in reverse flushing, no objective studies have proved the superiority of one solution over another. The use of nonsterilized tap water is condemned.
3. Cystocentesis.
   a. In instances in which reverse flushing proves to be ineffective in relieving urethral obstruction, cystocentesis should be performed (see Chapter 5, Collection of Urine).
   b. Cystocentesis will provide immediate, but temporary, decompression of the bladder.
   c. Reverse flushing frequently is successful after cystocentesis has been performed.
4. Combined use of cystocentesis and meperidine hydrochloride**.
   a. This technique has been advocated as a method of relieving urethral obstruction without manipulation of the penis and urethra.
   b. Preliminary evaluation of this technique indicates that its success is variable.

---

*Renacidin, Fort Dodge Laboratories, Fort Dodge, Iowa.
**Demerol Hydrochloride, Winthrop Laboratories, New York, N.Y.

c. Recommended dosages of meperidine (5 mg. per lb) may cause undesirable side effects including central nervous system excitement, ataxia, and salivation.
5. Amputation of the penis.
    a. Amputation of the penis has been recommended by some for the relief of urethral obstruction.
    b. This procedure should be avoided since the inflammation and scarring which occur following amputation predispose the patient to urethral stricture.
6. Smooth muscle relaxants.
    a. Numerous products with this action have been advocated for use in the treatment and prophylaxis of feline urethral obstruction.
    b. Subjective evaluation of these products indicates that they have little if any value for this purpose, although they may alleviate pain due to smooth muscle spasm of the urinary tract.

C. *Maintenance of urine outflow by use of an indwelling catheter*
1. Frequently, urethral obstruction recurs despite repeated episodes of reverse flushing.
2. A variable degree of urethral trauma frequently occurs with each attempt at flushing.
3. For these reasons, placing an indwelling catheter in the urethra is advantageous. If a flexible catheter is used for relieving the original obstruction, relief of the obstruction and placement of the indwelling catheter can be accomplished simultaneously.
4. Technique.
    a. A sterile lubricated catheter should be inserted into the urethra in a manner described for reverse flushing.
    b. Once the obstructing material has been dislodged, the catheter should be moved toward the bladder while an assistant exerts a slight degree of negative pressure with a syringe attached to the end of the catheter.
    c. The insertion of the catheter should be discontinued as soon as urine can be aspirated. This maneuver assures correct placement of the tip of the catheter just cranial to the neck of the bladder (see Chapter 5, Collection of Urine).
    d. The protruding portion of the catheter should be thoroughly dried.
    e. Several layers of adhesive tape about 1 cm. in width should be wrapped around that portion of the catheter which is adjacent to the tip of the penis.
    f. A suture should be placed through the tape and the prepuce in order to fix the catheter in place. Only a short segment of the taped catheter should remain exposed.
    g. The excess portion of the catheter should be removed.
    h. An Elizabethan collar should be applied around the cat's neck in order to discourage removal of the catheter.
5. The indwelling catheter should be allowed to remain in place for two to four days, depending on the character of the urine.
6. If the catheter becomes obstructed, it should be rinsed with sterilized saline.

D. *Fluid therapy*
1. Obstructed cats may be severely dehydrated (see Chapter 32, Fluid Therapy in Renal Failure, for a guide to deficit therapy).

2. Patients with prolonged obstruction may have impairment of the renal concentrating mechanism for a period of days to months. If polyuria is present, maintenance requirements of water will be greater than normal.
3. Severe metabolic acidosis may be present in instances where urethral obstruction is prolonged (see Chapter 32, Fluid Therapy in Renal Failure, for recommendations for alleviation of the acidosis). Urinary acidifiers are contraindicated in the acute phase of therapy because they will aggravate the acidosis.

E. *Control of bacterial infection*

Prophylactic or therapeutic antibacterial therapy should be chosen on the basis of culture and sensitivity testing (see Bacterial culture of urine, in Chapter 6; Treatment of bacterial Cystitis, in Chapter 38; and Chapter 33, Drug Therapy in Renal Failure).

F. *Surgical treatment*
1. Surgical treatment of urethral obstruction is indicated:
    a. In instances where nonsurgical therapeutic and prophylactic measures have not alleviated the problem.
    b. When permanent strictures develop in the distal portion of the urethra.
    c. Corrective surgery is contraindicated in patients with uremic crises since they are poor surgical risks. Only after the obstruction has been relieved and renal function reestablished should corrective surgery be considered. If the urethral obstruction cannot be removed and the patient is severely uremic, intermittent cystocentesis and peritoneal dialysis should be considered prior to surgical intervention.
2. The following surgical techniques have been successfully utilized for alleviating urethral obstruction; however, none have proven to be consistently successful.
    a. Perineal urethrostomy (Carbone technique).
    b. Perineal urethrostomy (Blake technique).
    c. Preputial urethrostomy.
    d. Antepubic urethrostomy.
3. Consult surgery texts and references for details concerning surgical technique.
4. Urethral stricture is a common complication following surgery. Although several modifications have been developed to reduce the incidence of postsurgical urethral stricture, reports indicate that this complication occurs in five to 20 per cent of the cases.

VIII. Prophylaxis

A. *Because of the frequency of recurrence of this disease in male cats, prophylactic therapy should be considered.*

Specific prophylactic procedures based on etiology are presently unavailable. Prophylaxis of the cystitis–urethral obstruction complex in the cat should be directed toward alleviating secondary factors that contribute to the complex.

B. *Prophylactic measures of probable benefit include:*
1. Inducement of polydipsia and polyuria.

a. Administer salt orally (tablet, capsule or granular form; ¼ to 1 Gm. daily).
b. Continue salt therapy indefinitely.
c. Be sure drinking water is available at all times.
d. These procedures result in the production of an increased volume of dilute urine, and as a result, crystallization and aggregation of particulate material is decreased.
2. Acidification of urine.
a. Any one of several acidifiers is satisfactory.
   (1) d,1-methionine
   (2) Ascorbic acid.
   (3) Mandelic acid.
   (4) Ethylenediamine dihydrochloride.
   (5) Ammonium chloride.
b. Dosage of acidifiers should be adjusted according to urine pH; pH should be maintained at 6.5 or below.
c. It may be necessary to administer acidifiers indefinitely.
d. Acidification of urine minimizes struvite crystal formation.
3. In some cats, it has been observed that use of dry cat food is associated with an increase in the quantity of urinary struvite crystals.
a. It may be advantageous to avoid feeding a diet composed exclusively of dry food.
b. If the use of dry food is unavoidable, mix it with water.

IX. Summary of treatment

A. Because the pathophysiology of this disease complex has not been established, only supportive and symptomatic methods of therapy are currently available.

B. Consistent effective management will not be available until treatment is designed to correct or eliminate etiopathogenic abnormalities of the disease.

X. Prognosis

A. The prognosis for male cats with urethral obstruction is usually guarded.

B. Although the patient may survive, recurrence of urethral obstruction is common.

C. Stricture of the urethral lumen is a frequent sequela in patients with recurrent obstruction.

REFERENCES

Archibald, J., Sumner-Smith, G., and Dingwall, J.: Surgical management of urethral obstruction in male cats. MVP, *52*:55–61, 1971.
Blake, J. A.: Perineal urethrostomy in cats. J.A.V.M.A., *152*:1499–1506, 1968.
Bone W. J.: Perineal urethrostomy in the male cat. Vet. Med./S. A. C., *64*:518–520, 1969.
Brodey, R. S.: Seasonal incidence of urolithiasis in male cats. Mod. Vet. Pract., *52*:20, March, 1971.
Carbone, M. G.: Phosphocrystalluria and urethral obstruction in the cat. J.A.V.M.A., *147*:1195–1200, 1966.
Carbone, M. G.: Modified technique for perineal urethrostomy, *151*:301–305, 1967.
Carbone, M. G.: Urethral surgery in the cat. Vet. Clin. N. Amer., *1*:281–298, 1971.
Christensen, N. R.: Preputial urethrostomy in the male cat. J.A.V.M.A., *145*:903–908, 1964.
Fabricant, C. G., Gillepsie, J. H., and Krook, L.: Intracellular and extracellular mineral crystal formation induced by viral infection of cell cultures. J. Infect. Immun., *3*:416–419, 1971.
Fabricant, C. G., and Rich, L. J.: Microbial studies of feline urolithiasis. J.A.V.M.A., *158*:976–980, 1971.

Fabricant, C. G., Rich, L. J., and Gillespie, J. H.: Feline viruses. XI. Isolation of a virus similar to myxovirus from cats in which urolithiasis was experimentally induced. Cornell Vet., 59:667–672, 1969.

Ford, D. C.: Antepubic urethrostomy. J. Amer. Animal Hosp. Assoc., 4:145–149, 1968.

Herron, M. A.: The effect of prepubertal castration on the penile urethra of the cat. J.A.V.M.A., 160:208–211, 1972.

Klide, A. M., and Soma, L. R.: Epidural anesthesia in the dog and cat. J.A.V.M.A., 153:165–173, 1968.

McCully, R. M., and Lieberman, L. L.: Histopathology in a case of feline urolithiasis. Canad. Vet. J., 2:52–60, 1966.

Meier, F. W.: Urethral obstruction and stenosis in the male cat. J.A.V.M.A., 137:67–70, 1960.

Mendham, J. H.: A description and evaluation of antepubic urethrostomy in the male cat. J. Sm. Anim. Pract., 11:709–721, 1970.

Miller, G. K.: Observations of the Blake perineal urethrostomy in cats. Vet. Med./S. A. C., 66:1170–1174, 1971.

Osbaldiston, G. W., and Taussig, R. A.: Clinical report of 46 cases of feline urological syndrome. Vet. Med./S. A. C., 65:461–468, 1970.

Rich, L. J.: Current concepts of feline urethral obstruction. Vet. Clin. N. Amer., 1:245–250, 1971.

Rich, L. J., and Fabricant, C. G.: Experimental production of urolithiasis in male cats. J.A.V.M.A., 158:974–976, 1971.

Rich, L. J., and Fabricant, C. G.: Urethral obstruction in male cats: Transmission studies. Canad. J. Comp. Med., 33:164–165, 1969.

Rich, L. J., Fabricant, C. G., and Gillespie, J. H.: Virus-induced urolithiasis in male cats. Cornell Vet., 61:542–553, 1971.

Rich, L. J., and Kirk, R. W.: Struvite crystals in urethral obstruction. J.A.V.M.A., 154:153–157, 1969.

Rich, L. J., and Kirk, R. W.: Mineral aspects of urethral obstruction. Amer. J. Vet. Res., 29:2149–2156, 1968.

Rich, L. J., and Norcross, N. L.: Feline urethral obstruction: Immunologic identification of a unique urinary protein. Amer. J. Vet. Res., 30:1001–1005, 1969.

Schecter, R. D.: The significance of bacteria in feline cystitis and urolithiasis. J.A.V.M.A., 156:1567–1573, 1970.

Sharpnack, S.: Feline urethral obstruction. In Current Veterinary Therapy. Vol. 4. Edited by Robert W. Kirk. Philadelphia, Pa., W. B. Saunders Co., 1971.

Wilson, G. P., and Harrison, J. W.: Perineal urethrostomy in cats. J.A.V.M.A., 159:1789–1793, 1971.

Chapter 40
CAPILLARIA PLICA

I. **Capillaria plica is a nematode of cosmopolitan distribution which is found in the urinary bladder, and uncommonly, in the renal pelves, of the dog, fox, wolf, and cat.**

   A. *Foxes are considered to be the definitive host.*

   B. *Capillaria felis-cati is a related (and possibly identical) nematode which occurs in the urinary bladder of the cat.*

   It has been reported in Australia and Egypt.

II. **Morphologic characteristics**

   A. *Adults are fragile, thread-like yellowish parasites, 1 to 6 cm. in length, which are difficult to see without magnification.*

   B. *The eggs of C. plica are oval in shape and have bipolar plugs.*

   They are colorless and have a slightly pitted shell (Fig. 40–1).

III. **Life cycle**

   A. *The life cycle of C. plica is controversial.*

   Both direct and indirect cycles have been postulated.

   B. *In the indirect life cycle, the earthworm is considered to be the intermediate host.*

   When infected earthworms are ingested by a susceptible host, it has been postulated that the larvae migrate through the intestinal wall and reach the urinary bladder via blood vessels.

IV. **Pathology**

   A. *Capillaria plica are considered to be relatively nonpathogenic by most investigators.*

   B. *Infected dogs and cats usually do not develop clinical signs.*

V. **Diagnosis**

   A. *A definitive diagnosis of Capillaria spp. infection of the urinary tract must be based on identification of the adult parasites, larvae, or ova (Fig. 40–1).*

   B. *On occasion, urine collected from a cage may be contaminated with fecal material.*

   In this situation, caution must be used in differentiating the ova of *C. plica* from the ova of other *Capillaria* spp. which parasitize the intestinal tract and respiratory tract.

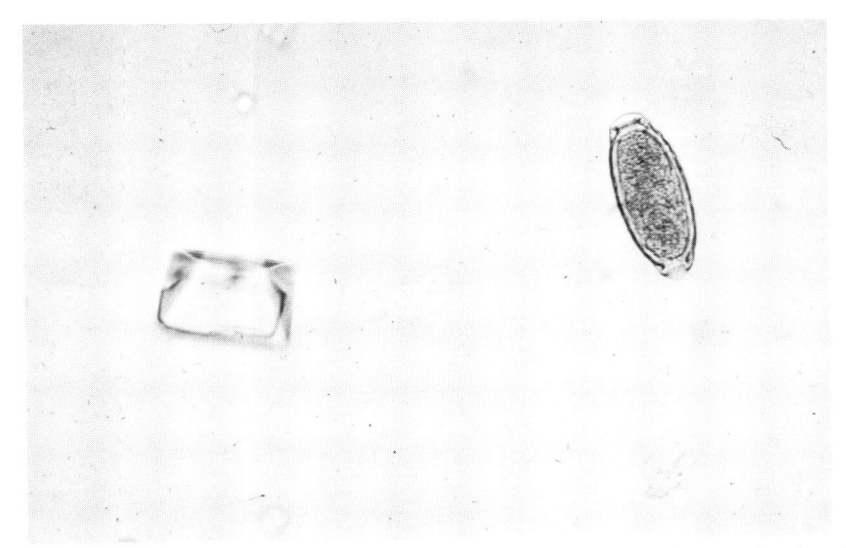

Figure 40-1. Photomicrograph of *Capillaria plica* ova in the urine sediment of a dog. (Courtesy of S. M. Gaafar and D. F. Brobst, School of Veterinary Science and Medicine, Purdue University.)

VI. Treatment

　A. *Very little information concerning the treatment of* C. plica *is currently available.*

　B. *Although no effective treatment for* C. plica *has been described, treatment is usually unnecessary.*

VII. Control. Investigators who have incriminated earthworms as the intermediate host for C. plica recommend eliminating patient contact with earthworms.

REFERENCES

Soulsby, E. J. L.: Textbook of Veterinary Clinical Parasitology. Vol. I—Helminths. Philadelphia, Pa., F. A. Davis Co., 1965.
Waddell, A. H.: Further observations on Capillaria feliscati infection in the cat. Aust. Vet. J., *44*:33–34, 1968.
Waddell, A. H.: Anthelmintic treatment for Capillaria feliscati in the cat. Vet. Rec., *82*:598, 1968.

Chapter 41
NEOPLASMS OF THE URINARY BLADDER

I. **Prevalence**

   A. *Neoplasms of the excretory pathway of the urinary system may originate in the renal pelves, ureters, urinary bladder, or urethra.*

   B. *In dogs:*
      1. They occur more commonly in the urinary bladder.
      2. Neoplasms of the urinary bladder account for less than 0.5 per cent of the neoplasms of the body.
      3. The frequency of occurrence of bladder neoplasms increases with age.

   C. *In cats:*
      1. Epithelial neoplasms of the excretory pathway of the urinary system are exceedingly rare.
      2. Less than 10 transitional cell carcinomas of the urinary system have been reported in the world literature.
      3. It has been hypothesized that the low concentration of carcinogenic tryptophan metabolites in cat urine may be related to the low incidence of urinary epithelial neoplasms in the cat as compared to other species.
         a. In dogs and human beings, primary neoplasms of the bladder epithelium are encountered more frequently.
         b. Primary neoplasms of the renal pelvic epithelium comprise approximately 10 per cent of the renal tumors in man.

II. **Etiopathogenesis**

   A. *All causes of spontaneous neoplasia of transitional epithelium of man and animals have not been defined.*
      1. Endogenous carcinogens, exogenous carcinogens, chronic inflammation, and viruses have been incriminated in the genesis of spontaneous and experimental tumors in man and animals.
      2. Prolonged exposure to aromatic amine chemicals is a known cause of transitional cell carcinomas of the urinary system of human beings.
      3. Malignant epithelial neoplasms have been experimentally produced in dogs by administration of carcinogens such as beta-naphthylamine.
      4. It has been hypothesized that the low frequency of occurrence of transitional cell neoplasms of cats, as compared to that of dogs and human

beings, may be related to species differences in the metabolism of potential endogenous and exogenous carcinogenic agents.
   a. Clinical and experimental data have revealed that exogenous aniline carcinogens produce transitional cell neoplasms of the urinary tract only in those species (dogs, rodents, man) which metabolize and excrete significant quantities of aniline derivative metabolites as free ortho-aminophenols in urine.
   b. Cats metabolize these carcinogens differently than do dogs, and it has been suggested that metabolites excreted in cat urine are non-carcinogenic.
5. Tryptophan, an essential aromatic amino acid, has been incriminated as a factor in the genesis of urinary transitional cell carcinomas in man and animals.
   a. Aromatic amine metabolites derived from tryptophan and excreted in urine of several types of animals are similar in biochemical structure to proved exogenous carcinogens of the urinary tract.
   b. These metabolites are ortho-aminophenols and occur as intermediate stages in the biochemical conversion of tryptophan to nicotinic acid.
   c. Since these metabolites are excreted in urine in a conjugated inactive form, it is thought that certain enzymes (beta-glucuronidase) found in transitional epithelium liberate them in active form following excretion into urine.
   d. Recent studies have revealed that human beings, cows, rats, and dogs excrete significant quantities of potential carcinogenic aromatic amine metabolites derived from tryptophan in their urine.
   e. Human beings with bladder cancer also have an abnormally high concentration of these tryptophan metabolites in their urine.
   f. Cats metabolize tryptophan by a process that does not involve production of ortho-aminophenols, and consequently have extremely small quantities of these metabolites in their urine.

B. *Although neoplasms of transitional epithelium may originate anywhere in the urinary tract of dogs and cats, they occur most often in the urinary bladder.*

1. Tumors originating from transitional epithelium of the renal pelvis, ureters, and urethra are less common, even though these structures are lined by the same type of epithelium as found in the bladder.
2. The higher incidence of primary epithelial neoplasms of the urinary bladder may be associated with storage of urine in this organ. Storage of urine in the bladder may enhance the action of carcinogenic agents by allowing increased contact time with tissue. The latter conclusion is supported by the following facts:
   a. Experimental production of epithelial tumors in the dependent portions of dog urinary bladders requires continuous oral administration of carcinogenic agents over a period of two to three years.
   b. Epithelial tumors develop in the urinary bladders of dogs only if carcinogenic agents excreted in urine have direct contact with transitional epithelium.
   c. Epithelial neoplasms of the ureters and renal pelves have been induced only following continuous administration of carcinogenic agents to dogs with partial obstruction to the ureters.

III. Classification

Spontaneous neoplasms of the urinary bladder may be:

A. *Primary or metastatic in origin.*

B. *Benign or malignant in biologic behavior.*

C. *Differentiated or undifferentiated in morphologic appearance.*

D. *Papillary or sessile in attachment to bladder wall.*

E. *Superficial or infiltrating in invasiveness.*

IV. Benign urinary bladder neoplasms of dogs

A. *Papillomas*
  1. Papillomas are less common than malignant neoplasms of the urinary bladder.
  2. Papillomas are more common in older animals, but they can occur at any age.
  3. Papillomas reportedly have a malignant biological behavior, although this conclusion is apparently based on very limited numbers.
  4. Papillomas may be single or multiple.
  5. Papillomas have a variable size (microscopic to several cm. in diameter).
  6. Papillomas arising in the region of the trigone may partially or totally obstruct the urethra or ureters (or both).
  7. Papillomas often are associated with signs of cystitis. As papillomas increase in size, contraction of the bladder wall may lead to fragmentation of surface fronds with resultant necrosis of the underlying tissue. This is often followed by ulceration, infection, and hemorrhage, resulting in hematuria.
  8. Papillomas may serve as a nidus for calculi formation if their necrotic surface becomes encrusted with mineral salts.
  9. Papillomas are composed of well differentiated transitional epithelium which shows no tendency to invade the mucosal basement membrane.

B. *Fibromas often occur singly and grow slowly, and therefore are usually asymptomatic.*

C. *Leiomyomas*
  1. Leiomyomas are often multiple and small.
  2. Larger tumors may protrude into the lumen of the urinary bladder, or protrude from its serosal surface, but usually don't produce clinical signs until they become large enough to cause mechanical interference with function of the bladder.

D. *Other benign tumors which may potentially occur in the urinary bladder include:*
  1. Neurofibromas.
  2. Rhabdomyomas.
  3. Angiomas.
  4. Myxomas.

V. Malignant urinary bladder neoplasm of dogs

A. *The most common primary malignant tumors of the urinary bladder of the dog are of epithelial origin.*

B. Carcinomas
1. Transitional cell carcinomas are most frequently encountered; squamous cell carcinomas, adenocarcinomas, and undifferentiated carcinomas occur less frequently.
2. Gross appearance.
   a. Transitional cell carcinomas may be solitary or multiple papillary projections involving the bladder mucosa, and/or they may occur as local or diffuse swellings of the bladder wall. The nonpapillary variety is most frequently encountered in the dog.
   b. Invasion of the bladder wall is common, especially with nonpapillary varieties. The mucosa and underlying muscular layers may be completely destroyed and replaced by tumor cells.
   c. Neoplastic tissue may extend into the urethra or ureters and result in obstruction and hydronephrosis.
   d. Metastasis is frequent.
      (1) The regional lymph nodes and lungs are the most frequent sites of metastasis.
      (2) Many other organs and tissues may be involved in some instances.

C. Sarcomas
1. Fibrosarcomas:
   a. Are uncommon.
   b. Frequently show diffuse invasive growth and metastasis.
2. Leiomyosarcomas are uncommon, but have been encountered.
3. Rhabdomyosarcomas are uncommon. Only three cases have been reported in dogs.

Figure 41-1. Survey radiograph of the lateral aspect of the abdomen of a 7-year-old male domestic shorthaired cat. Arrows outline an irregular area of increased density in the bladder lumen which was a myxomatous neoplasm of low grade malignancy. (J.A.V.M.A., *152*:247–259, 1968.)

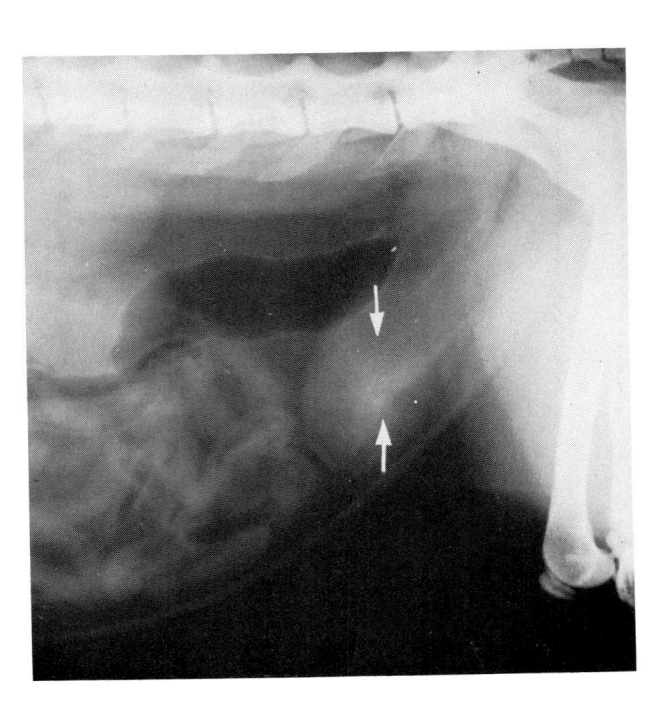

378 DISEASES OF THE LOWER URINARY SYSTEM

   4. Other sarcomas possible, but not as yet reported, in dogs include:
      a. Hemangiosarcomas.
      b. Osteosarcomas.
      c. Myxosarcomas. A myxosarcoma has been reported in a cat (Fig. 41–1).

  D. *Metastatic tumors of the urinary bladder*
   1. Metastatic bladder neoplasms are apparently uncommon.
   2. Malignant neoplasms may metastasize to the urinary bladder by:
      a. Extension of malignant primary tumors from adjacent organs, such as the prostate gland.
      b. Implantation from primary lesions located in kidneys or ureters.
      c. Embolic spread through lymphatic or vascular channels.
   3. Reported cases in dogs include:
      a. An adenocarcinoma originating in the prostate gland.
      b. A transitional cell carcinoma originating in the prostatic urethra.
      c. A hemangiosarcoma originating in the heart.

VI. Clinical findings

  A. *History*
   1. The most frequent complaint made by owners of dogs and cats with bladder tumors is that their pet has constant or intermittent hematuria. The hematuria may be mild or severe, but the quantity of blood in the urine is not a reliable indication of the size or the biologic behavior of the neoplasm.

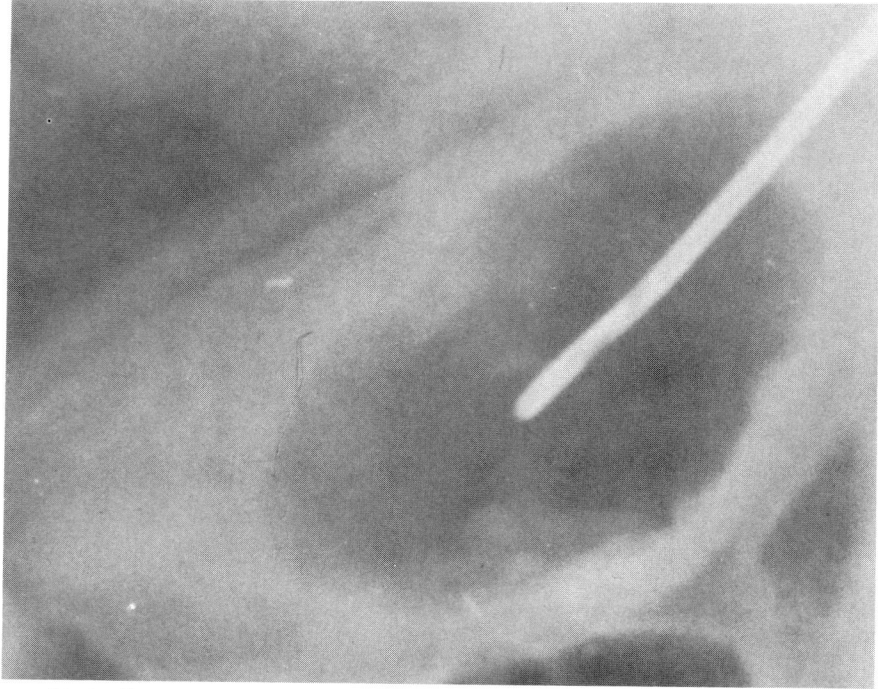

Figure 41–2. Pneumocystogram of a 3-year-old domestic short-haired cat. The bladder wall is markedly thickened, and the contour of the mucosal surface is extremely irregular. A diagnosis of chronic polypoid cystitis was established by microscopic examination of a biopsy specimen. A radiopaque catheter is in the upper right hand corner of the radiograph. (J.A.V.M.A., *152:*247–259, 1968.)

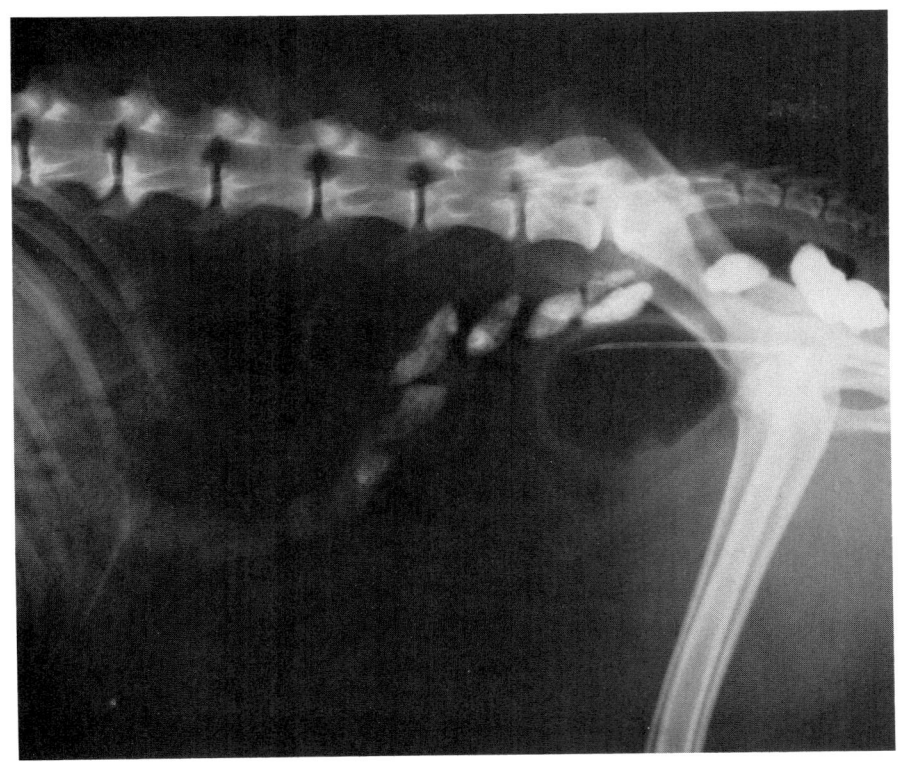

Figure 41-3. Pneumocystogram of a 9-year-old female mixed breed dog with polypoid cystitis. The bladder wall is thickened, and multiple polypoid growths project into the lumen of the bladder. A diagnosis of polypoid cystitis was made by microscopic examination of a surgical biopsy specimen of the bladder wall. A radiopaque catheter is located just below the dorsal bladder wall. Fecal material is radiopaque because barium had previously been administered orally. Notice the similarity to Figure 41-4.

    2. Increased frequency of urination is a less common complaint and occurs as a result of associated cystitis, reduction in bladder capacity because of the large size of the tumor, or loss of bladder distensibility as a result of neoplastic destruction of the bladder wall.

    3. Anorexia and weight loss are uncommon complaints.

B. *Physical examination*

    1. The clinical signs associated with bladder neoplasms are not pathognomonic.

    2. Neoplasms that are at an early and potentially curable stage usually do not produce abnormalities detectable by physical examination alone.

    3. Clinical signs commonly associated with urinary bladder tumors are essentially the same as those seen in many diseases that involve this organ, especially cystitis. Cystitis is a frequent complication of bladder neoplasia because bacteria readily invade the necrotic and ulcerated surface of the neoplasm and stimulate inflammation.

    4. Partial or complete obstruction of the urethra may cause:

        a. Dysuria.

        b. Decrease in the size of the urine stream.

        c. Overdistention of the bladder with urine.

d. Hydronephrosis.
e. Signs referable to renal failure.
5. Partial or complete obstruction of the ureters may cause:
   a. Hydronephrosis.
   b. Signs referable to renal failure.
6. The animal may be anemic as a result of one or more of the following:
   a. Decreased production of erythrocyte stimulating factor by hydronephrotic kidneys.
   b. Bone marrow depression associated with secondary chronic bacterial infection (i.e., anemia of infection).
   c. Severe hematuria.
7. Results of abdominal palpation are dependent on the size, shape, and location of the neoplasm.
   a. A thickened bladder wall may be caused by:
      (1) Tumors which diffusely invade the bladder wall.
      (2) Severe generalized chronic cystitis.
      (3) Compensatory muscle hypertrophy secondary to outflow obstruction.
   b. Solitary and multiple tumors that protrude into the lumen of the urinary bladder may be palpated as firm, nonyielding, nongrating masses within the bladder.

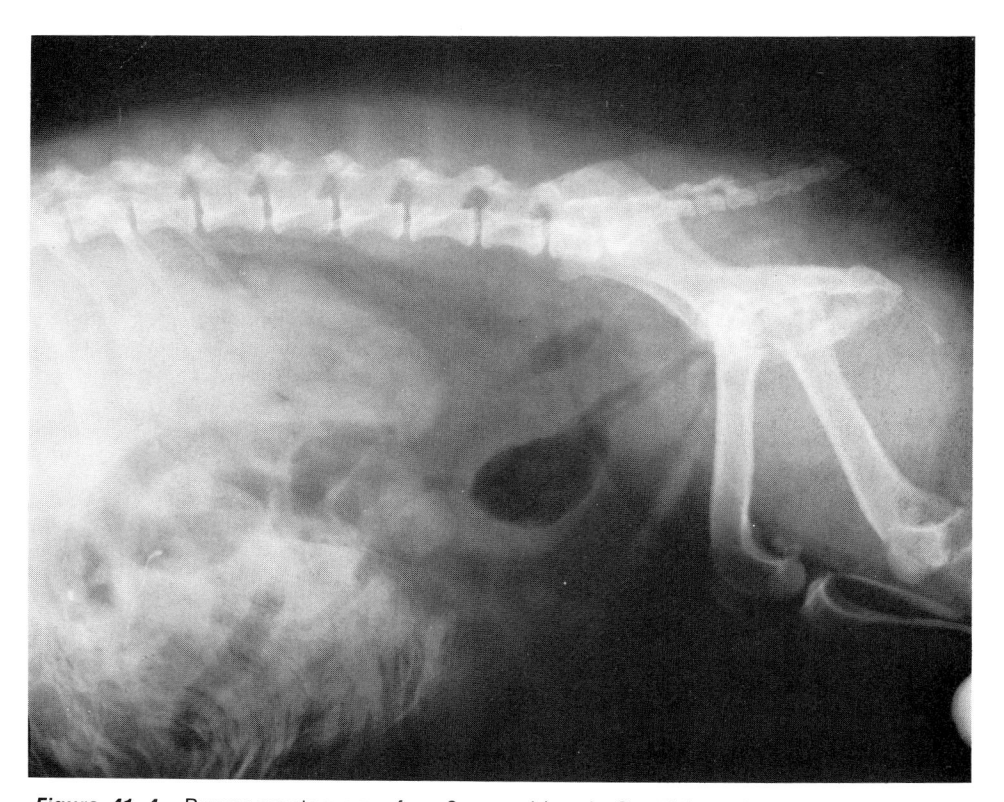

Figure 41-4. Pneumocystogram of an 8-year-old male Scottish terrier with a transitional cell carcinoma of the urinary bladder. The bladder wall is markedly thickened and the contour of the mucosal surface is irregular. A diagnosis of transitional cell carcinoma was established on the basis of microscopic examination of a surgical biopsy specimen. Notice the similarity to Figures 41-2 and 41-3. (J.A.V.M.A., *152:*247–259, 1968.)

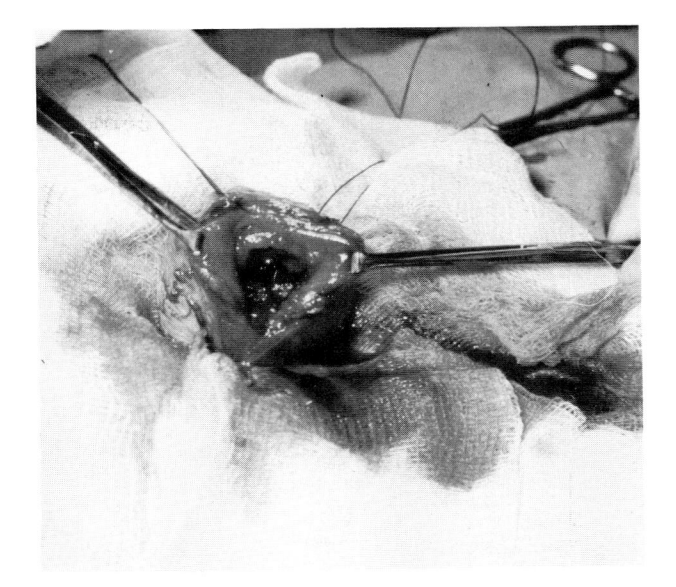

Figure 41-5. Thickened, contracted, neoplastic urinary bladder of the dog described in Figure 41-4. Neoplastic tissue involved the mucosa, submucosa, and tunica muscularis of the bladder wall. Neoplastic cells were also found in the urine sediment and internal iliac lymph nodes. Notice similarity to Figure 38-2. (J.A.V.M.A., *152*:247-259, 1968).

8. Signs referable to metastatic lesions may occur.
9. Most of the signs, with the exception of hematuria, do not develop until the neoplasm becomes well established.

C. *Laboratory findings*
   1. Urinalysis.
      a. The results of a urinalysis may be indicative of cystitis (i.e., alkaline pH, proteinuria, hematuria, pyuria, and bacteriuria).
      b. In uninfected or treated patients, red blood cells may dominate the microscopic findings in urine sediment.
      c. Neoplastic cells may be found in urine sediment, especially in association with carcinomas. The use of new methylene blue stain is recommended for identification of neoplastic cells in urine sediment.
   2. Hemogram.
      a. Hemograms are usually normal.
      b. A regenerative or nonregenerative anemia may be present, depending on the cause.
   3. Renal function tests. The results of renal function tests are normal unless there is obstruction to urine flow.

D. *Radiographic findings*
   1. Bladder tumors are often difficult to demonstrate radiographically, especially if they are diffuse.
   2. Radiographic findings are not pathognomonic as they may be the same as those seen in chronic cystitis (Figs. 41-2, 41-3, 41-4 and 41-5).
   3. Tumors that protrude into the lumen of the bladder may be visualized as space-occupying masses (Figs. 41-6 and 41-7).
   4. Double contrast cystography may enhance visualization of neoplastic lesions.
   5. Invasive tumors that cause thickening and deformity of the bladder wall may be detected by fractional superimposition cystography.

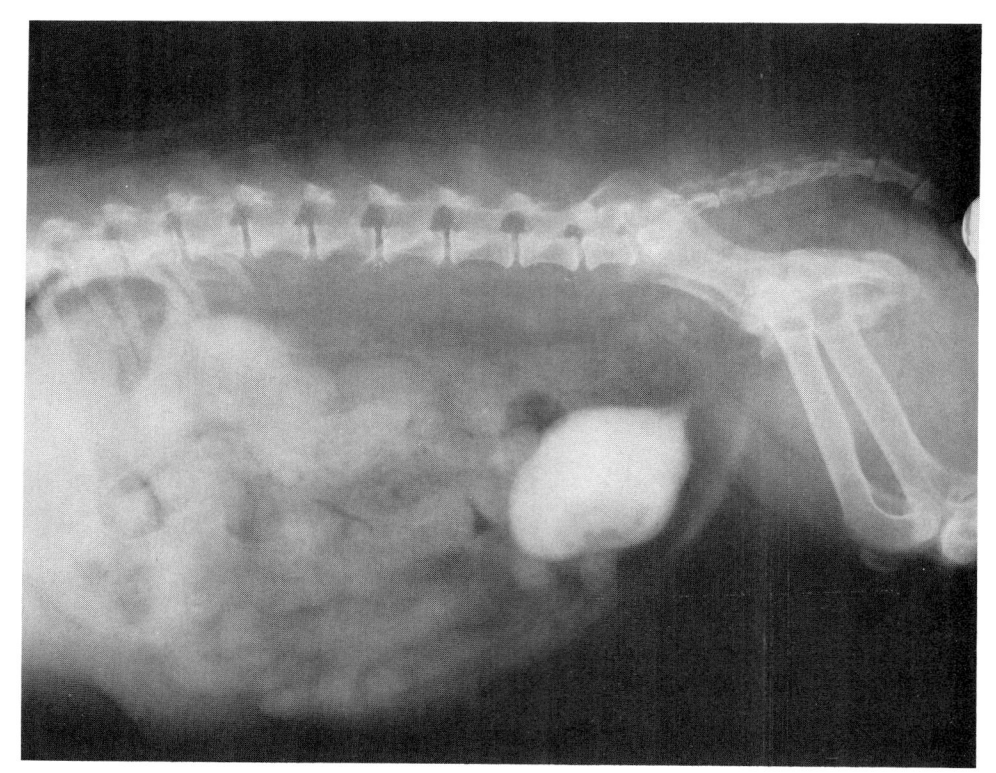

Figure 41-6. Positive contrast cystogram of the urinary bladder of a 13-year-old female Scottish terrier. A space occupying lesion, which appears as an area of decreased density, protrudes from the ventral aspect of the bladder wall. A diagnosis of transitional cell carcinoma was established by microscopic examination of the extirpated mass. (J.A.V.M.A., 152:247-259, 1968.)

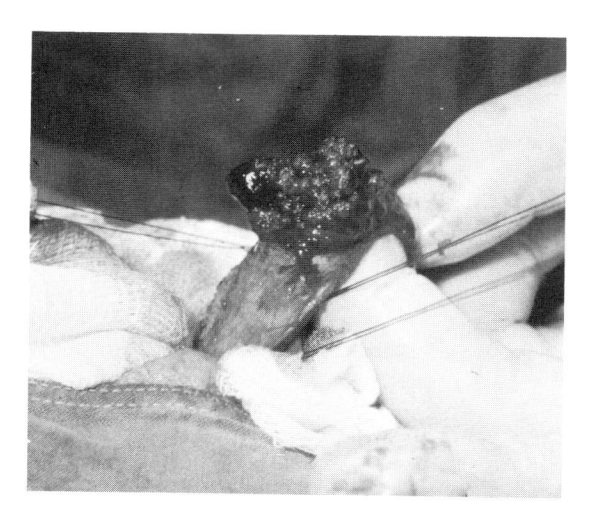

Figure 41-7. Transitional cell carcinoma of the urinary bladder of the dog described in Figure 41-6. The tumor was removed by partial cystectomy. (J.A.V.M.A., 152:247-259, 1968.)

NEOPLASMS OF THE URINARY BLADDER

6. Intravenous urography may reveal hydronephrosis and hydroureter if the ureters or urethra are obstructed.

VII. Diagnosis

  A. *A tentative diagnosis may be based on history, physical findings, radiologic interpretation, and laboratory findings.*

  B. *Bladder neoplasia is often an exclusion diagnosis which is established after other causes of hematuria have been eliminated (see Urinalysis, in Chapter 6).*

  C. *A definitive diagnosis must be based on microscopic detection and evaluation of neoplastic cells.*
  1. Neoplastic cells may be detected in urine sediment (Fig. 41–8).
  2. Cystoscopy and transurethral biopsy may be of value in medium- or large-size female dogs.
  3. Exploratory laparotomy.
      a. The occurrence of persistent hematuria due to unknown cause which does not respond to conventional methods of therapy for cystitis, and the presence of clinical findings consistent with neoplasia of the urinary bladder, is justification for surgical exploration of the bladder.
      b. Biopsy of the lesion, preferably by complete excision, may be indicated at the time of surgery since differentiation between diffuse neoplasia and cystitis is often difficult. The tissue may be necrotic, ulcerated, inflamed, and thickened in both conditions.
      c. The internal iliac and lumbar lymph nodes should be examined and, if necessary, biopsied at the time of laparotomy in order to confirm or eliminate the possibility of metastasis.

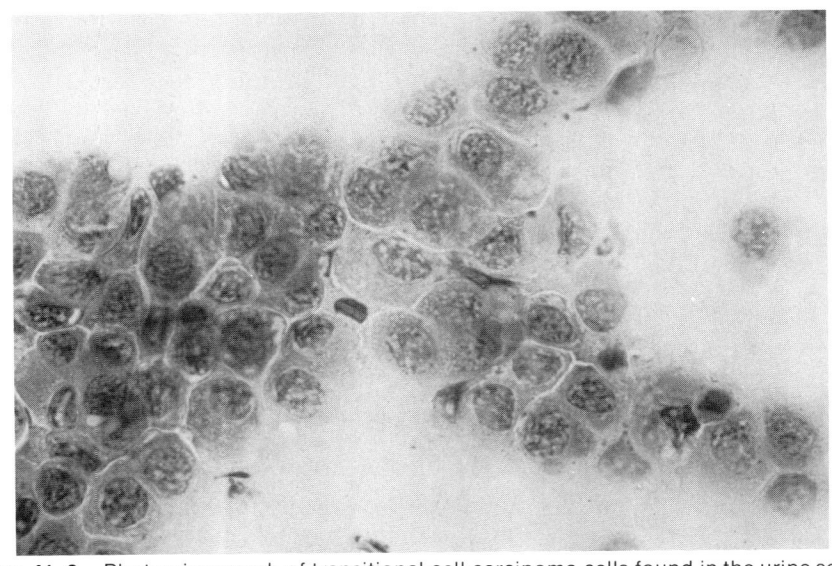

Figure 41–8. Photomicrograph of transitional cell carcinoma cells found in the urine sediment of an 8-year-old male Scottish terrier. Sheets and clumps of malignant cells were seen in the urine sediment on several occasions. New methylene blue stain: ×400. (J.A.V.M.A., *152*:247–259, 1968.)

VIII. Treatment

A. *Symptomatic treatment of hematuria due to bladder neoplasia is rarely justified and is usually unsuccessful.*

Nontreatment has little to offer a patient with bladder neoplasia, however, since the condition will remain the same at best and usually becomes worse.

B. *The poor results generally reported in the treatment of urinary bladder tumors of dogs may be related to one or more of the following:*
1. The initial diganosis is usually not established until the condition is far advanced.
2. Operative procedures may remove the tumor, but not the cause of neoplasia.
3. The surgeon's gloves and instruments are used to repair the surgical wound following contamination with neoplastic tissue.

C. *Partial cystectomy should be employed to extirpate tumors located in accessible areas of the bladder.*
1. The neoplastic tissue and a wide zone of healthy tissue, including the entire depth of the bladder wall, should be removed.
2. Ureteral transplantation may be necessary.

D. *Tumors that occupy the neck of the bladder, the trigone, or a great portion of the bladder wall cannot be removed by partial cystectomy.*

Total cystectomy preceded by transplantation of the ureters into an ileal conduit may be considered, but postoperative complications and loss of function make such an approach impractical for most house pets.

E. *The presence of metastatic neoplasms precludes surgical intervention in most instances.*

F. *Palliative therapy*
1. A poor response has been obtained in man and experimental animals following the use of chemotherapeutic agents such as 5-fluorouracil.
2. Irradiation has been unrewarding in human patients. Most urinary bladder neoplasms are relatively radio-resistant, and the dosage required to achieve significant regression is often associated with complications, including:
   a. Hemorrhage.
   b. Severe inflammation.
   c. Contracture of the bladder wall.

G. *Supportive therapy*

Treat the cystitis associated with neoplasia (see Chapter 38, Bacterial Cystitis).

H. *Prophylactic consideration*

Because of the tendency of bladder neoplasms to recur following surgery, periodic reevaluation of the patient is indicated.

IX. Prognosis

A. *The location, extent, histologic appearance, and depth of penetration are important factors that should be considered when establishing a prognosis.*

1. The site of the neoplasm is often as important a factor in determining the future course of events as is histologic type.
2. In general, tumors that have penetrated beyond the mucosal basement membrane are more likely to recur and metastasize than tumors confined to the mucosa.

B. *In cases in which complete surgical extirpation of solitary noninfiltrating benign tumors has been performed, a fair to good prognosis is justified.*

C. *In cases in which malignant neoplasms have been surgically removed, a guarded prognosis should be offered because of the great tendency of these tumors to recur and metastasize.*

D. *In cases in which no treatment is given, or in which the neoplasm has metastasized, a poor to grave prognosis should be offered.*

REFERENCES

Boyland, E.: The Biochemistry of Bladder Cancer. Springfield, Ill., Charles C Thomas, 1963.

Boyland, E., Kinder. C. H., and Williams, K.: The treatment of carcinoma in dog bladders with cytotoxic drugs. Invest. Urol., 2:446–452, 1965.

Harrold, M. W., Edwards, C. N., and Garvey, F. K.: Treatment of bladder tumors by direct instillation of 5-fluorouracil. Experimental observations in dogs. Invest. Urol., 2:47–51, 1964.

Leklem, J. E., Brown, R. R., Hankes, L. V., and Schmaeler, M.: Tryptophan metabolism in the cat. A study with Carbon-14 labeled compounds. Amer. J. Vet. Res., 32:335–344, 1971.

McDonald, D. F., and Lund, R. R.: The role of the urine in vesical neoplasia. I. Experimental confirmation of the urogenous theory of pathogenesis. J. Urol., 71:560–570, 1954.

Mostofi, K. K.: Potentialities of bladder epithelium. J. Urol., 71:705–714, 1954.

Osborne, C. A., Low, D. G., Perman, V., and Barnes, D. M.: Neoplasms of the canine and feline urinary bladder: Incidence, etiologic factors, occurrence, and pathologic features. Amer. J. Vet. Res., 29:2041–2055, 1968.

Osborne, C. A., Low, D. G., and Perman, V.: Neoplasms of the canine and feline urinary bladder: J.A.V.M.A., 152:247–259, 1968.

Scott, W. W., and Boyd, H. L.: A Study of the carcinogenic effect of beta-naphthylamine on the normal and substituted isolated sigmoid loop bladder of dogs. J. Urol., 70:914–925, 1953.

Stamps, P., and Harris, D. L.: Botyroid rhabdomyosarcoma of the urinary bladder of the dog. J.A.V.M.A., 153:1064–1068, 1968.

Weinberg, S. R., Waterhouse, K., Salerno, F., and Hamm, F. C.: Substitute urinary bladders constructed from an isolated segment of small bowel. Surg. Forum, 9:833–837, 1958.

Chapter 42
PATENT URACHUS

I. **The urachus is an embryologic structure whose function is to provide a channel of communication between the urinary bladder and the allantoic sac.**

Normally it becomes fibrotic and nonfunctional after birth.

II. **Anomalies of the urachus**

  A. *Although uncommon, urachal anomalies have been reported in the dog and cat.*

  B. *If the urachal canal remains patent from the urinary bladder to the umbilicus, urine is voided to the exterior by this route.*

  C. *The urachal canal may remain partially patent.*

  This results in the formation of a blind diverticulum at the vertex of the bladder, or a blind diverticulum that communicates with the exterior through an opening in the umbilicus.

  D. *Urachal cysts may form as a result of persistence of secreting urachal epithelium in isolated stretches of patent lumen.*

  These may form at any point between the umbilicus and the bladder. Urachal cysts may become infected with bacteria (Fig. 42–1).

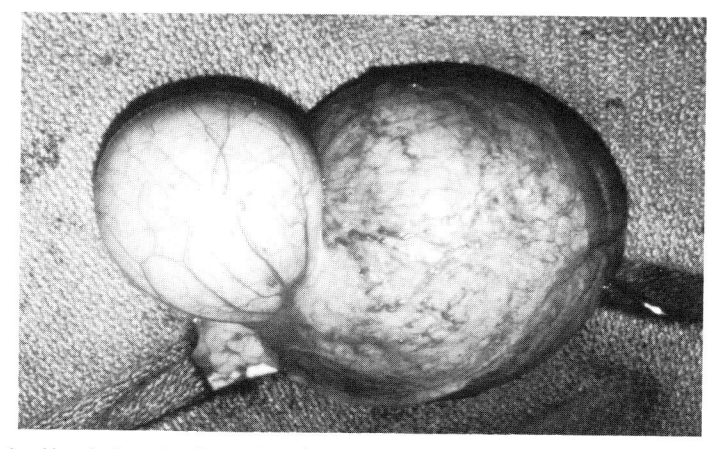

Figure 42–1. Urachal cyst adjacent to the urinary bladder of a 7-year-old female boxer dog. The cyst was an incidental finding during ovariohysterectomy. The cyst did not communicate with the lumen of the urinary bladder. (Courtesy of Dr. Richard W. Greene, The Animal Medical Center, New York, N.Y.)

PATENT URACHUS 387

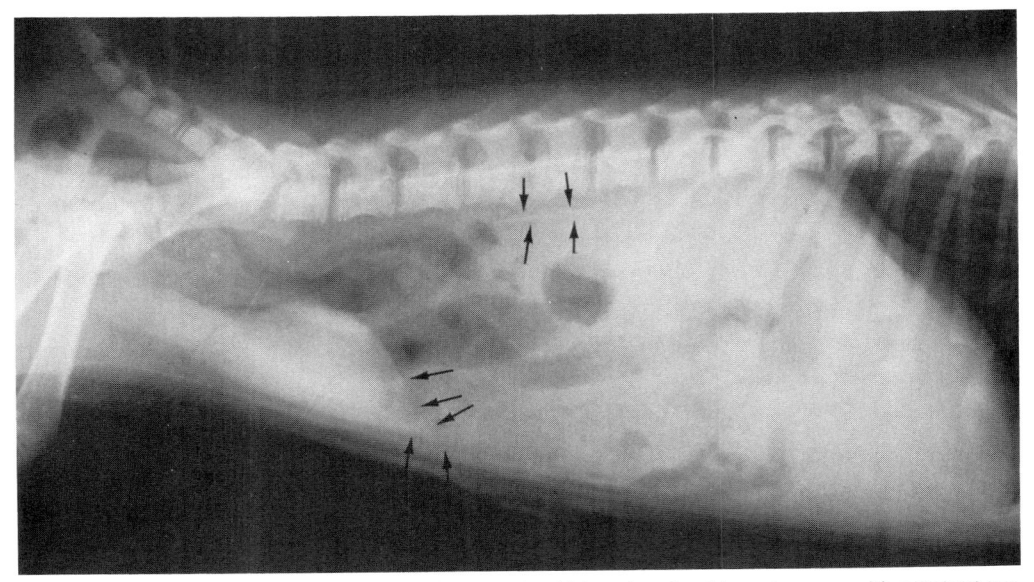

Figure 42–2. Intravenous urogram of a 5-week-old female mixed breed puppy with a patent urachus. Arrows outline the abnormal contour of the vertex of the urinary bladder. Arrows delineate a ureter ventral to the lumbar vertebrae. (J. Amer. Animal Hosp. Assoc., 2:245–250, 1965.)

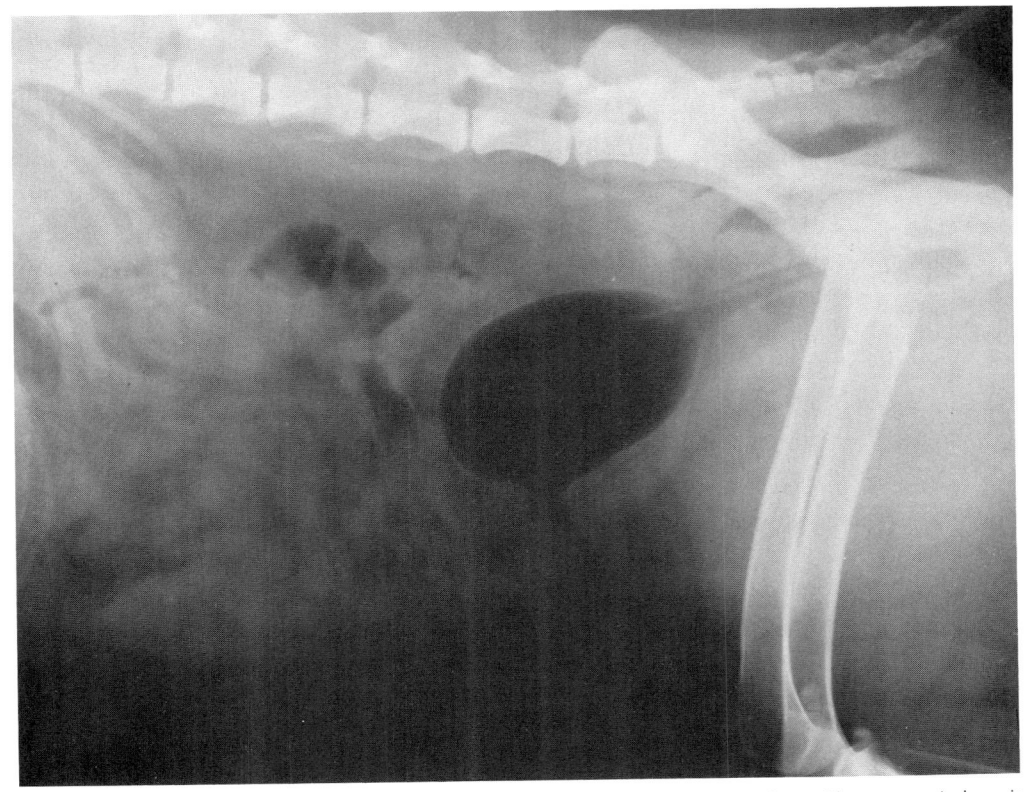

Figure 42–3. Pneumocystogram of a 2-year-old female Siberian husky dog with recurrent chronic cystitis. A diverticulum is present in the ventral wall of the bladder. A diagnosis of partially patent urachus was established on the basis of the location of the diverticulum and its microscopic appearance. (Courtesy of Dr. John P. Arnold, College of Veterinary Medicine, University of Minnesota.)

III. Physical findings associated with a patent urachus include:

A. Passage of urine through the umbilicus in a young animal.

B. Secondary omphalitis and cystitis.

IV. Diagnosis

A. History and physical examination usually allow establishment of the diagnosis.

B. Intravenous urography or retrograde cystography may be required to confirm the diagnosis (Figs. 42–2 and 42–3).

V. Treatment

A. Surgical excision of the urachal stalk is the treatment of choice.

B. Bacterial infection should be eliminated with appropriate antibiotics (see Chapter 38, Bacterial Cystitis).

VI. Prognosis. Surgical intervention is usually followed by complete recovery.

REFERENCES

Greene, R. W., and Bohning, R. H.: Patent urachus associated with urolithiasis in a cat. J.A.V.M.A., *158*: 489–491, 1971.

Osborne, C. A., Rhodes, J. D., and Hanlon, G. F.: Patent urachus in the dog. Anim. Hosp., 2:245–250, 1966.

Pearson, H., and Gibbs, C.: Urinary tract abnormalities in the dog. J. Sm. Anim. Pract., *12*:67–84, 1971.

Chapter 43

ABNORMAL LOCATIONS OF THE URINARY BLADDER

I. **The normal position of the bladder varies with the quantity of urine it contains.**

   A. *When full, it is completely in the peritoneal cavity.*

   B. *When empty, it is partly in the pelvic cavity.*

   C. *Peritoneal folds (ligaments) help to maintain the urinary bladder in its normal position.*

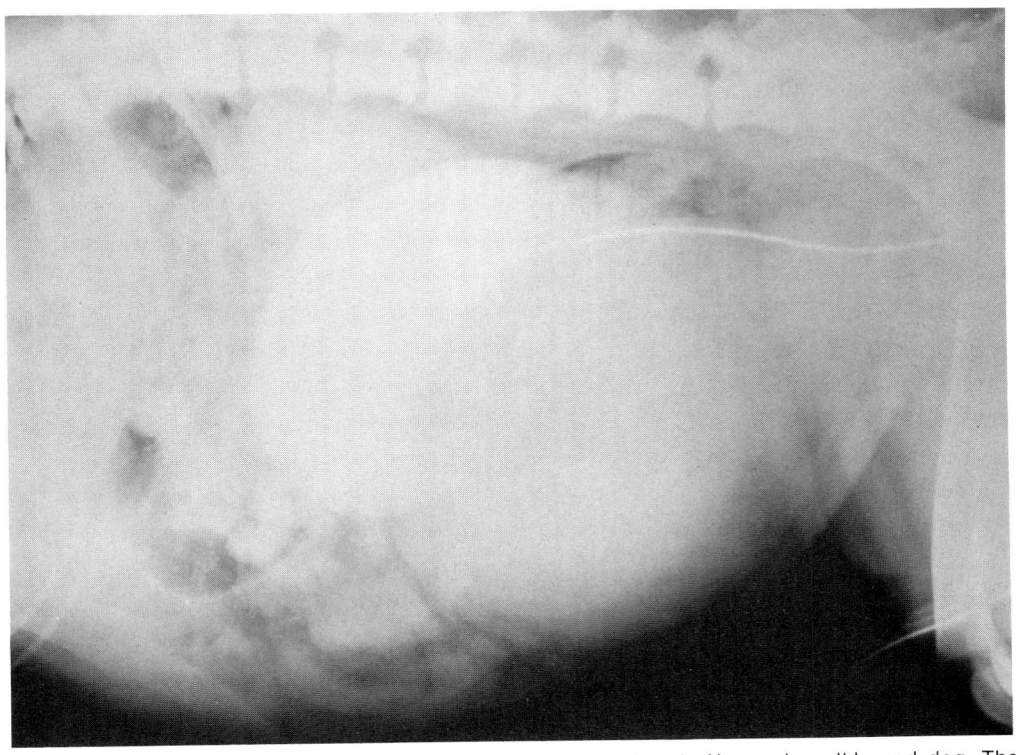

Figure 43-1. Positive contrast cystogram in a 7-year-old male Norwegian elkhound dog. The urinary bladder has been displaced by a cystic prostate gland. The prostatic cyst was successfully treated by marsupialization of the prostate gland and castration.

390   DISEASES OF THE LOWER URINARY SYSTEM

II. Abnormal positions

A. *Prostatic enlargement (hyperplasia, tumors, cysts, abscesses) displaces the bladder cranially (Fig. 43–1).*

B. *If the uterus or vagina has prolapsed, the urinary bladder may be pulled into the pelvic cavity.*

C. *The bladder may be fixed in an abnormal position as a result of peritonitis and adhesions.*

D. *Torsion*

1. Torsion of the urinary bladder is characterized by rotation of the bladder on its long axis.
2. Torsion may be partial or complete. When complete it causes obstruction of the urethra and ureters and is associated with retention of urine.
3. Torsion of the bladder may be associated with trauma or extravesicular tumors.

E. *Hernias*

1. Perineal hernias.
    a. Perineal hernias are most common in aged male dogs.
    b. The urinary bladder and the prostate gland may be forced into the hernial sac as a result of increased intra-abdominal pressure.

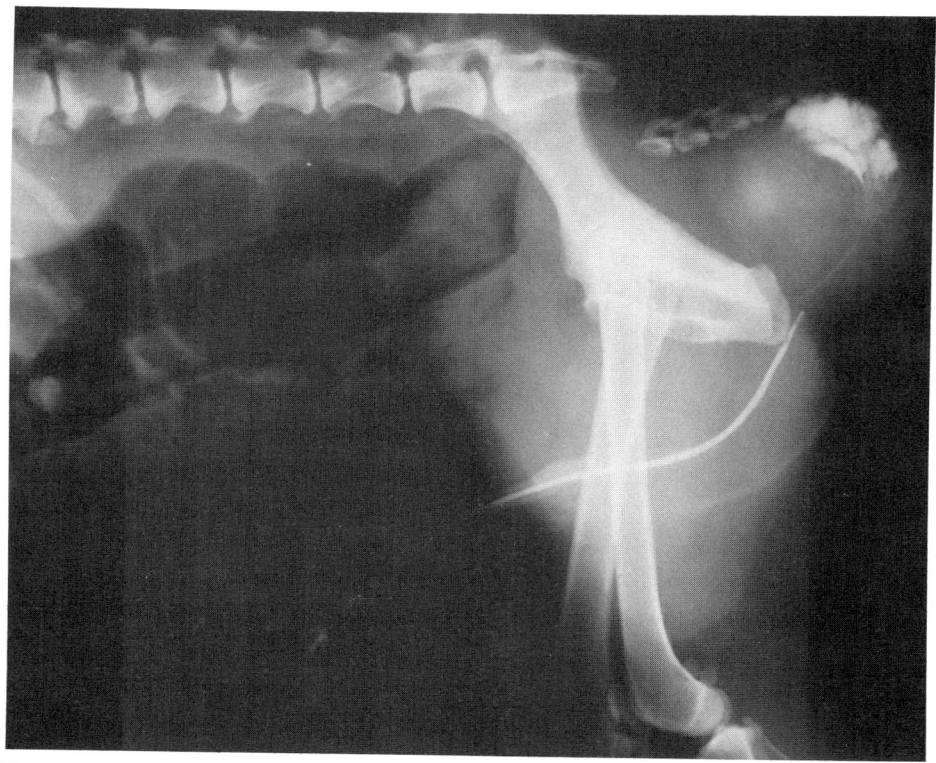

Figure 43–2. Retrograde cystogram of a 10-year-old male mixed breed dog with a history of straining to urinate and defecate. The urinary bladder has been displaced into a perineal hernia adjacent to the right side of the rectum. The dog had post renal uremia (BUN = 225 mg. per 100 ml.). (Courtesy of Dr. Robert M. Hardy, College of Veterinary Medicine, University of Minnesota.)

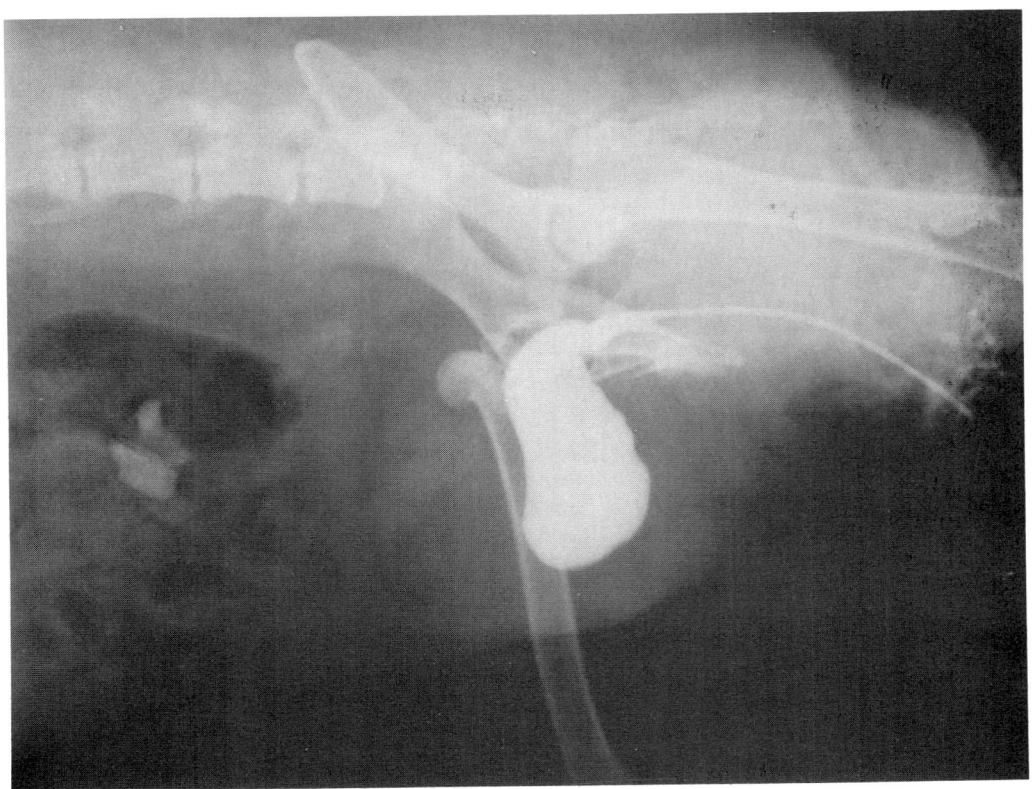

Figure 43-3. Positive contrast cystogram of a 6-year-old female springer spaniel dog. The urinary bladder is in a ventral abdominal hernia. The dog also had dislocations of the left sacroiliac articulation and right coxofemoral articulation, multiple fractures of the bony pelvis, and a fracture of the right tibia.

       (1) Tenesmus usually occurs as a result of constipation or obstipation.
       (2) The urinary bladder must be relatively empty before it can be displaced into the hernial sac.
       (3) Urine retention secondary to occlusion of the bladder neck or urethra may occur (Fig. 43-2).
       (4) The bladder may move in and out of the hernia, or it may become fixed in the hernia as a result of adhesions.
  2. Ventral abdominal hernias:
    a. Are usually associated with trauma (Fig. 43-3).
    b. Usually contain other abdominal viscera, in addition to the urinary bladder, in the hernial sac.
  3. Inguinal hernias:
    a. Are most common in females. They occur infrequently in males.
    b. Are often associated with pregnancy or advanced age. The occurrence of inguinal hernias in aged and pregnant female dogs may be related to one or more of the following:
       (1) Females have a relatively short inguinal canal.
       (2) The hernias may be related to an anatomical weakness. A familial tendency has been suggested.

(3) Inguinal hernias may be associated with increased intra-abdominal pressure.
(4) They may be related to loss of muscle tone in aged animals.
c. May be bilateral or unilateral.
d. May be asymptomatic.
e. May be recurrent.
f. May become irreducible and associated with obstruction to urine outflow.

F. *Prolapse*
1. The urinary bladder may prolapse through the urethra of female dogs on rare occasions.
   a. Possible contributing factors include:
      (1) The relatively short and wide urethra of female dogs.
      (2) Weakening of supporting ligaments of the bladder.
      (3) Increased intra-abdominal pressure.
      (4) Weakened urethral sphincters.
   b. Prolapse of the bladder is usually associated with retention of urine.
   c. Following prolapse, infarction of the bladder wall may occur as a result of occlusion of blood vessels.

III. Clinical findings

Abnormal locations of the urinary bladder may be:

A. *Clinically asymptomatic if urine flow is not obstructed.*

B. *Detected by physical examination as a swelling in the hernial sac.*
The size of the swelling varies with the volume of urine in the bladder.

C. *Associated with frequent attempts to urinate if urine flow is partially or totally obstructed.*
Obstruction to urine flow may be associated with:
1. Abdominal pain.
2. Cystitis secondary to urine retention.
3. Postrenal uremia.
4. Varying degrees of hydronephrosis if the patient survives.

IV. Diagnosis. A diagnosis of displacement of the bladder may be based on:

A. *History and physical findings.*

B. *Reduction in the size of a hernia following manual expression of urine from the bladder or catheterization of the bladder. If the bladder is obstructed, cystocentesis may yield urine.*

C. *Cystography or intravenous urography.*

D. *Exploratory surgery.*

V. Treatment

A. *If urine flow is obstructed and the bladder cannot be returned to its normal position, aspirate the contents with needle and syringe.*

B. *Eliminate the underlying cause when possible.*
   1. Surgical repair, castration, and estrogen therapy (or both) should be considered for perineal hernias.
   2. Ventral abdominal and inguinal hernias should be surgically repaired.
   3. Treatment of prostatic enlargement is dependent on the cause.

C. *Supportive*
   1. Treat cystitis if present (see Treatment of bacterial cystitis, in Chapter 38).
   2. Cystopexy.

Chapter 44
URINARY INCONTINENCE

I. Definition

Urinary incontinence may be defined as the loss of voluntary control of micturition which results in frequent or constant involuntary passage of urine. Because urinary incontinence occurs as the result of several fundamentally different disease mechanisms, it must be considered a sign of urinary bladder and urethral dysfunction and not as a diagnosis.

II. Urinary incontinence must be differentiated from:

A. *Dysuria*
  1. Dysuria is characterized by painful and difficult micturition, or both.
  2. It most commonly occurs in association with diseases (inflammation or calculi) of the urinary bladder and urethra.

B. *Pollakiuria, which is characterized by abnormally frequent passage of urine (essentially a synonym of dysuria).*

C. *Polyuria, which is characterized by the passage of a large volume of urine per unit of time.*

III. Pathogenesis

On the basis of the pathogenesis, it is clinically useful to classify diseases of the dog and cat associated with urinary incontinence as neurogenic incontinence, nonneurogenic incontinence, paradoxical incontinence, and miscellaneous incontinence.

A. *Neurogenic incontinence*
  1. Paralytic bladder.
     a. A paralytic bladder may be caused by diseases which damage the nerve supply (pudendal, pelvic, and hypogastric nerves) to the urinary bladder and sphincters. Such diseases include:
     (1) Fractures, luxations, or subluxations of vertebrae.
     (2) Protruding or ruptured intervertebral discs.
     (3) Inflammation (myelitis, ossifying pachymeningitis, or osteomyelitis) due to any cause (Figs. 44-1 and 44-2).
     (4) Primary or secondary neoplasia of the spinal cord or surrounding structures (Fig. 44-3).
     (5) Congenital anomalies of the vertebrae or spinal cord (e.g., spina bifida).
     b. Lack of voluntary micturition, marked overdistention of the urinary bladder, and involuntary dribbling of urine are the hallmarks of a paralytic bladder. Because the patient cannot micturate normally, the

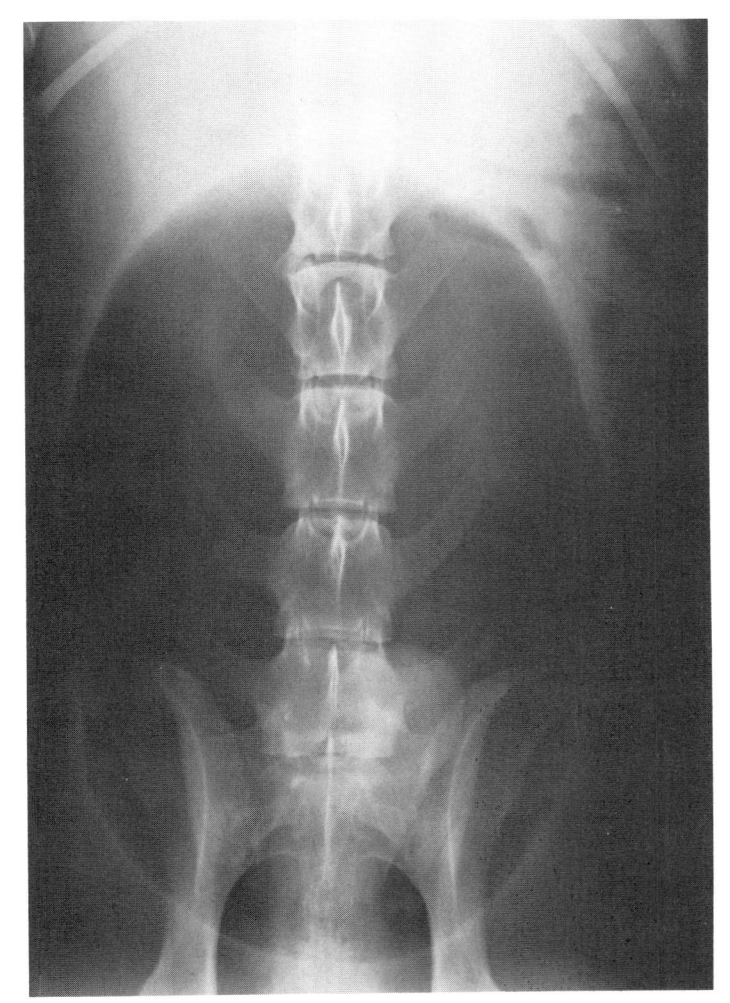

Figure 44–1. Pneumocystogram of a 4-year-old male great Dane dog with ossifying pachymeningitis. The dog had overflow urinary incontinence which developed as a result of loss of innervation to the bladder. Seven liters of urine were removed from the bladder prior to injection of air.

       urinary bladder becomes overdistended with urine. When intravesical urine pressure exceeds urethral resistance to urine flow, urinary incontinence occurs. Urine may readily be expressed from the bladder by digital palpation.
    c. Overflow urinary incontinence is often complicated by bacterial cystitis because of stagnation of urine.
    d. Paralysis of the urinary bladder may be associated with fecal incontinence since the same nerves supply the bladder and the anus.
2. Cord bladder.
    a. Cord bladders are caused by lesions of the CNS which are located between the brain and the spinal reflex center of micturition in the sacral cord. Some causes include:
       (1) Spinal shock secondary to trauma.
       (2) Destructive lesions of the spinal cord.

396 DISEASES OF THE LOWER URINARY SYSTEM

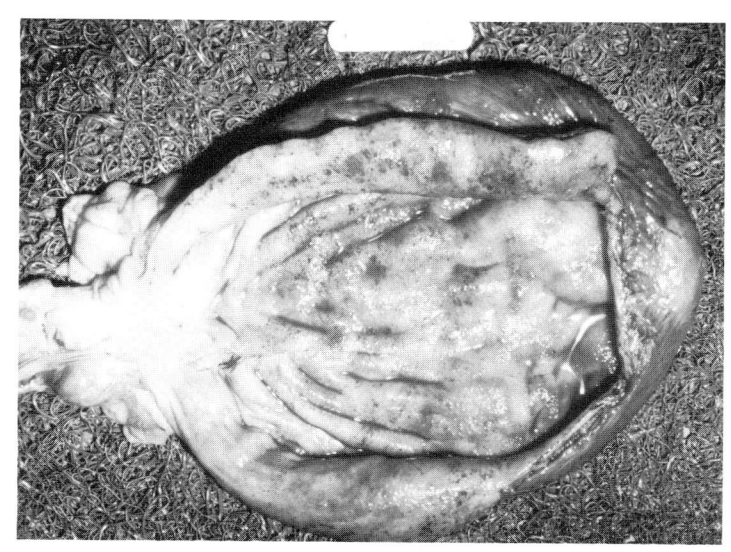

Figure 44-2. Massive enlargement of the urinary bladder of the great Dane described in Figure 44-1. Loss of innervation to the urinary bladder resulted in overflow incontinence and secondary cystitis.

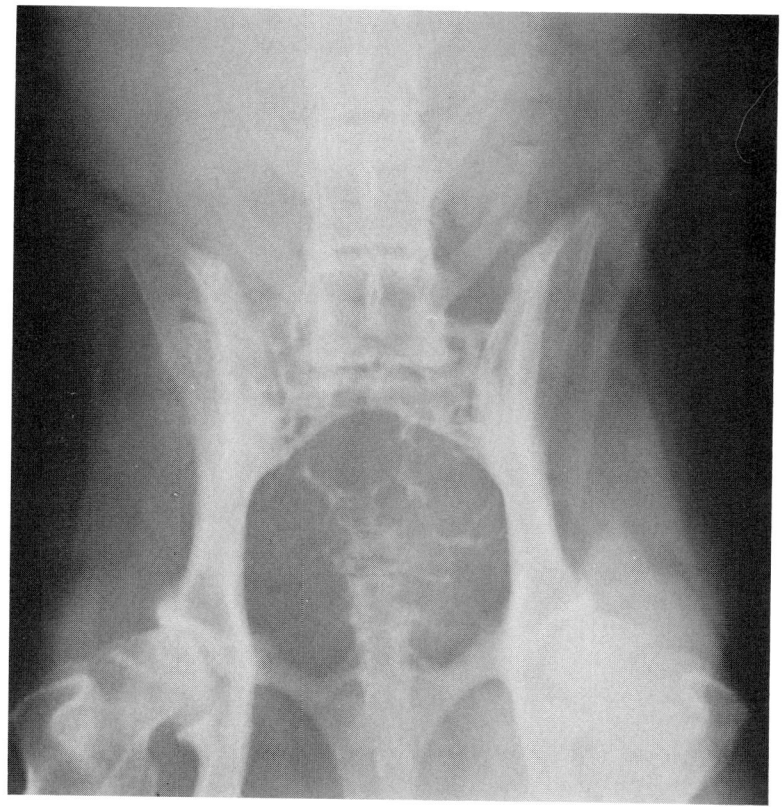

Figure 44-3. Survey radiograph of the bony pelvis of an 8-year-old female boxer with a multiple myeloma. There is complete lysis of the sacrum without evidence of reactive osteoblastic activity. The dog developed overflow urinary incontinence as a result of destruction of innervation of the urinary bladder. (J.A.V.M.A., *153*:1300–1319, 1968.)

b. Initially there is a temporary paralysis of the bladder similar to that seen in patients with a paralytic urinary bladder. If the spinal reflex center for micturition is not damaged, it may periodically stimulate the bladder to contract without the patient's awareness.

B. *Nonneurogenic causes*
1. In patients with nonneurogenic urinary incontinence, the nerve supply to the urinary bladder and the urinary bladder itself are normal. For this reason the bladder does not become overdistended with urine and the patient can micturate normally.
2. Nonneurogenic causes of urinary incontinence include:
   a. Ectopic ureter(s) (see Ectopic ureters, in Chapter 35).
   b. Congenital anomalies of the urethra and urethral sphincter(s) (see Chapter 45, Diseases of the Urethra).
   c. Patent urachus (see Chapter 42, Patent Urachus).
   d. Endocrine imbalance following ovariohysterectomy.
      (1) This type of incontinence occurs in spayed female dogs.
      (2) Although the exact mechanism(s) responsible has not been established, replacement therapy with estrogens usually results in remission of the incontinence. Oral administration of 0.1 to 1.0 mg. per day of diethylstilbestrol for 3 to 5 days, followed by a maintenance dosage of 1.0 mg. per week may be used. Alternatively, parenteral administration of ¼ to 1 mg. of ECP* per patient may be used. The latter must be repeated at intervals of several weeks to several months.

C. *Paradoxical incontinence*
1. Paradoxical incontinence occurs in patients with partial obstruction of the urethra.
2. It is most likely to be encountered in male dogs. Potential causes include:
   a. Urethral calculi.
   b. Strictures.
   c. Neoplasms.
3. The obstructive lesion in the urethra must be sufficiently severe to prevent normal micturition, but not so severe as to cause anuria.
   a. When the bladder becomes overdistended with urine, intravesical pressure eventually exceeds the resistance imparted by the urethral lesion and urinary incontinence results.
   b. The bladder wall may become atonic as a result of prolonged overdistention.
4. Paradoxical incontinence should be suspected if:
   a. The urinary bladder is overdistended.
   b. The patient cannot normally micturate.
   c. Involuntary dribbling of urine and dysuria are present.
   d. Urine cannot be readily expelled from the urinary bladder by digital palpation.
   e. Difficulty is encountered in catheterizing the patient.
5. Localization of the urethral lesion may be established by catheterization and with the aid of contrast urethrography.

---

*Estradiol cypionate, The Upjohn Co., Kalamazoo, Michigan.

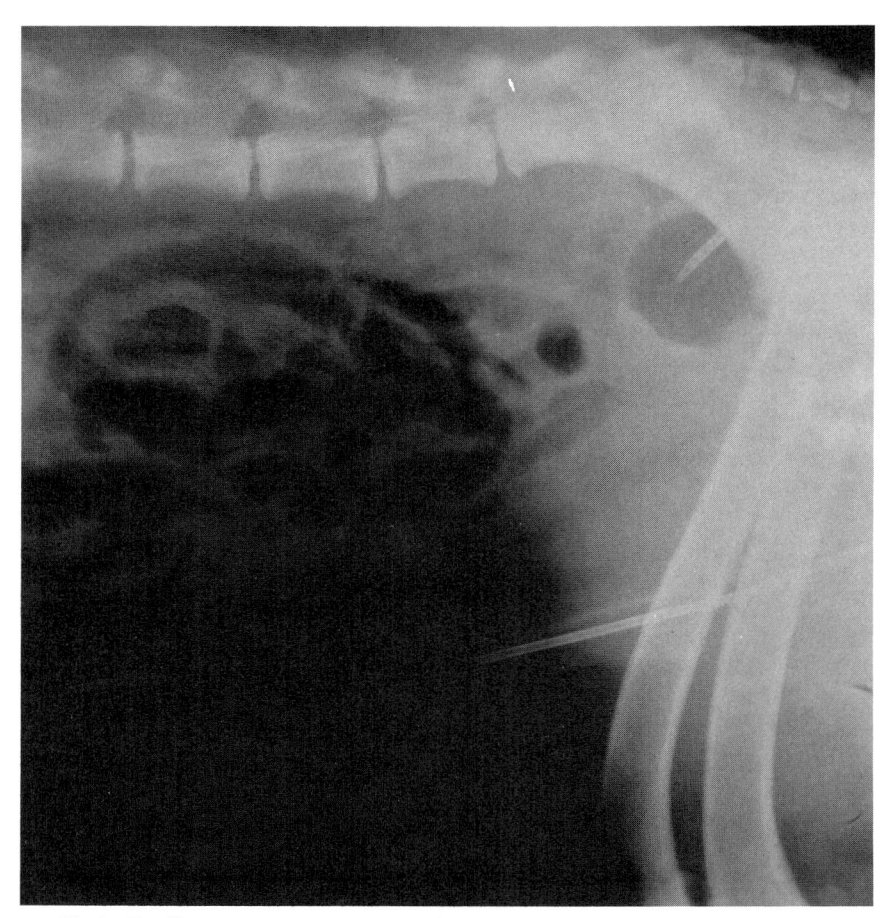

Figure 44-4. Positive contrast cystogram of a 7.5-month-old male Irish setter with urinary incontinence. The lumen of the bladder is abnormally small. The bladder wall is nonfunctional as a result of destruction and replacement of smooth muscle with inflammatory cells and fibrous connective tissue.

   D. *Miscellaneous causes*
   1. Primary diseases of the urinary bladder, such as severe inflammation or neoplasia, may impair normal bladder function by replacing the smooth muscle of the bladder wall with connective tissue or neoplastic tissue (see Chapter 39, Cystitis, and Chapter 41, Neoplasms of the Urinary Bladder).
      a. The bladder wall becomes permanently indistensible and insensitive to the normal pressure stimulus of micturition (Figure 44-4).
      b. Lack of normal micturition, abdominal palpation of a small, firm urinary bladder, overflow dribbling of urine, and demonstration of small bladder capacity by injecting air or fluid characterize this type of urinary incontinence.
   2. Iatrogenic surgical damage to the bladder neck or proximal urethra may result in urinary incontinence.

IV. Diagnosis

   A. *Because successful treatment is dependent upon establishing the specific cause of urinary incontinence, every attempt should be made to establish a specific diagnosis.*

TABLE 44–1. Classification of Urinary Incontinence

Type	Normal micturition	Involuntary dribbling of urine	Overdistended bladder	Small, contracted bladder	Ability to catheterize bladder
Neurogenic	Absent	Present	Present	Absent	Easy
Nonneurogenic	Present	Present	Absent	Absent	Easy
Paradoxical	Absent	Present	Present	Absent	Difficult
Miscellaneous	Absent	Present	Absent	Present	Variable

    B. The results of the history and physical examination usually allow urinary incontinence to be placed into a neurogenic, nonneurogenic, paradoxical, or miscellaneous category.

(Table 44–1.) A specific diagnosis must then be based on pertinent findings of the history and physical examination, and radiographic and laboratory procedures.

    C. Control of urinary incontinence by replacement therapy with a low dosage of estrogens is necessary to confirm a diagnosis of endocrine imbalance following ovariohysterectomy.

    D. Refer to specific disease entities mentioned under Pathogenesis for additional information.

V. Treatment

    A. Every effort should be made to eliminate the primary cause.

    B. Permanent damage of the nerve supply to the urinary bladder and advanced generalized inflammation or neoplasia of the bladder wall are usually unresponsive to therapy. Neurogenic incontinence which occurs as a result of acute trauma may spontaneously improve over a period of weeks to months.

    C. Supportive treatment
        1. Eliminate or control secondary cystitis when present.
        2. Liberal quantities of an emollient cream should be applied to the skin to prevent dermatitis from urine scald.
        3. In patients in which overdistention of the urinary bladder occurs, the bladder should be manually expressed two or three times per day.
            a. Care must be used to avoid rupturing the bladder by exerting too much pressure.
            b. Regular elimination of urine from the bladder helps to prevent cystitis and atonicity of the bladder wall, both of which may occur as a result of prolonged overdistention.
            c. Catheterization of a nonfunctional urinary bladder should be avoided unless there is no other alternative, because bacterial cystitis is a frequent complication.

VI. Prognosis.
The prognosis for patients with urinary incontinence is dependent upon the biological behavior of the causative disease.

Chapter 45

DISEASES OF THE URETHRA

I. Congenital anomalies

    A. *Many variations have been reported including:*
        1. Absence of the urethra.
        2. Urethral duplication.
        3. Hypospadias (opening of the urethra on the ventral surface of the penis or perineum) (Fig. 45–1).
        4. Diverticula.
        5. Accessory meatus.

    B. *Congenital anomalies of the urethra occur infrequently in dogs and cats.*

    C. *A diagnosis can usually be established on the basis of a physical examination.*

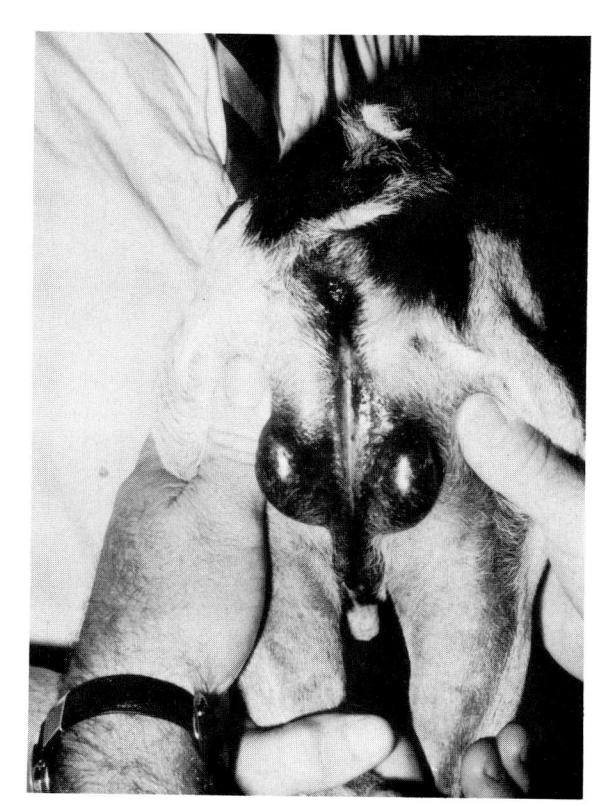

Figure 45–1. Extensive hypospadias and anomalous scrotum in an 11-year-old male mixed breed dog. The external urethral orifice is located just ventral to the anus. The dog had urinary incontinence.

II. Trauma to the urethra

A. Etiology
1. Injury induced by catheterization.
2. Auto accidents, especially when associated with pelvic fractures or fracture of the os penis.
3. Urethral calculi.
4. Bite wounds.

B. Diagnosis
1. A diagnosis can usually be established on the basis of the history and physical examination.

C. Complications
1. Urethral stricture and dysuria.
2. Urethral dilation.
3. Anuria and uremia.

D. Treatment should be directed toward eliminating or correcting the primary cause.

III. Neoplasms of the urethra

A. The paucity of reported cases suggests that urethral neoplasms are uncommon in dogs and cats.

B. Primary tumors include:
1. Transitional cell carcinomas.
2. Leiomyomas.
3. Squamous cell carcinomas.

C. Secondary tumors include:
1. Transmissible venereal sarcomas.
2. Malignant lymphomas.

D. History and clinical signs
1. Dysuria or anuria may occur secondary to partial or total occlusion of the urethral lumen.
2. Hematuria may be present.

E. Diagnosis and treatment
1. Clinical signs usually suggest urethral obstruction as a diagnostic probability.
2. Urethral obstruction due to calculi may be differentiated from urethral obstruction due to other causes by physical examination and radiography (see Chapter 8, Radiographic Evaluation of the Urinary System).
3. Establishing whether a tissue mass represents neoplastic or nonneoplastic involvement must be made on a histopathologic basis. Cystoscopy and transurethral resection, or transurethral biopsy may be feasible in medium-sized and large female dogs. In male dogs, surgical exposure of the lesion may be necessary.

F. Prognosis. The prognosis is dependent on the biological behavior and location of the neoplasm.

IV. Urethral obstruction in the male cat (see Chapter 39, Cystitis–Urethral Obstruction Complex in the Cat).

REFERENCES

Bloom, F.: Pathology of the Dog and Cat. The Genitourinary System with Clinical Considerations. Evanston, Ill., Amer. Vet. Publ. Inc., 1954.

Cass, A. S., and Hinman, F.: Constant urethral flow in female dog. I. Normal vesical and urethral pressures and effect of muscle relaxant. J. Urol., 99:442–446, 1968.

Cass, A. S.: Constant urethral flow in female dog. IV. Determination of functional urethral diameter. J. Urol., 104:273–276, 1970.

Davis, J. E.: The study and measurement of urethral resistance. I. The effect of isolation and relocation of the urethra and bladder neck upon continence and micturition. Invest. Urol., 2:342, 1965.

Knecht, C. D., and Slusher, R.: Extrapelvic anastomosis of the bladder and penile urethra in a dog. J. Amer. Anim. Hosp. Assoc., 6:247–251, 1970.

Piermattei, D. L., and Osborne, C. A.: Nonsurgical removal of urethral calculi from male dogs. J.A.V.M.A., 159:1755–1757, 1971.

Pollock, S.: Urethral carcinoma in the dog. J. Amer. Vet. Rad. Soc., 9:95–98, 1968.

Tanagho, E. A., and Lyon, R. P.: Urethral dilatation versus internal urethrotomy. J. Urol., 105:242–244, 1971.

APPENDICES

I. Table of normal values (mature animals)

A. Urine specific gravity

	Dog	Cat
Mean	1.025	1.030
Usual range	1.018 to 1.050	1.018 to 1.050
Maximum limits	1.001 to 1.060+	1.001 to 1.080+

B. Approximate urine volume (ml./kg. body wt./day. Normal environmental conditions)

	Dog	Cat
Range	25 to 41	22 to 30

C. Osmolality (mOsm./Kg. water – dog)

	Urine	Plasma
Usual range	500 to 1200	300
Maximal limits	2000 to 2400	—

D. Renal function tests (dogs)

Effective renal plasma flow .... 266 ± 66 ml./min./sq. m. body surface
13.5 ± 3.3 ml./min./kg. body wt.
Glomerular filtration rate .... 84.4 ± 19 ml./min./sq. m. body surface
4 ml./min./kg. body wt.

E. Blood chemical values (mature animals)

	Dog	Cat
Blood Urea Nitrogen (mg./100 ml. serum)	10 to 30	20 to 30
Creatinine (mg./100 ml. serum)	1 to 2	1 to 2
Total protein		
(Gm./100 ml. plasma)	6.0 to 7.5	6.0 to 7.5
(Gm./100 ml. serum)	5.0 to 7.0	5.2 to 6.6
Albumin (Gm./100 ml. serum)	3.0 to 4.8	1.7 to 2.4
Globulins (Gm./100 ml. serum)	1.3 to 3.2	2.4 to 4.8
Glucose (mg./100 ml. blood)	60 to 100	70 to 118
Total Cholesterol (mg./100 ml. serum)	125 to 250	75 to 151

Cholesterol Esters (mg./100 ml. serum)	75 to 200	45 to 120
Calcium (mg./100 ml. serum)	9 to 11.5	9 to 11
Inorganic phosphorus (mg./100 ml. serum)	2.5 to 5.0	4.5 to 8.1
Sodium (mEq./L.)	137 to 149	147 to 156
Chloride (mEq./L.)	90 to 110	115 to 130
Potassium (mEq./L.)	3.7 to 5.8	4.0 to 4.5
Alkaline phosphatase (Bodansky units/100 ml. serum)	3 to 6	0 to 7
Amylase (Somogyi units/100 ml. serum)	423 to 562	
(Harding units/100 ml. serum	1600 to 2400	
Glutamic pyruvic transaminase (Sigma Frankel units/100 ml. serum)	10 to 40	10 to 40
Bicarbonate (mEq./L. blood)	21 to 27	21 to 27
Blood pH	7.31 to 7.42	? to 7.4

F. *Hemogram (mature animals)*

	Dog Range	Dog Ave.	Cat Range	Cat Ave.
RBC (millions/cmm.)	5.5 to 8.5	6.8	5.0 to 10.0	7.5
Hb. (Gm./100 ml.)	12.0 to 18.0	15.0	8.0 to 15.0	12.0
PCV (ml./100 ml.)	37.0 to 55.0	45.0	24.0 to 45.0	37.0
WBC (thousands/cmm.)	6 to 17	11.5	5.5 to 19.5	12.5
Lymphocytes (%)	12 to 30	20	20 to 55	32
Nonsegmented WBC (%)	0 to 3	0.8	0 to 3	0.5
Segmented WBC (%)	60 to 77	70	35 to 75	59
Eosinophils (%)	2 to 10	4.0	2 to 12	5.5
Basophils (%)	Rare	0	Rare	0
Monocytes (%)	3 to 10	.5.2	1 to 4	3.0

G. *References*

1. Bentinck-Smith, J.: A roster of normal values. *In* Current Veterinary Therapy IV. Edited by Robert W. Kirk. Philadelphia, Pa., W. B. Saunders Co., 1971.
2. Bloom, F.: The Blood Chemistry of the Dog and Cat. New York, N.Y., Gamma Publications, Inc., 1960.
3. Cornelius, C. E., and Kaneko, J. J.: Clinical Biochemistry of Domestic Animals. New York, N.Y., Academic Press, 1963.
4. Schalm, O. W.: Veterinary Hematology. 2nd ed. Philadelphia, Pa., Lea & Febiger, 1965.
5. Smith, H. W.: The Kidney. Structure and Function in Health and Disease. New York, N.Y., Oxford University Press, 1951.

II. Conversion factors

A. $\text{mEq./L.} = \dfrac{\text{mg./100 ml.} \times 10 \times \text{valence}}{\text{atomic weight}}$

B. $\text{mg./100 ml.} = \dfrac{\text{mEq./L.} \times \text{atomic weight}}{10 \times \text{valence}}$

C.
Element	Valence	Atomic Weight
Na^+	1	23
K^+	1	39
Ca^{++}	2	40
Mg^{++}	2	24
Cl^-	1	35.5
HCO_3^-	1	61 (Eq. wt.)

III. Electrolytes lost in body excretions (generalities)

A. *Vomitus*
  1. Gastric juice; primarily loss of water, hydrogen ion, chloride and sodium. Also some loss of potassium.
  2. Intestinal juice; contains a significant quantity of bicarbonate.

B. *Diarrhea; primarily loss of water, sodium, chloride, potassium, and bicarbonate.*

C. *Evaporation from respiratory tract; primarily loss of electrolyte free water.*

D. *Pathologic polyuria due to generalized renal disease; primarily loss of water, sodium, chloride, and bicarbonate. In some cases, a sufficient quantity of potassium may be lost in urine to cause hypokalemia. The latter is uncommon in dogs and cats.*

GENERAL REFERENCES

Allen, A. C.: The Kidney. Medical and Surgical Diseases. New York, N.Y., Grune and Stratton, 1962.
Archibald, J.: Urinary system. *In* Canine Surgery. Edited by J. Archibald. Santa Barbara, Calif., Amer. Vet. Publ., Inc., 1965.
Bernstein, L. M.: Renal Function and Renal Failure. Baltimore, Md., The Williams and Wilkins Co., 1965.
Bloom, F.: Pathology of the Dog and Cat. The Genitourinary System with Clinical Considerations. Evanston, Ill., Amer. Vet. Publ., Inc., 1954.
Cecil-Loeb Textbook of Medicine. Edited by P. B. Beeson and W. McDermott. 13th edition. Philadelphia, Pa., W. B. Saunders Co., 1971.
Current Veterinary Therapy. Vol. 4. Edited by R. W. Kirk, Philadelphia, Pa., W. B. Saunders Co., 1971.
Gultman, P. H.: Renal Pathology. *In* The Beagle as An Experimental Dog. Edited by A. C. Anderson and L. S. Good. Ames, Iowa, Iowa State University Press, 1970.
Jubb, K. V. F., and Kennedy, P. C.: Pathology of Domestic Animals. Vol. 2. 2nd edition. New York, N.Y., Academic Press, 1970.
Kirk, R. W., and Bistner, S. I.: Handbook of Veterinary Procedures and Emergency Treatment. Philadelphia, Pa., W. B. Saunders Co., 1969.
Lucke, V. M.: Renal Disease in the Domestic Cat. J. Path. Bact., 95:67–91, 1968.
Markowitz, J., Archibald, J., and Downie, H. G.: Experimental Surgery. 5th edition. Baltimore, Md., The Williams and Wilkins Co., 1964.
Osborne, C. A., Low, D. G., and Johnson, K. H.: Renal Disease. Vet. Clin. N. Amer., *1*:323–353, 1971.
Robbins, S. L.: Pathology. 3rd edition. Philadelphia, Pa., W. B. Saunders Co., 1967.
Smith, H. W.: The Kidney: Structure and Function in Health and Disease. New York, N.Y., Oxford University Press, 1951.
Symposium on the Kidney. Amer. J. Med., *36*:641–818, 1964.
The Kidney. Edited by F. K. Mostofi and D. E. Smith. Baltimore, Md., The Williams and Wilkins Co., 1966.

Index

Page numbers in *italic* type indicate illustrations. Page numbers followed by the letter "t" indicate tables.

Acetonuria, causes of, 49
Acid-base balance, detecting alterations in, 295
Adenoma, 255
Alkaline phosphatase, serum concentrations in renal failure, 59
Amphotericin B, toxicity of, 313
Amyloid, 220
    deposition of, significance of, 220
Amyloidosis, renal, 148, 219, 220–227
    and nephrotic syndrome, *229*
    clinical findings, 224
    diagnosis, 225
    pathogenesis of, 220
    pathology, 221, *221, 222, 223*
    primary, 220
    prognosis, 226
    secondary, 220
    treatment, 225
Anemia, in renal failure, 138, 286
Angioma(s), 255
    of urinary bladder, 376
Antibacterial therapy, in bacterial cystitis, 358
"Antiseptics," urinary tract, in bacterial cystitis, 359
Aplasia, renal, diagnosis, 153
    prognosis, 153
    treatment, 153
Aqueous vasopressin test, in pitressin concentration test, 68
Atrophy, hydronephrotic, 200

Bacitracin, toxicity of, 313
Bacteria, in urine, 54
Bacterial culture, laboratory technique in, 56
    needle biopsy sample and, 56
Bacterial cystitis, 355–360
    ancillary measures in treatment of, 360
    antibacterial therapy in, 358
    chronic, *356, 358*
    clinical course, 357
    diagnosis, 357
    etiologic agents in, 356
    factors predisposing to, 355
    history in, 356
    normal defense mechanisms of bladder in, 355

Bacterial cystitis (*Continued*)
    pathogenesis of, 355
    physical examination in, 357
    routes of infection, 355
    treatment, 358
    urinary tract "antiseptics" in, 359
Bacterial endocarditis, clinical syndrome, 232
    definition, 232
    diagnosis, 233
    renal disease associated with, 233
    treatment, 234
Barbiturates, in renal disease, 314
Bilirubinuria, 49
Biopsy, absolute contraindications, 114
    at laparotomy, 113
    care after, 113
    complications after, 114
    fine needle, 113
    limitations in, 115
    keyhole, 109, *110*
    percutaneous renal, 107–117
        choice of site, 109
        equipment, 108
        indications for, 107
        pre-biopsy considerations in, 108
        restraint in, 109
        specimen of, *115*
        techniques in, 109
        with manual localization of the kidney per abdomen, 112
Biopsy needle, Franklin modified Vim-Silverman, 108, *108*
Biopsy samples, artefacts, 117
    processing and staining of, 116
Bladder, urinary, abnormal locations of, 389–393
    abnormal positions of, *389*, 390, *390, 391*
    clinical findings, 392
        diagnosis, 392
        hernias and, 390, *390, 391*
        torsion and, 390
        treatment, 392
    contusions and abrasions of, 343
    location, 7
    manual compression of, complications, 26
        technique, 25
    neoplasms of, 374–385
    normal positions of, 389

409

410 INDEX

Bladder (*Continued*)
  urinary, physical examination of, 24
    prolapse of, 392
    rupture of, 343, *345, 347*
      catheterization in, 347
      clinical findings, 344
      diagnosis, 348
      etiology, 343
      pathophysiology, 343
      radiographic findings, 346
    shape and structure of, 7
    trauma to, 343
    with multiple polypoid lesions, *102*
Blastomycosis, 254
Blood, normal chemical values, 403
  normal hemogram values, 404
Blood pH, in renal disease, 59
Blood urea nitrogen, 73, 122
  factors influencing concentration, 74
  relationship to glomerular filtration rate, 74, 75
Blood urea nitrogen test, basis for, 73
  clinical use of, 76
  disadvantages of, 76
  interpretation of results, 75
  methodology, 75
Bone marrow, in chronic uremia, *137*
  normal, *137*

Calcium, serum concentrations of, in renal disease, 58
Calculi, (see urolithiasis, uroliths)
Calories, maintenance requirements for hospitalized dogs and cats, *298*
Capillaria plica, 372–373
  diagnosis, 372
  life cycle, 372
  morphologic characteristics, 372
  ova of, *373*
  pathology, 372
  treatment, 373
Carcinoma(s), of urinary bladder, 377
  renal, 255, *256, 258*
  renal cell, nephrectomy in, 259
  squamous cell, of urethra, 401
  transitional cell, *380, 381, 382*
    of urethra, 401
Cardiac glycosides, in renal failure, 314
Cardiovascular system, and renal failure, 136
Castration, pre-puberal, in cystitis-urethral obstruction complex, 363
Casts, as indication of renal disease, 53
  bile stained, 54
  epithelial, 53
  fatty, 54
  granular, 53
  hyaline, 53
  mixed, 54
  RBC, 54
  renal failure, 54
  types of, 53
  waxy, 54
  WBC, 54
Catheter(s), correct placement of, *29*
  Foley, 27, *34*

Catheter(s) (*Continued*)
  indwelling, maintenance of urine outflow by, 368
  size, composition and types of, 26
  urinary, care of, 27
    feline, 27
Catheterization, blind, technique in, 35
  complications of, 29
  indications for, 26
  of female cat, 36
  of female dog, 33, *34*
  of male cat, 35
  of male dog, 30
  overinsertion of, *32*
  technique of, 28
  use of endoscopes in, 34
Cellulitis, *367*
Chloride deficit, in renal disease, 57
Cholesterol, concentrations in renal disease, 59
Chondroma, 255
Coccidioidomycosis, 254
Constipation, in renal failure, 139
Contrast agents, 91
Contrast radiography, 91
Creatinine, clinical use of, 78
Creatinine clearance, endogenous, 81, 122
Creatinine concentration, factors influencing, 77
Creatinine test, basis for, 76
  interpretation of results, 77
  methodology of, 77
Cryptococcosis, 254
Cyst(s), renal, 196–197
  retention, diagnosis, 197
    pathology of, 197
    prognosis, 197
    significance of, 197
    treatment, 197
  solitary renal, diagnosis, 196
    prognosis, 196
    significance of, 196
    treatment, 196
  urachal, 386, *386*
Cystinuria, clinical findings, 159
  diagnosis, 159
  history in, 159
  treatment, 159
Cystitis, bacterial, 355–360
  chronic polypoid, *378, 379*
Cystitis-urethral obstruction complex, 361
  alkaline urine in, 363
  bacterial infection in, 362
  clinical examination, 364
  diagnosis, 365
  etiology, 361, *362*
  history in, 364
  ingestion of dry cat foods and, 363
  laboratory findings, 365
  mineral intake in, 363
  pre-puberal castration and, 363
  prognosis, 370
  prophylaxis, 369
  treatment, 365
    control of bacterial infection in, 369
    emergency, 366
    fluid therapy in, 368
    summary of, 370
    treatment, surgical, 369

Cystitis-urethral obstruction complex (*Continued*)
  viral infection and, 364
  vitamin A deficiency in, 363
Cystocentesis, as method for collecting urine specimen, 56
  equipment used in, 37
  objectives of, 36
  technique in, 37
Cystogram, double contrast, *102*
Cystography, double contrast, complications of, 103
    indications for, 103
    interpretation, 101
    mediums available, 100
    technique, 100
  definition, fractional superimposition, 103
    indications for, 104
    technique, 103
    positive contrast, 99
Cystolithiasis, 327
Cystometry, 18
Cystoscopy, 118–120
  definition of, 118
  equipment used, 118
  indications for, 119
  in dogs, technique, 119

Dehydration, in renal disease, 293, *294*
  in renal failure, 144
Diabetes insipidus, history in, 150
  renal, 150
  urinalysis in, 150
Diabetes mellitus, abnormalities of, 235
  clinical findings in, 149, 236
  definition, 234
  diagnosis, 237
  etiology, 235
  laboratory data, 149, 236
  prognosis, 237
  treatment, 237
Dialysis, peritoneal. See *Peritoneal dialysis*.
Dietary restrictions, in treatment of renal failure, 271
Digestive system, and renal failure, 138
Dioctophyma renale, 209–212
  clinical findings, 211
  control of, 212
  diagnosis, 212
  life cycle, 209
  male and female, 210–211
  morphologic characteristics, 209
  ova of, *209*
  pathology, 210
  treatment, 212
Dirofilaria immitis, 213
Disease(s), urinary, clinical history in, 20–22
  diagnostic aspects, 121–123
  hemograms in, 121
  history and physical examination, 121
  radiology in, 123
  renal biopsy in, 123
  renal function tests in, 121
  serum and urine enzymes in, 123
  serum electrolytes in, 122
  urinalyses in, 121

Diuresis, in acute nephrosis, 173
  osmotic, contraindications to, 278
    indications for, 278
    mechanism of action, 275, 279
    procedure for 10 to 20% dextrose, 275
    procedure for 20% mannitol, 277
Drug dosage, in renal failure, modification of, 311
Drug excretion, major routes in dogs and cats, 312t
Drug therapy, in renal failure, 310–315
  recommendations for, 311
Drug toxicity, in renal failure, 310
Dysuria, 394

Ectopic ureter, 334
  diagnosis, 335
  prognosis, 337
  treatment, 337
Edema, nephrotic, 228
Electrolytes, detecting alterations of in renal disease, 294
  lost in body excretions, 405
  maintenance requirements for hospitalized dogs and cats, *298t*
Endocrine system, and renal failure, 140
End-stage kidney(s), 189–195
  definition, 189
  diagnosis, 194
  gross appearance, *190*, 191, *191*, *192*, *193*
  history, 193
  microscopic appearance of, 192
  pathophysiology, 189
  physical findings, 193
  prognosis, 194
  significance of, 195
  treatment, 194
Enterocolitis, in renal failure, 139
Epithelial cells, types of, 52
Erythropoeitin, 16
Excretory urography, 79, 92
  limitations of, 93
  technique, 94
  use of in diagnosis, 93

Fibroma(s), 255
  of urinary bladder, 376
Fibrosarcoma, 257
Filiforms, description and use of, 27
Fluid therapy, in renal disease, patient response to, 299
  in renal failure, 291
    plan for, 297
    principles of, 291
    types of, 291
  products used in, 302
  routes and rates of administration, intramedullary, 309
    intraperitoneal, 308
    intravenous, 307
    oral, 306
    rectal, 309
    subcutaneous, 308
Followers, description and use of, 27
Formalin, in preserving urine, 41

INDEX

Gastritis, hemorrhagic ulcerative, in renal failure, 139
Gentamicin, toxicity of, 313
Glomerular filtration rate, determination of, 80
Glomerular lipoidosis, 219
Glomeruli, primary diseases of, 214–219
Glomerulonephritis, acute, 214
   chronic, 215
   definition, 214
   membranous, 215, 216, *217*
   spontaneous, 217
   subacute, 214
   types of, *215*
Glomerulus, normal, 217
Glucosuria, 48
   causes of, 48
   primary renal, diagnosis, 159
      history, 158
      laboratory results, 158
      prognosis, 159
      treatment, 159

Halothane, in renal disease, 314
Hematuria, 50
   causes of, 51
Hemic system, and renal failure, 138
Hemodialysis, in treatment of renal failure, 284
Hemoglobinuria, causes of, 51
Hemogram, erythrocyte numbers in, 39
   hemoglobin in, 39
   packed cell volume in, 39
Hepatitis, infectious canine, 238
Hernias, and abnormal position of urinary bladder, 390
Histoplasmosis, 254
Hormones, in kidney function, 16
Horseshoe kidneys, clinical findings, 158
   etiology, 157
   pathophysiology, 158
Hydronephrosis, 198–208
   bilateral, *198, 199, 200,* 204
   clinical findings, 206
   definition, 198
   diagnosis, 207
   etiology, acquired, 198
      congenital, 198
   obstruction of urine outflow and, 202
   of left kidney, *205*
   pathogenesis, 200
   pathology, 203
   prognosis, 207
   treatment, 207
   unilateral, 204, *205, 206*
      severity of morphological changes in, 203
Hydronephrotic kidney, 201, 202
Hyperadrenalcorticism, history in, 149
   laboratory data in, 149
   physical findings in, 149
Hypercalcemia, degrees of damage caused by in man, dogs, rats, and cats, 58
Hypercholesterolemia, as finding in renal disease, 59
Hyperparathyroidism, secondary renal, in renal failure, 140
Hyperphosphatemia, in renal disease, 58
   in renal failure, 140

Hypertension, in renal failure, 136
Hypertrophy, left ventricular, in renal failure, 138
Hypocalcemia, in renal disease, 58
Hypocalcemic tetany, in chronic renal failure, 287
Hypoplasia, renal, clinical signs, 153
   diagnosis, 154
   renal cortical, 148
Hypospadias, 400, *400*

Incontinence, urinary, 394–399
   classification of, 399
   definition, 394
   diagnosis, 398
   miscellaneous causes, 398
   neurogenic, 394, *395, 396*
   nonneurogenic, 397
   paradoxical, 397
   pathogenesis, 394
   prognosis, 399
   treatment, 399
Infarction, renal, 219
Interstitial nephritis, chronic, blood chemistry in, 148
   hemogram in, 148
   history in, 147
   pertinent laboratory data, 148
   physical findings in, 147
   urinalysis in, 148
Inulin, description of, 80
Ischemia, renal, versus nephrotoxins, 169

Juxtaglomerular apparatus, 6

Kanamycin, toxicity of, 313
Ketamine, in renal disease, 314
Ketonuria, 49
Kidney(s), cut surface of, *4*
   end-stage. See *End-stage kidney(s).*
   gross organization of, 5
   horseshoe, clinical findings, 158
      etiology, 157
      pathophysiology, 158
   location and gross appearance, 3
   morphological and functional adaptation to injury, 131
   neoplasms of, 255–260, *256*
      metastatic, 259
   neoplastic, *243, 244*
   nephron and collecting duct system of, 4
   normal dog, *190*
   palpation of in physical examination, 23
   physical examination of, 23
   response of to injury, 130
Kidney function, 11
   and nonrenal hormones, 17
   mechanisms of, 12
      countercurrent system, 15
      elaboration of hormones, 16
      glomerular filtration, 13
      tubular reabsorption, 13
      tubular secretion, 16

Kidney function (*Continued*)
  normal, requirements for, 11
Kidney size, estimating, results of studies, 86
    value of, 85
    radiographic estimate of, 85

Laboratory tests, findings in diseases of urinary system, 39–61
Leiomyoma(s), 255
  of urethra, 401
  of urinary bladder, 376
Leiomyosarcoma, 257
Leptospira canicola, 238
Leptospira icterohemorrhagiae, 238
Leptospirosis, diagnosis, 240
  etiology, 238
  history, 238
  laboratory findings, 239
  physical examination, 239
  prognosis, 241
  renal alterations during, 240
  treatment, 240
Leucocytosis, in pyelonephritis, 186
Lhasa apso dogs, familial renal disease in, diagnosis, 162
    history and clinical features, 161
    laboratory features, 161
    necropsy, 162, *162*
    prognosis, 162
    treatment, 161
Lipiduria, in cats and dogs, 55
Lipoidosis, glomerular, 219
Lipoma, 255
Liposarcoma, 257
Liver disease, polyuria and, 151
Lymphoma, malignant, clinical findings, 244
    diagnosis, 246
    etiology, 241
    laboratory findings, 245
    pathophysiology, 241
    prevalence, 241
    prognosis, 247
    pseudohyperparathyroidism with renal failure and, 247
    radiographic findings, 246
    treatment, 246

Metabolic acidosis, in renal failure, 59, 144
Metastatic tumors, of urinary bladder, 378
Micturition, frequency of, in urinary disease, 21
  mechanisms of, 17
  physiology of, 17
    muscles involved, 17
    nerves involved, 17
    normal requirements, 17
  spontaneous, collection of urine sample during, 25
Mucormycosis, 254
Myeloma, multiple, *396*
Myxoma, 255
  of urinary bladder, 376, *377*
Myxosarcoma, 257

Negative contrast agents, 92
Neomycin, toxicity of, 313
Neoplasm(s), of kidney, 255–260, *256*
  of urethra, 401
    diagnosis and treatment, 401
    history and clinical signs, 401
    prognosis, 401
  of urinary bladder, 374–385
    benign, 376
    classification, 376
    clinical findings, 378
    diagnosis, 383
    etiopathogenesis, 374
    history, 378
    laboratory findings, 381
    malignant, 376
      carcinomas, 377
      sarcomas, 377
    physical examination, 379
    prevalence, 374
    radiographic findings, 381
    treatment, 384
Nephritis, chronic interstitial, 147, 182–183
  definition, 182
  etiology, 182
  prevalence, 183
Nephroblastoma, 257
Nephrography, indications for, 97
Nephrolithiasis, *322*, 327
Nephron(s), 4
  microdissection from kidneys of dogs, 131, *132*
Nephrosis, acute, oliguria in, 178
    polyuria in, 179
    prognosis, 179
    symptomatic and supportive therapy of, 178
  clinical findings, 172
  definition of, 169
  diagnosis, 175
  ischemic, and chemical, 169–181
    etiopathogenesis of, 170
    specific therapy of, 177
  laboratory findings, 174
  nephrotoxic, specific therapy of, 177
    etiopathogenesis of, 172
  radiographic findings, 174
  renal biopsy findings, 174
  treatment, 175
Nephrotic syndrome, 228–231
  clinical findings, 229
  definition, 228
  diagnosis, 230
  etiology, 228
  pathogenesis, 228
  prognosis, 231
  transudative ascites in, *230*
  treatment, 231
Nephrotoxic drugs, examples of, 313
Nervous system, and renal failure, 143
Neurofibromas, of urinary bladder, 376
Nonprotein nitrogen, determination of, 78
Norwegian elkhound, familial renal disease in, diagnosis, 160
    history and clinical features, 160
    laboratory findings, 160
    necropsy, 161, *161*

Norwegian elkhound (*Continued*)
   familial renal disease in, prognosis, 160
      renal biopsy, 160
      treatment, 160

Obstructive ureteropathy, clinical findings in, 331
   prognosis, 332
   significance of, 331
   treatment, 332
Obstructive uropathy, 350–351
   definition, 350
   etiology, 350
   pathophysiology, 351
   ureters and renal pelves, 350
   urethral, 350
   urinary bladder, 350
Occult blood, detection of, 49
Oliguria, 300
   causes of, 42
   in acute nephrosis, 173
Osmolality, as renal function test, 64
   vs. specific gravity, 65
Osmolarity, definition of, 65
Osmole, definition of, 65
Osmometers, in clinical medicine, 66
Osmotic diuresis, contraindications to, 278
   indications for, 278
   mechanisms of action, 275, 279
   procedure for 10 to 20% dextrose, 275
   procedure for 20% mannitol, 277
Osteodystrophy, in chronic renal failure, 58, 286
Osteoma, 255

Papilloma(s), 255
   of urinary bladder, 376
Parasites, miscellaneous, 213
Parathyroid hyperplasia, *139*, 142
Patent urachus, 386–388, *387*
Penis, exposure of, in catheterization, *31*
   feline, normal position of, *36*
Penicillin G, toxicity of, 313
Peritoneal dialysis, contraindications to, 284
   equipment needed, 280
   indications for, 284
   in treatment of renal failure, 279
   mechanism of action, 280
   patient complications, 283
   technical complications, 282
   technique for, 281
Phenolsulphonphthalein dye, urinary excretion of, 122
Phenolsulphonphthalein excretion, and endogenous creatinine clearance, 82
Phenolsulphonphthalein excretion test, basis for, 70
   determination of quantity of dye excreted, 72
   dosage, 71
   indications, 71
   interpretation of results, 73
   procedure for, 72
Phosphorus, serum concentrations of, in renal disease, 58

Pitressin concentration test, aqueous vasopressin test in, 68
   basis for, 68
   contraindications to, 69
   indications, 68
   interpretation of results, 69
   procedure for, 68
   repositol vasopressin test in, 69
Plasma bicarbonate deficit, in renal disease, 57
Pneumocystography, 97
   indications for, 98
   technique, 98
Pollakiuria, 394
Polyarteritis nodosa, definition, 248
   etiology, 248
   in kidneys of dogs and cats, 248
   necrotizing vasculitis and, 248
Polycystic disease, 155, *155*
   clinical findings in, 156
   diagnosis, 156
   gross pathology, 156
   histopathology, 156
   prognosis, 156
   treatment, 156
Polydipsia, 20
   in renal failure, *139*
Polymyxin B, toxicity of, 313
Polysystemic diseases, renal diseases and, 232–254
Polyuria, 20, 302, 394
   and liver disease, 151
   causes of, 41
   in renal failure, 139
Polyuria-polydipsia complex, causes of, 147–152
Postrenal uremia, in obstructive uropathy, 351
Potassium, concentration of in renal disease, 57
Prolapse, of urinary bladder, 392
Proteinuria, 46
   Bence Jones, 48
   pathologic, 47
   physiologic, 47
   polysystemic, 48
   postrenal urinary, 48
   renal, 47
Pruritus, renal failure and, 136
Pyelonephritis, 184–188
   chronic, 148
   clinical findings, 186
   definition, 184
   diagnosis, 187
   incidence, 184
   parathyroid gland in, *139*
   pathogenesis, 184
   pathology, 185, *185*
   prognosis, 187
   treatment, 187
Pyometra, abnormal renal function and, 250
   and endometrial hyperplasia, 249
   clinical findings, 250
   definition, 249
   diagnosis, 251
   glomerular changes associated with, 249
   glomerulonephritis associated with, 249
   history in, 151, 250
   laboratory data in, 151, 251
   physical findings in, 151, 250
   polydipsia and, 250
   polyuria and, 250

Pyometra (*Continued*)
  prognosis, 252
  renal function impairment associated with, 249
  renal lesions in, 249
  treatment, 252
  uterine lesions in, 249
Pyonephrosis, *322*
Pyuria, 52

Refractometers, in clinical medicine, 66
Renal circulation, 5
Renal clearance, and glomerular filtration rate, 79
  concept of, 79
Renal cysts, 196-197
Renal cortical hypoplasia, 156
  diagnosis, 157
  laboratory features, 157
  prognosis, 157
Renal disease, acid-base alterations in, 295
  acute, 165-168. See also specific disease, e.g., *Nephritis, acute.*
    definition, 165
    diagnosis, 167
    etiology, 165
    history, 166
    laboratory findings, 166
    pathology, 167
    physical findings, 166
    prognosis, 167
    treatment, 167
  congenital and inherited, 153-164
  detecting acid-base alterations in, 295
  detecting electrolyte alterations in, 294
  end stage, 147. See also *Interstitial nephritis, chronic.*
    history in, 147
  patient response to fluid therapy in, 299
Renal failure, access to water in treatment of, 273
  acute vs. chronic, 128
  altered acid-base balance in, 144
  altered electrolyte balance in, 144
  altered fluid balance in, 144
  anabolic steroids in treatment of, 273
  anemia in, 138
  cardiovascular system and, 136
  causes of, 127
  common signs of, 136
  constipation in, 139
  degree of dysfunction in, 262
  dehydration in, 144, 293, *294*
  dietary restrictions in treatment of, 271
  differentiation of chronic from acute, 263
    history in, 263
    laboratory aids in, 264
    physical examination in, 264
    radiography in, 264
    renal biopsy in, 265
  digestive system and, 138
  drug therapy in, 310-315
  drug toxicity in, 310
  endocrine system and, 140
  end stage, kidneys in, 145

Renal failure (*Continued*)
  enterocolitis in, 139
  fluid therapy in, types of, 291
  hemic system and, 138
  hemodialysis in treatment of, 284
  hemorrhagic ulcerative gastritis in, 139
  hyperphosphatemia in, 140
  hypertension in, 136
  importance of accurate diagnosis, 266
  intensive diuresis in treatment of, 275
  left ventricular hypertrophy in, 138
  metabolic acidosis in, 144
  mouth ulceration in, 138
  nervous system and, 143
  osmotic diuresis in treatment of, 275
  peritoneal dialysis in treatment of, 279
  oliguric vs. polyuric, 299
  osteodystrophy in, *140*, *141*, 142, *142*
  pathophysiology of, 127-134
  polydipsia in, 139
  polyuria in, 139
  postrenal, 127, 261, 268
  potential causes of death in, 143
  potential for reversal of lesions in, 263
  prerenal, 127, 261, 267
  primary, 127, 262, 268
    conservative medical management, 269
    nephrectomy in, 269
    oliguria in, 269
  pruritus and, 136
  prognosis of, 261-265
    basis for, 261
    definition of, 261
    etiopathogenesis of, 261
  respiratory system and, 136
  reversible vs. irreversible, renal reserve capacity in, 129
    response of kidneys to injury in, 130
  secondary renal hyperparathyroidism in, 140
  skin dehydration and, 136, *136*
  sodium bicarbonate in treatment of, 271
  sodium chloride in treatment of, 270
  stress avoidance in treatment of, 274
  summary of recommended therapy, 287
  treatment of, 266-290
  types of, 127
  types of treatment, palliative, 267
    specific, 266
    supportive, 267
    symptomatic, 267
  uremic frost and, 136
  urinary system and, 139
  vitamin supplements in treatment of, 273
Renal function tests, 62-84
  perspective of, 62
  precise measurements in, 63
  purpose of, 62
Renal transplant, in treatment of renal failure, 285
Renal trauma, clinical findings, 338
  diagnosis, 340
  etiology of, 338
  pathophysiology of, 338
  prognosis, 341
  treatment, 340
Renal tumors, benign, 255
Renin, 16

Repositol vasopressin test, in pitressin concentration test, 69
Respiratory system, and renal failure, 136
Retrograde pyelography and ureterography, 97
Rhabdomyomas, of urinary bladder, 376
Rhabdomyosarcoma, 257

Sarcomas, of urinary bladder, 377
  venereal, of urethra, 401
Sclerosing glomerular disease, 218
Serum amylase, concentrations of in uremic dogs and cats, 59
Serum electrolytes, evaluation of, 56
Serum proteins, and renal disease, 60
Skin dehydration, renal failure and, 136, *136*
Sodium bicarbonate, in treatment of renal failure, 271
Sodium chloride, in treatment of renal failure, 270
Sodium deficit, in renal disease, 57
Sounds, description and use of, 27
Specific gravity, vs. osmolality, 65
Spirocerca lupi, 213
Systemic lupus erythematosus, associated renal disease, 253
  clinical findings, 253
  definition, 253
  diagnosis, 254
  increase in serum globulins and, 60
  prognosis, 254
  treatment, 254
Systemic mycoses, 254

Tetracyclines, toxicity of, 313
Thrombosis, of abdominal aorta, *222*
Thymol, in preservation of urine, 40
Toluene, in preservation of urine, 40
Torsion, of urinary bladder, 390
Toxocara canis, 213
Trauma, to urethra, 401
  to urinary bladder, 343
Tumors. See also *Neoplasms*, and specific disease, e.g., *Sarcomas, of urinary bladder.*
  benign renal, 255
  primary malignant, 255
    diagnosis of, 258

Urachal cyst, 386, *386*
Urachus, anomalies of, 386, *386*
  patent, 386–388, *387*
    diagnosis, 388
    physical findings, 388
    prognosis, 388
    treatment, 388
Uremia, 12, 127
  and anuria, 292
  and oliguria, 292
  and polyuria, 292
  BUN concentration and, 135
  chronic, bone marrow in, *137*
  clinical signs of, 135

Uremia (*Continued*)
  deviations of water, electrolyte, acid-base, and caloric balance in, 292
  extrarenal manifestations of, 135–146
  postrenal, 262, 268
    in obstructive uropathy, 351
    treatment of, 268
  prerenal, 176, 261, 267
    treatment of, 267
  primary, 176, 262, 268
    treatment of, 268
Uremic syndrome, etiology of, 135
Uremic toxins, 135
Ureter(s), calculi in, 332
  diseases of, 330–337
  ectopic, 334, *336*
  hydronephrosis in, *204*
  location, 6
  neoplasia of, 332
  obstruction of, *330*
  physical examination of, 23
  structure, 7
  trauma to, 332
  traumatic rupture of, clinical findings, 342
    diagnosis, 342
    hydronephrosis and, *342*
    prognosis, 343
    radiographic findings, 342
    treatment, 343
Ureterolithiasis, 327
Ureteropathy, obstructive, 331
Urethra, congenital anomalies of, 400
  diseases of, 400–402
  female canine and feline, 8
  male canine, 7
  male feline, 8
  neoplasms of, leiomyomas, 401
    transitional cell carcinoma, 401
  physical examination of, 24
  rupture of, 349
  trauma to, 401
  venereal sarcomas of, 401
Urethral calculi, removal of, *326*
Urethrography, indications for, 105
  technique, 105
Urethrogram, positive contrast, *104*
Urinalysis, bilirubinuria in, 49
  collection of specimen for, 40
  formalin in timing of, 41
  glucosuria in, 48
  interpretation of, 40
  ketonuria in, 49
  occult blood in, 49
  proteinuria in, 46
  quantitative vs. qualitative, 41
  specific gravity in, 43
  thymol in preservation of, 40
  toluene in preservation of, 40
  urine color and, 42
  urine pH in, 46
  urine transparency in, 43
  urine volume and, 41
Urinary bladder. See *Bladder, urinary.*
Urinary disease(s). See *Diseases, urinary;* also specific disease, e.g., *Bacterial cystitis.*
Urinary incontinence. See *Incontinence, urinary.*
Urinary system, anatomy of, 3–10
  physical examination of, 23–24

Urinary system (*Continued*)
  physical injuries to, 338–349
  physiology of, 11–19
  radiographic evaluation of, 85–106
  preradiographic considerations, 85
  radiographic studies in, patient preparation for, 87
    survey films, 88, *88, 89, 90*
Urine, alkaline, in cystitis-urethral obstruction complex, 363
  bacteria in, 54
  bacterial culture of, methods of obtaining urine specimens for, 55
  collection of, 25–38
  color of, 42
  decreased specific gravity of, causes, 45
  expulsion of, 12
  gross appearance of in urinary disease, 22
  increased specific gravity of, 45
  metazoan parasite ova in, 54
  methods of removing from bladder, 25
  normal values, 403
  pH of, 46
  specific gravity of, 43
    as renal function test, 63
  transparency of, 43
  volume of, 41
  yeast and fungi in, 54
Urine color, abnormal, causes of, 42
  normal, 42
Urine concentration test, basis for, 66
  contraindications to, 67
  interpretation of results, 67
  procedure for, 66
Urine dilution test, basis for, 69
  indications, 70
  interpretation of results, 70
  procedure for, 70
Urine osmolality, 122
Urine output, in diagnosis of urinary disease, 21
Urine sediment, description of, 50
  method for obtaining, 50
  nonorganized, 55

Urine specific gravity, 122
Urine volume, decreased, causes of, 42
  increased, pathological causes of, 41
  normal values for, 41
  polyuria and, 41
Urolithiasis, 319–329
  breed predilection, 320
  clinical history in, 321, 323
  diagnosis of, 323
  physical examination in, 322, 323
  prophylactic treatment after, 327
  sex predilection, 321
  site predilection, 321
  treatment, 323
Uroliths, bladder, 323, *324*
  composition of, 319
  etiology of, 320
  renal, 323, *324*
  ureteral, *331*
  urethral, 322, *325*, 326
Uropathy, obstructive, 350–351

Vagina, canine, normal, *33*
Vancomycin, toxicity of, 313
Viral infection, and cystitis-urethral obstruction complex, 364
Vitamin A deficiency, in cystitis-urethral obstruction complex, 363
Vesico-ureteral reflux, definition of, 332
  diagnosis of, 334
  pathophysiology of, 332
  significance of, 333
  treatment of, 334

Water, maintenance requirements for hospitalized dogs and cats, *298t*
Water consumption, excessive, 147
  in diagnosis of urinary diseases, 20
White blood cell count, 39